The Split Mind

Schizophrenia from an Insider's Point of View

Kevin Lee

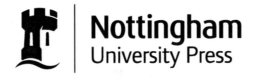

Nottingham
University Press

Nottingham University Press
Manor Farm, Main Street, Thrumpton
Nottingham, NG11 0AX, United Kingdom

NOTTINGHAM

First published 2011
© Kevin Lee

British Library Cataloguing in Publication Data
The Split Mind - Schizophrenia from an Insider's Point of View
Kevin Lee

ISBN 978-1-907284-74-8

Disclaimer

Every reasonable effort has been made to ensure that the material in this book is true, correct, complete
and appropriate at the time of writing. Nevertheless the publishers, the editors and the authors do not
accept responsibility for any omission or error, or for any injury, damage, loss or financial consequences
arising from the use of the book.

Typeset by Nottingham University Press, Nottingham
Printed and bound by Lightning Source, England

Contents

Dedication

For Ray

FOREWORD

"The Split Mind" is a hybrid of a memoir and reference book on the subject of schizophrenia. There are currently over 50 million people who suffer from this debilitating disease. Schizophrenia is an illness that warps the individual's perspective of the real world. It is classified as a disability because all affected patients will also lack the ability to function within their community. Further, schizophrenia is ranked among the ten top causes of a disability, within developed nations worldwide.

Isolation may be common among all persons who suffer from a disability, either mental or physical. It can be cured through the virtues of understanding and compassion. Acknowledging the fact that schizophrenia is a sickness, like cancer, that can affect persons of all types of backgrounds, should be a common understanding. Having compassion for persons who are sick should also be a universal undertaking.

The modes of treatment for schizophrenia will be lifelong. Thankfully, there are numerous individuals who have made this possible. These individuals have dedicated their lives to helping persons who, through misfortune, have developed an illness. I possess the ability to function because of the work of scientists, in many different nations around the world, who have painstakingly developed methods of treatment for my illness. The many doctors, psychiatrists, and other medical professionals are also vital to the recovery process from schizophrenia. Without these persons, I would have neither the ability, nor the strength to record my personal account with this disorder.

1

Introduction

As a member of the human race, I feel that it is my personal responsibility to share my experiences with the rest of the world. I would also like to educate the general public and dispel any myths that have been associated with my illness. I have schizophrenia. I was first diagnosed with this disease when I was 20 years old, although in retrospect, I have suffered from problematic symptoms during some of my earliest memories in life. It was only after I reached 20 years of age when the disease took full control over my personhood. The disease changed my perspective of the world, and it created an entirely new mode of existence for me. It destroyed my personal history and wrote in a new and fictitious future. The main problem with this future was that it interfered with my daily functioning. It also blurred my perception of the actual world. The disease caused me to become delusional, and these delusions would eventually take full control over my entire perspective of life. At times, I would be extremely delusional, but I never realized this fact until much later in my life.

First and foremost, I would like to share my life experiences with my peers and their loved ones. I hope that by sharing my experiences, I can help others deal with their illness and cope with their personal problems. I would also like to share my experiences with those who are curious about what it is like to live with schizophrenia. Perhaps a better understanding of mental illness will cure the current prevalence of social stigmas that exist against it. Persons suffering from a mental illness are not lesser human beings. We are similar to the average person, except for the fact that we have poor health. We have an illness, and illnesses in themselves do not discriminate. People from all walks of life can become affected by a mental illness. Furthermore, many others are born into the world with a mental disability. Unfortunately, I had to learn this the hard way.

With respect to physical disabilities, an injury to the spinal cord can often lead to a loss of control over one's limbs. Persons who are physically disabled may rely on tools, like wheel chairs, for help with their day to day living. In contrast, persons with mental disabilities will require medications for daily life. Both forms of disability are due to problems within the individual's central nervous system. In the former case, the spinal cord no longer functions normally. In the latter case, the brain no longer functions normally.

In both cases, the individual may also require assistance from a third party, for the remainder of his life. Many persons in our society will label these individuals as disabled or challenged. Technically, these labels may be valid. However, from a social perspective, I feel that these labels degrade the individual into a lesser human being. Yet, the root of this degradation can be expected. It may be natural to view individuals who have lost the ability to use their legs, or those who have lost the ability to think rationally, as persons with disabilities. However, in my opinion, this is a dispassionate perspective. This perspective essentially condemns the individual into life as a lower class citizen.

The stigma connected to mental disabilities not only affects the psyche of the patient, but it can also affect his entire family. However, the shame that may be attached to a disability arises through pure ignorance. In fact, illness is a very natural part of human existence. Every human body is vulnerable to illness. Every individual is susceptible to sickness and disease. Furthermore, I can only think of a few things that are actually indestructible within our universe. Therefore, the act of discriminating against persons with a mental disease reflects on a kind of unwarranted prejudice within our civilization, based purely on hate and intolerance.

When the individual views a disability as a limitation, he will be guilty of a form of hypocrisy. By focusing on the limits of other persons, we are essentially directing focus off our own limitations. The limitation of the hypocrite comes in an inability to feel compassion for another fellow human being. In actual fact, the concept of human inequality is absurd and based on nonsense. Every human being is unique, and our differences do not provide a reasonable foundation for any forms of discrimination or personal bias. One individual may be physically strong, while another individual may be stronger intellectually. A third individual may possess neither quality. However, the trait of imperfection is common to all human beings. Each individual differs with respect to his talents and shortcomings. Accordingly, I believe that our society should focus less on the concept of disability, when we think about persons with either a mental or physical illness.

The view that disabilities are personal defects essentially puts a limit on the growth of human civilization as a whole. In our history, patients with disabilities did not have access to the technology and scientific progress that we have today. Advancements in the fields of science and engineering have enabled sick individuals to live a better and a more independent way of life. The existence of medicines, which effectively treat illnesses like schizophrenia, are now a part of our modern world. It was only during our distant past when the schizophrenia patient faced a much bleaker way of life.

Indeed, at one point in our history, there were no effective modes of treatment for persons with mental illness. Under these circumstances, the illness would usually take control over the individual's entire life and personhood. I would agree that the fear associated with this loss of control might be partially justified. Thus, many societal stigmas, based on fear, can be quite natural. However, at present day, there are medicines available that can effectively treat many forms of mental disease. In view of that, the negative image attributed to persons with mental illness should also evolve.

All in all, the stigma associated with mental illness has many serious ramifications on our society. For one thing, persons impacted by a mental illness may not openly discuss their problems, because of discrimination. In this case, the individual may fail to objectively address his problem, and his family members may do the same. A lack of social acceptance towards mental illness also creates a general barrier in the treatment and rehabilitation of all affected patients. In contrast, if people were free to discuss subjects like mental illness in an open capacity, most patients would not live in seclusion, nor would they be isolated from the rest of their community.

An open acceptance of mental illness would advance human civilization in every possible way. Most importantly, it would serve to unite a divided community. Mental illness also has indirect effects on persons with good mental health. As a result, the social stigma generated towards mental illness will have much wider repercussions on our society, than what is generally known.

At this point, the skeptic may ask, "Isn't the individual utterly responsible for his mental health?" My reply would be no, because no person possesses the ability to avoid illness in an absolute fashion. It is true that we can take precautions against the development of some specific illnesses. However, if we possessed the ability to avoid all forms of illness, it would also be true that no person would ever suffer from any illness during his entire lifetime.

The skeptic may also ask, "What about persons who develop lung cancer through smoking cigarettes?" Indeed, many individuals who smoke cigarettes will go on to develop lung cancer. Nonetheless, many other persons, who do not smoke, will also develop some form of cancer within their lifetime. With this in mind, I believe that there are many other factors, beyond personal life choices, which account for the development of many diseases.

These factors will most likely include specific biological characteristics and genetic traits. At present, no one knows the true cause of schizophrenia. Less informed persons may believe that the individual's past choices and behaviours will lead to the development of schizophrenia. Scientists, on the other hand, are constantly discovering evidence which implicates a genetic cause. If our scientists are right, then it may also be true that I would have always developed schizophrenia, independent of what life choices I may have made in the past.

I never wanted, nor asked to become ill. Then again, every other sick individual would say the same thing. Personally, I believe that the illness chooses the person. No individual has the power to choose his genetic or biological makeup. My genetic makeup makes me susceptible to develop schizophrenia, while my neighbour's essentially makes him immune. The random nature of illness seems to suggest the inescapable fact that biological factors are most significant to a state of sickness or good health.

If my last statement is true, then it is also true that schizophrenia, as a disease, has chosen me. If my genetic profile were different, it may be possible that I would have never acquired schizophrenia during my entire lifetime. However, my genetic makeup makes me susceptible to develop schizophrenia. This susceptibility was pre-programmed into my biological makeup. Moreover, I believe that this is true concerning persons who go on to develop other illnesses, like cancer. If I am right, then there are persons with a differing genetic makeup, who will never develop schizophrenia or cancer no matter what life choices they may make.

Rationally, I would have to agree with our scientists when they state that the cause of schizophrenia is mainly due to genetics. I believe this for many reasons. First, my biological makeup has determined many other personal characteristics of mine. The colour of my hair, my height, and my athletic capacity are all pre-determined by specific genetic and biological traits. I will never naturally grow blond hair, be six feet tall, or become a professional hockey player. I have inherited these biological attributes by nature. I could list a countless amount of other personal characteristics that are determined solely through genetics. Therefore, although I believe that all persons possess the power to control their lifestyle, being immune to sickness and disease may be beyond any person's control.

Secondly, many scientific discoveries suggest the possibility that a genetic predisposition exists in all individuals who eventually go on to develop schizophrenia (Weiten, 1995). Likewise, no scientific evidence exists which connects the cause of schizophrenia solely to the individual's life choices.

Thirdly, if schizophrenia is not caused through genetics, and it is rather due to the individual's lifestyle, then many more persons, who are mentally healthy, should also develop schizophrenia. I believe that most of the choices that I have made in my past are not unique, and that they are common among many of my peers. My peers can include other persons in my community, other persons who are relatively the same age as me, or other males around the world. In fact, I believe that it is possible to find other persons in the world who have made lifestyle choices that are nearly identical to my own. I may also be right to assume that some of these individuals will never go on to develop schizophrenia. If this is true, then the cause of my illness may be more complex than being solely due to one's life choices. Many scientists and doctors around the world would agree with this latter possibility.

Whatever the cause of schizophrenia, I believe that our society would benefit more if it focused on the treatment and cure for this disease. It is true that in our history, the treatment and rehabilitation of persons with schizophrenia was not always possible. However, at present day, the treatment and rehabilitation of persons with schizophrenia is extremely viable. The current treatments available should enable most patients to live a higher standard of life. Instead of being committed into a hospital for an indefinite period of time, more patients are being treated and discharged to live freely within their community. In addition, newer and more improved forms of medications are being continually developed, as our scientific knowledge progresses. The availability of more enhanced antipsychotic medications will provide some patients with the ability to live an even higher standard of life, through self-determination. I also believe that our scientists will eventually discover some form of cure for schizophrenia, at some point in our future.

With all of the newer forms of medications available, what more is there left to be said about diseases like schizophrenia? Some persons may believe that the patient is diagnosed, treated, and then resumes his normal life. Unfortunately, this is often not the case, and most disabilities will affect the individual for his entire lifetime. A further question may revolve around the true efficacy of antipsychotic medications. The answer to this question can be complicated. It is true that the medicines prescribed by our doctors do relieve some of the symptoms exhibited by schizophrenia patients. However, the efficacy of these medicines will vary on a case-by-case basis. Therefore, although a particular medication may be effective in relieving a symptom like paranoid thoughts, the patient can still suffer from other symptoms. As a result, it is quite probable that the patient will try more than one medication before he finds the most effective medicine for his body type. The reason for this is due to the individual's unique biological makeup. Everyone has unique genetic and biological attributes, and accordingly, while one medication may work for one person, it may not necessarily work for another. Finding a medicine that will relieve the individual's symptoms, with a minimal amount of side effects, will almost always vary on an individual basis.

Undoubtedly, the treatment for schizophrenia can be a frustrating process. All antipsychotic medicines can potentially treat the symptoms of schizophrenia. Nevertheless, some are also capable of producing extremely unbearable side effects. Some side effects may be generally tolerable, but most are not. Thus, most patients with schizophrenia will also share a common experience, in relation to an intolerable side effect of a prescribed medication. Some of the early generation antipsychotic medications produced bodily pains as a side effect. Other side effects can include anxiety and weight gain. Even though there has been substantial progress towards the treatment of schizophrenia, the patient can still reject his mental health care system because of these side effects. As a result, the refusal to take antipsychotic medications is a very real problem for many schizophrenia patients.

The human rights for freedom and liberty may complicate this issue. With these constitutional rights, every citizen will also possess the right to refuse medical treatment. At first glance, this particular freedom may seem a bit irrational. Nevertheless, rights based on the principle of freedom are constitutional elements, in most developed nations. When the individual refuses medical treatment, he is essentially exercising his right to act as an autonomous agent. This right may be comparable to the right to conduct an abortion. Under both circumstances, the individual necessarily has the right to determine what happens to his or her body, over the demands of his society.

There are two main reasons why a schizophrenia patient may refuse medical treatment. One common reason may be due to the exceedingly intolerable side effects of a particular antipsychotic medication. In this case, the patient has lost confidence in his community's mental health care system.

The second, and more problematic reason, may be due to the concept of denial. The problem of denial occurs when the patient fails to acknowledge the fact that he is suffering from some form of illness. This problem is also very common among many schizophrenia patients. When a sick individual denies a psychiatric diagnosis, he believes that he is making a sound and rational decision. This individual may believe that his doctors are guilty of a misdiagnosis, and that he is truly not ill. Therefore, the individual trusts his own personal beliefs over the opinion of a certified medical professional.

The individual's illness itself may have some bearing on the problem of denial. Imagine that a stranger were to approach and tell you that you are mentally ill. How would you react? I believe that many persons, with good mental health, would critically analyze and then deny this supposition. This is because the majority of healthy persons hold the firm belief that they are not psychotic. In fact, for many persons, it may be quite difficult to admit that this latter belief may be wrong, even in cases when it is. The majority of healthy persons will have no objective reason to believe that they lack any control, whatsoever, over their mental faculties. As a result, some may not even entertain the possibility that they may be ill.

In the latter case, the individual usually possesses enough sound evidence to conclude that he is neither insane, nor suffering from a mental illness. The fundamental problem in denial remains in the fact that the individual will usually disavow many forms of sound evidence, even when this evidence is completely rational. In my case, I entered into a state of disbelief and mistrust, due to my paranoid thoughts. When I was severely ill, I believed that there were persons in the world who were out to get me in some way. I then further deduced that my doctor's diagnosis was a part of this conspiracy. This erroneous belief seemed to be fully rational, in my mind, at that point in time. As a result, the irrational beliefs held by a mentally sick individual may give him enough reasons to deny a medical diagnosis. In essence, a conflict of belief ensues between the patient and his doctor, and this will result in the patient's refusal for medical treatment.

When a patient enters into a state of denial, the existence of social stigmas may also be relevant. Under these circumstances, the patient may not accept his doctor's diagnosis, because he fears the social shame that may be associated with it. More specifically, the individual fears that he will be labelled as a person that is mentally ill. In this case, the individual denies his doctor's diagnosis because he fears the possibility that he may be negatively stereotyped and discriminated upon, because of his illness.

Under this specific circumstance, I believe that the patient would have no reason to enter into a state of denial, if there were no societal stigmas associated to mental disease. The patient would then, subsequently, have no reason to refuse medical treatment. To solve this problem, the individual's society must be educated in the subject of mental illness, which should then address any problems related to stigma and intolerance.

In contrast, when a patient refuses medical treatment because of his experiences with an intolerable side effect, the problem is less serious. In this case, the patient does acknowledge that he is suffering from some form of mental illness. His decision to refuse treatment is centred more on feelings of frustration, which are directed towards methods of psychiatric treatment in general. Thankfully, many different treatment options are readily available for schizophrenia patients today. The addition of more treatment options should further address problems related to an intolerable side effect.

Schizophrenia can be defined as a chemical imbalance. This imbalance is due to some biological defect within the brain. In principle, the main goal of all antipsychotic medications is to modify the chemical equilibrium within a schizophrenia patient's brain.

Patients who refuse treatment will continue to suffer from a chemical imbalance. They will also suffer from psychosis, as a direct result. Conversely, if the individual consents to psychiatric treatment, this chemical imbalance can be corrected. If his illness is chronic, the patient must comply with antipsychotic treatments for the rest of his life. This is the first step that the patient must take towards a successful rehabilitation from a mental illness. The patient must fully comply with his doctor's counsel, before any type of recovery can take place.

The treatment process for mental illnesses, like schizophrenia, is not limited solely to the prescribing of medications. Counselling is also significant to the recovery process. When the patient returns to a rational state, psychological counselling can help with problems related to excessive emotions and negative life experiences. In some instances, psychological counselling can also treat some forms of mild symptoms. A good counsellor will mainly help the patient with any psychological issues that may arise due to his illness. Psychological counselling can also help the patient maintain a more sound and rational frame of mind, when facing forms of adversity.

Regular visits to a mental health professional are also necessary to monitor the patient's condition. It is possible that a problem with a prescribed antipsychotic may occur at some point in the future. The patient can experience newer unwanted side effects or a change in the drug's potency. Even when the patient has been stable on a prescribed medicine for many years, it is still necessary to monitor his treatments. In other cases, a change in the individual's prescription can actually produce more beneficial effects than his previous mode of treatment.

Social rehabilitation is the final step in the patient's recovery from a mental illness. When the patient's symptoms are properly treated, he will then need to re-enter himself back into his community. Family members and friends can help with this undertaking. According to many researchers, the active socialization of mentally sick individuals is essential to their psychological and emotional well-being. The act of socialization can reinforce a positive lifestyle and help shape rational decision making in the patient. Social rehabilitation can also help the patient establish positive characteristics related to confidence and self-esteem. The concepts of dependence, independence, and interdependence are other important concepts that the patient will realize, once he re-enters himself back into a community based lifestyle.

These are the most essential steps that a patient must take towards a full recovery from schizophrenia. It is important to accept the fact that mental illnesses can affect any individual, in any part of the world. Dealing and coping with a mental illness may truly be a difficult course of action. A greater understanding of mental illness, with respect to the patient's family members, friends, and community, will further aid him in his rehabilitation process. A general understanding of mental illness can also shed some of the stigmas that have been associated with schizophrenia, and this will serve to strengthen our society as a whole.

2

My History

From some of my earliest memories, I remember having experiences with paranoid thoughts. For the most part, I believed that these thoughts were normal and possibly common among all human beings. In retrospect, however, I now realize that this belief was wrong. On other occasions, I would sometimes analyze my paranoid thoughts to be unusual, though I would typically dismiss these intuitions. Many of my paranoid thoughts also followed stressful events. Emotions like anger and shock sometimes preceded some of my most severe paranoid thoughts.

The medical community defines these unusual thoughts as delusions. In fact, mentally healthy persons can also produce paranoid thoughts. Their thoughts will usually be less severe in nature though. A common paranoid thought can occur when an individual witnesses a group of persons that are whispering to each other. Under this circumstance, the individual may believe that these persons are conversing about him. However, in many cases, this perception can be wrong. I would categorize this as a normal, yet paranoid thought.

The average person can also generate thoughts of grandeur. For example, the individual may believe that he is more talented at singing than he truly is. This is an example of a grand thought. Thoughts of grandeur may also be common among mentally healthy individuals. Nevertheless, the magnitude of their grand thought is minor, when compared to a schizophrenia patient's delusion of grandeur. The majority of my paranoid and grand thoughts were extreme and irrational. They were schizophrenic delusions. The average mentally healthy person will never experience a similar degree of irrationality, with respect to any of his paranoid or grand thoughts.

During some moments, I held the belief that my schizophrenic delusions were thoughts that may be common among other persons. At those times, I would subsequently dismiss the possibility that I could be suffering from a mental illness. This assumption would cause a problem for me later in life, at a time when I would become increasingly more ill.

Today, I now understand that many of my previous extreme thoughts were schizophrenic delusions. My delusions of grandeur always followed stressful events. However, I was not consistently delusional whenever I experienced intense levels of stress. During my youth, I experienced delusions of grandeur and paranoia mainly at random.

Throughout the early stages of my illness, my delusions would usually last for no longer than 15 seconds. After this period, my mental state would then return into a more regular state. The most radical delusion of grandeur that I have experienced caused me to hold the belief that I was God, the almighty Creator. I remember that I held this belief after I experienced periods of overwhelming stress. I also believed that I was God when I experienced manic emotions. All of my schizophrenic delusions evolved through an altered perception of the real, physical world. In my mind, the disease caused me to lose my personal identity as a human being, and conclude that I was God during these brief moments.

On other occasions, I would eventually come to realize that a number of my schizophrenic delusions were somewhat irrational. In fact, I always had a gut feeling that some of my most extreme thoughts were wrong. This may be due, in large part, to my education in religion. According to my religious beliefs, God exists somewhere beyond the physical world. I also believe that I am His creation. Therefore, some of my thoughts of grandeur would conflict with concepts that I had believed in throughout most of my life.

Now let me clarify what actually induced my delusions of grandeur. During any random social situation, things would often not make sense to me. Whenever I entered into this state of confusion, I would occasionally react further by entering into what I call a state of disbelief. My states of disbelief centred on my metaphysical existence. During these moments, I held the belief that I was not physically present within my environment. At this point, I would then fluidly enter into a surreal or dreamlike state.

My train of thought would furthermore continue, and I would then enter into an omniscient-like point of view. In essence, I lost a first person perspective of life and viewed my environment through a third person's perspective. This unusual psychological experience shifted my focus beyond the real, physical world. On some occasions, I would enter into a state of mental euphoria. This feeling would then lead me to believe that I was God. Whenever I entered into this dreamlike state, I would find it difficult to focus my attention on anything else. Further, the belief that I was God almost always preceded thoughts when my attention was focused back onto the real, physical world.

On some occasions, I would try to rationalize and make sense of these strange experiences. However, I always failed in this respect. According to my irrational mind, the only reason why I experienced this godlike awareness was based on the notion that I was something more than a regular human being.

My experiences with this extremely self-conscious dreamlike state would also often lead me back into a state of confusion. At times, I could not make any sense of my schizophrenic delusions. Based on my observations of other persons, I also came to believe that these self-conscious, surreal experiences were unique to me. However, I never came up with any sound reasons why this happened to me alone. My only seemingly rational thought was based on the belief that I was a unique entity. Following this faulty reasoning, I would subsequently ignore the majority of my other life experiences, which may have contradicted this evaluation.

As the frequency of my delusions increased, these extreme thoughts would usually serve to reinforce the belief that I was a supernatural being, who had taken a human form. The majority of my life experiences led me to conclude that I was not evil, and that I was, in fact, a good or benign spirit. Moreover, according to my religious beliefs, I knew that there is only one, almighty, and benevolent God. In time, I would then irrationally deduce the notion that since no other persons experienced any similar states of a dream-like over awareness, I was not in fact a normal human being and accordingly I must be God. This is roughly how stressful events, defective thoughts, and a state of surreal awareness ended up producing the delusion that I was God. A schizophrenic delusion always results through a combination of irrational thoughts and paranoid perceptions. Patients will also seldom conceive the possibility that their delusions may be fictitious.

My earliest memory of a delusion of grandeur occurred when I was approximately four years old. At that time, an aunt and uncle of mine had come to my home for a short visit. They along with my mother and father and I were standing in my living room. After a couple of minutes, my mother told me to show my uncle around the house. I was quite surprised about this request for several reasons. First, I wondered why my mother had asked me to do this, instead of doing it herself. Secondly, I also wondered why she asked me to do this solely for my uncle, and not for my aunt and uncle together. After pondering these thoughts, my mother became impatient. She then raised her tone and repeated her request. It was at this point when I experienced my earliest memory of a schizophrenic delusion.

When my mother raised her voice at me, I experienced an increasing amount of psychological stress which caused me to think in a rapid fashion. The rapid nature of my thoughts then shifted back on to my self-perception, and a raised awareness. Eventually, my thoughts led to a brief moment where I held the belief that I was God.

This shift in perspective may be difficult to understand, for persons who have always observed the world through a healthy frame of mind. When my mother raised her voice at me, my brain reacted in an automatic fashion and I entered into a surreal, dreamlike state. It may be difficult to understand why I would then come to believe in the notion that I was God. In fact, the activation of this surreal state seemingly enabled me to perceive the world through a bird's eye view. In my mind, I was not only aware of my own thoughts, but I was also aware of the thoughts of other persons within my physical environment. The only explanation that I could come up with why I alone experienced this omniscient-like perspective was based on the possibility that I was a supernatural being.

My delusions of grandeur occurred mainly because of three critical factors. Primarily, I would be experiencing a high degree of stress. Upon experiencing a stressful situation, my perspective would then shift into a surreal-like state. This perspective would essentially change from a first person's perspective, into a third person's point of view and then back again. My evaluation of this experience would then lead me to conclude that I was God.

During my youth, I would usually enter into a state of confusion, immediately after experiencing a delusion. No matter how hard I tried, I never came up with any explanation why I consistently entered into this surreal, dreamlike state. Today, I now realize that these strange experiences were due to a disease. At present, I am also able to realize that these thoughts were delusions, and not true representations of the actual world.

Another delusion of grandeur that I keenly remember occurred during the ninth grade, while I was attending high school. That day I decided to miss one of my classes and I went to a local video arcade instead. After some time, one of the vice-principals from my school stepped into that arcade. He went there to identify students who were truant from class. All of the students inside immediately ran for the exits. A friend of mine and I locked ourselves inside a bathroom. We then waited patiently until our vice-principle left the arcade.

Another friend of mine and I then stayed in the arcade, and we continued to play video games. My heart was still beating quickly due to my feelings of anxiety. As a consequence, I was constantly looking around the arcade, in the fear that my vice-principal may return. At that time, I entered into a mild paranoid state.

He never did return to the arcade. However, at that time, paranoid thoughts were still running rampant throughout my mind. The anxiety that I felt caused me to look around the arcade apprehensively. After a short period, my friend and I left the arcade and we started to walk back towards our school.

I am not quite sure why, but my feelings of anxiety persisted, and I continued to look behind us while we were walking in a back alleyway. This is when I saw a group of about 10 older and physically larger teenagers following us. One of them shouted, "Come here". My friend was a bit overweight and I quietly told him to keep on walking. My intention was to give him a head start, before I would start to run myself. I walked back towards this group and they asked for my money. After showing them my empty wallet, I looked around to make sure that my friend had gotten away. In fact, he did not get away, and he ignorantly walked back towards us. In reality, he did not truly comprehend what was happening. At this point, I was ready to run away from this situation, but I knew that if I did, my friend would not be able to outrun this group along with me.

The biggest hooligan in the group then picked me up by my jacket. He had a smile on his face, and after a long period of eye contact, he threw me to the ground. Suffice it to say, he beat me up, and it looked like he was enjoying this experience. It was at this time when I experienced another surreal, dreamlike state. For a couple of seconds, I experienced feelings of shock and disbelief. I could not understand why anyone would want to assault another human being, for no real reason. At that moment, it felt like I was existing in a daydream, and not in the physical world. After the first punch, I fell to the ground. The shock then hit me, and because of this psychological stressor, I experienced a delusion of grandeur. For a few seconds, I held the belief that I was Jesus Christ and I concluded that this was the reason why I was in that situation, getting beat up at that very moment.

During that stressful moment, an increase in adrenaline may have caused this extreme perception. I could not come up with any sensible reason why a group of larger teenagers would want to pick on two smaller and weaker youths. I then experienced a moment of over awareness, and viewed this situation through an omniscient-like perspective. My thoughts then progressed into a delusion of grandeur. My rapid thoughts eventually led me to believe that I was Jesus Christ, and that these persons were assaulting me in order to cleanse the sins of other persons around the world. At that moment, my delusion of grandeur seemed to be as normal as any other thought within my mind.

This crime affected me quite deeply. I was angry at the fact that someone would enjoy the act of assaulting an innocent human being and that there were individuals in the world who would devalue another human being to such a high degree. The next year I committed a crime of my own. To this day, I am not completely sure why I acted in this manner. Perhaps it was due to some experiences with my peers at that point in time. The reason may also be due to an experience during my youth, when someone accused my mother of this crime.

When I was approximately seven years old, my mother and I were walking into a store in the mall, and the door alarm started to ring. A security guard escorted us to a room in the back and he started to question my mother. The questioning lasted for about three hours before we were permitted to leave the store. It turns out that my mother was returning a pair of jeans from another store, with the security tag intact. This is what caused the door alarm to go off.

At that time, I did not know why that security officer had questioned my mother for such a long time. First of all, my mother had a store receipt along with her. Secondly, we were not walking out of that store when the alarm went off; we were actually walking into the store. Thirdly, the merchandise in question came from a different shop. Eventually, the security guard returned the merchandise to my mother and we left the mall. As a youth, I did not fully understand why this was happening to us. That was also a very stressful experience for me. In fact, no police officers ever questioned my mother, and she was never charged with any crime. That event is a vivid memory of mine, even to this day.

Some years later, I ended up shoplifting some merchandise from several stores in the same mall. I was approximately 14 years old at that time. I committed this act in a rebellious fashion, though at that time, I did not have anything specific to rebel against. After some time, a similar undercover security officer made a citizen's arrest. He escorted me into a questioning room, and I cooperated with him.

I remember that when he first apprehended me, he treated me like a low class criminal. After a few minutes, he then seemed to demonstrate some compassion for me. I think he knew that I was not truly a criminal, and that I was only an immature youth. No stores pressed charges against me that day.

For some reason, I shoplifted again a short time later. This time, I was in a store and I noticed that a Caucasian woman was staring at me, though the corner of her eye. She probably did this because I was a teenager. However, from my perspective, she may have also been racist. This thought made me quite angry. Something inside of me then caused me to act, again, in a rebellious fashion. I ended up putting a package of gum into my pocket, essentially because this woman was staring at me. When I left the store, she followed me outside and took a hold of my arm. I did not resist, though I also did not speak a single word to her. When a police officer came, I was fully cooperative. In an indirect fashion, I told the officer that the security guard may be racist. I am not sure if the officer had agreed with me, though in any case, she let me go without any further questioning.

Looking back, I believe that I had committed the crime of shoplifting as a reaction to some of my paranoid thoughts. During many times in my youth, I would sometimes believe in the idea that total strangers were focusing their attention on me. At times, I may have acted impulsively, in order to test this supposition.

I also somehow came to the belief that if I was caught committing a crime, this would confirm my thought that everyone was focusing their attention on me. In my mind, this would also confirm the possibility that many of my delusions of paranoia were real. In fact, I remember that during random points in my life, I did things that were out of character, in order to test and evaluate my experiences with paranoia.

When I was not delusional, I would hold the natural belief that I was an average human being. Therefore, the conflict in identity that I consistently experienced, when delusional, would often leave me in a state of confusion. At times, I suspected that something could be wrong with me mentally. Even though I was able to rationalize this possibility, I never really elaborated on this thought. Perhaps I feared the possible result of this analysis. At other points during my life, something inside of me wanted to solve this conflict in identity. The fact that I had been caught while committing a crime gave me one more reason to believe that I was an average human being, and not a supernatural figure.

I also remember a delusion of grandeur that occurred when I was graduating from high school. That year was especially difficult for me for personal reasons. Several years back, during my graduating year at elementary school, my cousin Ray passed away. We were very close, and the graduating theme in elementary school that year caused me to become depressed. My period of personal grief and mourning had returned in a swift and sudden fashion.

I recall that, on many occasions that year, I would continually perceive the world through a fragmented and surreal state of mind. My consciousness would shift from the real world, into a dreamlike state, and then back again quite frequently. The stress that I experienced also had a massive impact on my studies. My mood swayed back and forth that year as well. On some occasions, I would be quite happy with the thought of graduation. At other times, feelings of depression would overpower me. This emotional state influenced me to the point where I did not want to face much of the world that year. I spoke to a school counsellor, and then reduced my course load by half.

A delusion of grandeur of mine, at that time, occurred while I was writing a customary graduation write up for my school's annual. My conflicting emotions of joy and sadness were quite difficult to deal with. This stress affected my psychological state, and in due course, it caused me to hold the belief that I was God. This belief often affected my self-perspective for much of that year, and accordingly, I wrote my graduation message in the belief that I was God. Yet, when I look back at what I had created that day, my message was neither irrational, nor was it out of place. In fact, I believe that it demonstrated compassion, and that it was created through some unique leadership qualities.

Thus, psychological stress seems to be a common element among all of my delusions of grandeur. I have no real memories of any non-stressful events that caused me to generate a delusion of grandeur. However, it is also very likely that I have experienced many delusional thoughts that I cannot recall today. Before Dr. Lupton diagnosed me with schizophrenia, I found it very difficult to accept the possibility that my delusions were abnormal thoughts. On the other hand, I knew that, through my observations of other persons, most individuals do not hold the belief that they are God.

In any case, I never really came across any solid evidence which would have led me to believe that I was mentally unstable during much of my youth. At times, I would try to believe that my strange thoughts could be natural and not a symptom of a mental illness. Eventually, I came to the belief that my strange delusional thoughts were part of a unique, yet normal state of mind.

As a youth, my delusions of grandeur usually lasted no longer than several seconds. After experiencing a delusion, my perspective of the world would return back into a more regular state. After some time, and a prolonged history of delusional thoughts, the transition from my delusional states to a rational frame of mind began to feel more fluid and effortless. While severely ill, I never even realized that any transition was taking place. Therefore, in time, even my most extreme delusions would begin to feel as natural as any other thought within my mind.

Later in life, while in a prolonged delusional state, I usually could not make much sense of my experiences. I would then enter into a state of confusion and my overall awareness would decline. After these episodes, I would usually forget the fact that I had entered into a confused state, although I would remember the delusion itself. Accordingly, poor memory would pose as a problem for me in the future, because I would basically forget any negative evaluations that I held with respect to my extreme schizophrenic delusions.

Stressful events also triggered my delusions of paranoia. Instead of focusing on the nature of my existence, these delusions were based more on my physical environment. When I experienced paranoid thoughts, I would often believe that everyone within my physical environment was either talking about me, or focusing their attention on me. Similar to delusions of grandeur, paranoid delusions are also based on false perceptions and faulty interpretations of these perceptions. Purely at random, I would hold the belief that strangers were focusing their attention on me. At times, these delusions produced some fearful responses in me. At other times, these perceptions encouraged feelings of vanity.

For the most part, whenever I entered into a state of paranoia, I would usually be unaware of the fact that any change in my frame of mind had ever occurred. This is one major difference between my paranoid thoughts and my delusions of grandeur. Even from my earliest memories, the transition between rational thought to a state of paranoia felt quite natural. Therefore, because of this effortless transition and a lack of awareness, I eventually came to believe that my paranoid thoughts were regular in every possible way.

From the best of my memories, I mainly experienced extreme forms of paranoid thoughts later in life, in comparison to my extreme delusions of grandeur. In addition, after some time, my paranoid delusions became much more vivid than any of my delusions of grandeur. Hence, my paranoid delusions also had greater effects over my lifestyle. In my mind, the belief that I was God was a very radical belief. In contrast, the belief that everyone was focusing on me was much more realistic, and thus more stressful. The stress that I experienced also had vast impacts on my daily behaviour.

Whenever I experienced a delusion of grandeur, I would usually forget my belief that I was God after a short period of time. Accordingly, the temporal length of my grand delusions was usually shorter than my paranoid delusions. In most cases, I would re-enter into a regular state of mind at a faster pace after my delusions of grandeur. Instead of lasting for a few seconds, some of my paranoid delusions lasted for much greater lengths of time.

My earliest memory of an extreme paranoid thought occurred when I was eight years old. During my third grade at elementary school, I believed that many of my classmates were focusing their attention on me, as opposed to our teacher's instruction. These delusions usually lasted for approximately 30 seconds, after which my attention would then focus back onto our teacher's lessons. As my age and the severity of my disease increased, the duration and radical nature of my paranoid delusions would also increase. In time, I found it increasingly more difficult to focus my attention back into a regular state, after experiencing a paranoid delusion. The fact that I had to exert some mental energy to accomplish this was also new to me. However, my efforts, in this regard, would later become ineffectual.

I started to experience problems with concentration, due to my paranoid delusions, when I was approximately 15 years old. During my grade 10 year, I often found it difficult to remain attentive during class and concentrate on my studies. At that time, I also lacked a degree of awareness, and thus, I never really realized that I was shifting into a state of paranoia. Nonetheless, I still possessed some ability to function academically.

My experience with paranoia was most severe, though, during my college years. A couple of semesters into my studies, I went to class and found it progressively more difficult to concentrate on my professor's lecture. After a few classes, these paranoid thoughts would soon have a greater effect over my academic functioning. On some occasions, I believed that all of the students in my class were focusing their attention on me. On other occasions, I believed that my professors were focusing their attention on me, for the entire lecture.

My first reaction to this delusion put me into a state of shock and disbelief. Initially, I would try to scrutinize my paranoid thoughts. However, after much effort, I could not come up with any reason why everyone would be focusing their attention on me. Soon enough, I would also lose the ability to refocus my attention back onto the actual world. While in this prolonged delusional state, I pretended to be attentive during class. However, the only thing that I could truly focus on was my paranoid delusions. For several days, I would continue to experience these delusions, and likewise, I would persistently try to ignore them. After some time, my paranoid thoughts became much more difficult to control, and this started to have a massive impact on my ability to function as a student.

During those episodes, I was never aware of the fact that my thoughts were abnormal in any way. Furthermore, I eventually lost the ability to analyze any of my previous thoughts or experiences. On many occasions, my experiences with paranoia would cause me to enter into a state of confusion. At other times, I would enter into a defensive state. I never tried to speak out in class while experiencing these delusions, though after some time, my facial expressions may have expressed my confusion. After entering into a prolonged delusional state, I eventually became aware of my odd facial expressions, and I then considered the possibility that something may be wrong with me. At that time, whenever I experienced any negative emotions due to my delusions, I would still possess the ability to acknowledge that this was inconsistent with my true character.

After some time, I realized that some of my professors had also noticed my odd facial expressions, though they never reacted to my demeanour. They mainly continued with their lecture. At times, when I perceived that they were not focusing their attention on me, my mind would then switch back into a regular state. During my college years, I rarely contemplated about my strange experiences after class. I speculate that this lack of insight and awareness could indicate the probability that I was severely ill at that point in time.

When I became severely more ill, there were no specific triggers behind my schizophrenic delusions, and I began to experience paranoia in all types of situations. In due course, this paranoid state of mind would force me to withdraw from my college studies. For the most part, I knew that I was having problems with concentration, and I wanted to see if some time off would remedy this situation. In actuality, my paranoid delusions had taken full control over my mind, and I found it exceptionally difficult to concentrate on anything else. At this time, I lacked the ability to concentrate on anything other than my delusions, and this caused me to remain in a state of confusion as a direct result.

In time, I stopped socializing with my friends, and after some more time, I would not even leave my house. The severity of my disease caused me to become excessively irrational. My inability to function academically gave me one more reason to suspect that something may be wrong with me mentally.

Another radical experience with paranoia occurred when I was twenty years old. A friend of mine unexpectedly came over to my house and took me out for lunch. I was reluctant to leave my home, because I feared the possibility that I would experience further problems with paranoid thoughts. In all likelihood, I knew that I would become paranoid at some point during that outing. My experiences with paranoia, thus, caused feelings of anxiety within me. At that time, whenever I felt uncomfortable, my thoughts would mainly focus on my volition to return home, where I would be free from entering into a paranoid state while in public.

When my friend ordered a meal, my feelings of anxiety had steadily persisted. I ordered a coffee, but I ignored him for the most part. Paranoid delusions then began to take control of my mind, and they elevated feelings of anxiety into fear. The buzzing of voices inside of that restaurant also affected my psyche. I started to believe that everyone was focusing on our table, and that they were having conversations about me. This delusion impacted me greatly. I reacted in fear, and this caused me to further withdraw from that social situation. When I returned home, I barricaded myself inside of my bedroom because of this experience.

The harshest paranoid delusion that I have ever experienced occurred approximately one week after this incident. At that time, I had cut off all of my social ties, including family members. My daily routine was limited to watching television and listening to music on the radio. I was in a prolonged state of paranoia, and my social fears remained. Then without warning, I experienced the feeling that random radio and television personalities were either talking to me or talking about my life. I also believed that all of the songs on the radio and programs on television were based on some random aspect of my life. Subsequently, my paranoid thoughts became unusually more severe.

At times, I was able to recognize that these radical perceptions were out of the ordinary. Moreover, I could not come up with any reasons why so many people would be focusing on my life. In the end, I would experience paranoid delusions in all social situations. They escalated to the point where I believed that every person, within my physical environment, was focusing on my life. I would then enter into a constant state of confusion. The thought that I could be wrong or delusional never crossed my mind.

I found it difficult to think about anything other than my delusions, as the severity of my illness increased. In time, I would end up losing full control over my mind, and accordingly, I would then be unable to focus my attention back onto the real world. Likewise, the belief that I was God soon became a rational reason why everyone in the world was focusing on my life.

My experience with these changes in personal identity, however, had produced warning signals within me. At a rudimentary level, I knew that my thoughts had conflicted at times. I also became aware of the fact that my delusions of grandeur would usually surface in a sporadic fashion. This is when I finally decided to ask for help. After watching a local news program, my feelings of paranoia had returned and I believed that the media were reporting stories about my life. When the chance became available, I decided to speak with my sister about these strange thoughts. At first, she dismissed what I had to say. In her mind, she did not even conceive the possibility that I may be ill. Above all, she believed that I was joking with her. However, after I told her about my radical thoughts for the second and third times, she finally came to believe that something could be wrong.

My sister then contacted a psychiatrist, and this started the preliminary stages of my treatment process. After a lifetime of exposure to schizophrenic delusions, I only had the courage to tell someone after there was little doubt in my mind that something was truly wrong. My inability to function at school gave me a further reason to believe that some form of mental illness may be affecting me.

I can only analyze the effects of my schizophrenic delusions, after the fact. I know that my delusions had caused me to enter into a state of confusion, on many occasions. In particular, after experiencing some of my delusions of grandeur, I would become confused and then enter into a state of disbelief. During these moments, I had trouble deciding whether I was dreaming or an active member within the real world.

Thoughts of disbelief would often mediate my shift of perspective from a delusional mental state, back onto the physical world. When this occurred, I would ignore the fact that I had just experienced an extremely unusual thought. As a result, entering into a state of disbelief essentially acted as a personal coping mechanism. I would forget about my experience with radical thoughts, and this enabled me to normalize my condition and refocus my mind back onto my physical environment. At times, I did not even acknowledge the fact that I ever perceived any radical thoughts at all.

This was only a short-term solution though. I was able to temporarily forget about my strange thoughts, but I was not able to forget about them in any permanent fashion. This influenced my knowledge and interpretation of real world events. As I reached adulthood, every so often I would briefly recollect and reflect upon my previous delusions of grandeur and paranoia. In my mind, these memories felt no different from any other memory that I possessed. In time, this gave me a reason to believe that my delusions were no less irregular than any other thought within my mind.

When I thought about my shifts in personal identity from human into a supernatural being, I would often experience troubles while trying to analyze and examine these shifts. As such, deficits in cognition also impeded my ability to realize that my delusions were extreme thoughts, after the fact.

As my disease progressed, I found it increasingly more difficult to actively ignore any of my delusional states. This had a real impact on my functioning. Most of my previous schoolteachers thought of me as an intelligent and creative student. While in elementary school, I took part in a special program for gifted children. Correspondingly, my high school teachers may have attributed the cause of my low grades to laziness over inability. During my high school years, I also preferred to attribute laziness as the cause of my academic problems, over any other possibility. I do not think that my teachers, friends, or family ever truly suspected that I was suffering from schizophrenic symptoms, during my elementary and high school years.

The symptoms that I experienced also had an impact on my social life. I always had an introverted personality, but I now know that my schizophrenic thoughts had caused me to withdraw from many other social situations. The delusions that I experienced also affected my self-esteem. Whenever I entered into a state of confusion after experiencing a delusion, I would feel less confident to assert myself in the fear that I could act in a strange fashion. Indeed, it was very possible that I could have acted out of context under these circumstances. The main problem was that my true self-identity had come into question, and this influenced my thoughts and actions in all situations. The fact that my thoughts had often contradicted each other also gave rise to the feeling that I could not always depend on my faculty of reason. Therefore, my experiences with delusions also had a great impact over many of my everyday actions and behaviours.

I firmly believe that the effects of my illness also gave me a reason to start a lifestyle of substance abuse. I remember that as a child, I always detested the smell of cigarette smoke. Even so, I started to smoke when I was 15 years of age, and I continue to smoke today. There could be many reasons behind my decision to smoke cigarettes. Peer pressure and personal stress may be two major reasons. In fact, cigarette smoking and substance abuse is highly common among persons with schizophrenia (Torrey, 1995). Perhaps my delusional state of mind may also be relevant. The radical delusions regarding my personal identity, and other strange thoughts, may have produced a desire in me to experiment with substances that affect the human psyche. At present, I believe that a combination of all of these elements had some influence over my choice in this respect. This choice, nevertheless, is entirely inconsistent with the feelings that I had about smoking throughout most of my childhood.

In high school, I was enrolled in honours courses until I reached the tenth grade. After the tenth grade, my ability to concentrate was impacted to the point where I could not maintain a good academic record. In grade 11, my academic standing dropped drastically throughout all of my courses. In fact, my state of mind had deteriorated, and the dreamlike states that I experienced had increased in duration and number. At that time, I was too ill to realize the true reason why I was unable to function academically. I then began to live a day-to-day lifestyle, with no plans for my near future. I also lost all motivation to make my life better. After some more time, I entered into a new social sphere and I started to smoke marijuana.

There are two main reasons that may best explain why I started to smoke marijuana. Firstly, the drug provided an escape from my mental reality. This is probably the most common reason why all users experiment with illicit drugs. My mental reality, at that time, consistently shifted from a surreal state to a state of confusion, due to my delusions. Furthermore, I sometimes had enough insight to realize that the content of some of my thoughts were strange and irregular. However, my inability to concentrate and focus on my studies may have been the most significant reason why I started to smoke marijuana. At that point, I did speculate that something could be wrong with me mentally. Nonetheless, it may have also been possible that my radical thoughts and problems with concentration could have been due to stress. In fact, the collapse of my mental state hit me like a falling brick. I was unable to concentrate, and I was also constantly entering into dreamlike states at random points throughout the day. I then came to believe that a break from all external stressors might cure my condition.

I experimented with marijuana in order to gain another perspective on my poor state of mind. I held the ignorant belief that this drug would help me analyze my current predicament. Therefore, I mistakenly believed that this drug would help me discover the true reason why I was no longer able to concentrate during class and achieve high grades. At the time, I also believed that I had nothing to lose by experimenting with an illicit substance.

Many schizophrenia patients will also choose to abuse illicit substances, for the reason of self-medication. In some cases, alcohol and street drugs can decrease feelings of anxiety and depression, and improve energy levels in the individual (Torrey, 1995). Realistically, some individuals with schizophrenia would have chosen to abuse an illicit substance, even if they were never ill. On the other hand, it is also true that many persons would have never chosen to abuse an illicit substance, if they were not affected by a mental illness.

I strongly believe that I fit into the latter category. My choice to self-medicate did provide some escape from my delusions of grandeur and paranoia. In this respect, smoking marijuana did essentially provide a short-term cure from my schizophrenic symptoms. The effects of marijuana on my mental state also gave me a limited ability to analyze some of my delusional states. Therefore, my experiences with marijuana enabled me to further conceive the possibility that some of my delusions could be abnormal mental states.

I also mistakenly believed that my academic abilities would not deteriorate any further, even if I were to experiment with marijuana. Thus, I did not really consider the possibility that it may have negative effects on my psyche. This could be the main reason why I had continued to smoke it for over one year. In fact, the drug never provided me with any real insight as to why I was performing so poorly academically. It merely provided an escape from my diminished and delusional mental state.

I quit smoking marijuana after my grade twelve year. I did not complete my studies on time though, and I ended up taking an extra year to complete the rest of my high school credits. At that time, I remember that I felt better mentally, because I was free from many external stressors. The demands of graduating from high school and gaining entrance into university studies were no longer relevant to me. My concentration also subsequently improved.

During that period, I still experienced paranoid symptoms, though to a lesser degree. Nevertheless, I found comfort in my new social situation, and I also made some new friends. I was doing better both academically and socially because of this new environment. In retrospect, I was entirely free from any demands and expectations with respect to achieving academic success.

During my high school years, I held three separate part-time jobs within the service industry. I also found employment within an office setting, while attending night school and during my first semesters at college. Leaving the high school environment had a positive effect on me. I felt healthy enough to handle the extra work, and I also felt rejuvenated. Things were going good at first, and I did not experience any major problems with delusions at this point in my life. During my college studies, I was quite happy emotionally. On the weekends, I went to work and then I came home and spent time on my studies. I was not overly fatigued, and I felt ready to achieve anything that I had previously dreamed about as a child.

This feeling of liberation from my paranoid state of mind was what I was seeking throughout most of my high school years. My improved mental state would not last long nonetheless. After some time, a thief stole my car and this violation had an emotional toll on me. My car was also vandalized on many occasions in the past, and this proved to be an additional source of stress. I then entered into some extreme delusional states again. In essence, I began to suspect that many acquaintances of mine were responsible for these crimes. This included both family members and friends. Today, I know that my suspicions were wrong, and that I was in a state of paranoia. Further, I have reason to believe that the theft of my car was purely a random crime. The persons that I did suspect at that time are not persons that I would suspect, had I had access to a rational frame of mind. Thus, personal stressors consistently caused me to enter into a delusional frame of mind, throughout most of my entire life.

That paranoid episode did not last very long. I was able to manage my thoughts, and I continued to attend classes and work on a part-time basis. I also felt healthy enough to finance a new car. I did not know it at the time though, and I would soon become very ill. The illness affected me to the point where I could not maintain my studies or part-time job. In very little time, my delusions would start to overwhelm me and become much more difficult to manage. The illness rapidly took full control over my mind, and I would not experience a state of good mental health for another several years.

3

Onset of the Disease

Up until the point where I believed that persons on television were speaking to me, I never really thought about what my life would be like, should I be suffering from some form of mental illness. When my paranoid delusions became more frequent, it was then when I decided to ask for help. I remember that in one of my college classes, I viewed that environment as a kind of farce. I started to giggle and laugh in an uncontrollable fashion during that class. From my delusional perspective, the interactions between my professor and classmates were funny in some way. My delusions caused me to believe that these persons were there solely to entertain me, in the same manner that a stand-up comedian entertains his audience. I held this belief soon after I first stepped into that classroom. Actually, I walked into that classroom as regular college student. However, after I was sitting comfortably in that class, I would start to perceive something immensely different.

I could not come up with any reason why anyone would want to entertain me at that particular place and time. My professor probably believed that I was a student who was purposely disrupting his lecture. He may have also held the belief that I came to class intoxicated on some form of illicit substance. After a short time, I became aware of my strange behaviour, and I then quickly became embarrassed. It was at that point when I began to suspect that something could be very wrong with me. I found it utterly impossible to stop laughing that day in class. Soon enough, my classmates noticed my bizarre behaviour, and my professor also came over to check up on me. The look on his face made me realize that my behaviour was strange and irregular. I then immediately left the class and went home. The next day, I decided to withdraw from all of my classes and take a break from my college studies.

At that time, the disease had taken much more control over my mind. Whenever I experienced delusions now, my mind would remain in a delusional state for almost the entire day.

I was also laid off from my part-time job at an engineering firm. During that summer, I remember that I experienced problems with concentration on the job. I made simple mistakes on duties that required very little thought. The relationship between my employer and I also declined. All of these events seem to indicate that my health was deteriorating in a constant fashion. The illness eventually interfered with my ability to work constructively, and I found it difficult to maintain any social relationships away from home.

At the peak of my illness, I would be trapped in a delusional state during all times of the day. This delusional state replaced my perspective of the actual world. I could not function, and I spent much of my time in bed either listening to music or watching television. About a week after I spoke to my sister about my paranoid delusions, she sought some professional help. I remember that I was quite open to speaking with a medical professional. After all, I was neither working, nor studying, nor was I doing anything productive during day.

It was early September when two psychiatrists, Dr. Lupton and Dr. Adrian, and a nurse named Sharon came to my home. I was 20 years old at that time. They began to ask questions related to my daily activities. When Dr. Adrian spoke to me and asked how I was doing, I would reply quietly and politely, and then turn my head away. In fact, I did this after all of their questions. I tried to answer their questions to the best of my abilities, despite the fact that I was experiencing problems with attention. At times, I would also start to giggle. In my mind, I believed that these medical professionals came to my home, also to entertain me in some way. I then realized that something could be wrong with me, due to the tone in their voices. Both doctors would speak about me in the third person perspective, while talking with my mother. Although this bothered me, I realized that their actions may have further indicated the possibility that something could be wrong with my mental health.

In truth, I was not really present in any of the conversations that were held that day. My mind was somewhere else, and I showed little reaction to their presence. I then started to giggle at random and in an uncontrollable fashion. At times, their conversation felt ridiculous to me. Occasionally, I would also enter into a state of confusion, and I would then try to come up with some reason why these persons were in my home, having a conversation about me. After about ten minutes, Dr. Lupton diagnosed me with schizophrenia. I asked for her reasons behind this diagnosis, and she told me that my recent experiences could be symptoms of the disease. Thus, I listened. I took a leap of faith and believed in the opinion of two strangers who were entirely unknown to me. It was quite remarkable that I was able to do this through my irrational frame of mind. In actuality, I was not fully convinced with their diagnosis. However, I also could not dismiss the fact that I was experiencing problems with cognition and extreme thoughts. After some time, I felt that there was a high probability that Dr. Lupton could be right. After further deliberation, I decided to cooperate with her treatment plan, and I travelled to an inpatient facility, as per her orders.

That night was a very frightening experience for me. I did not know what to expect. Initially, I spoke with the receptionist. After she recorded my personal information, I suddenly realized that I was not going home that night. The thought of losing my freedom is what scared me the most. I did not know if I would be released from that unit in a couple of days, or a couple of years. I also had no idea of what was going to happen next, and I feared the possibility that their modes of treatment may have some permanent debilitating effects.

The inpatient facility was very clean and the interior looked like a hybrid of a hospital ward and a community centre. A male nurse took me to my room. The room was empty apart from two beds. I sat on a bed, and stared at a sign on the wall. It was a no smoking sign. My future started to look a great deal more clouded to me. I also started to doubt the fact that I was sick or suffering from a disease. This degree of doubt gave me one final reason to envision myself as a normal human being.

My state of mind then entered into a dream-like state of disbelief. During some moments, I did not believe that I was actually physically present at that psychiatric ward. At other times, I did realize that I was present within a mental health unit, and I would then enter into a state of mild shock. Afterwards, I held the belief that I was actually healthy, and that Dr. Lupton's opinion was erroneous. I wanted to believe that I was about to wake from a hazy dream. I then continued to stare at that blank wall. Over an hour had passed, and that was when I finally realized that I was not dreaming.

After some time spent in meditation, I eventually drew the courage to step out of my room and explore the rest of the hospital. I was quite surprised to see elderly patients there. In fact, there were patients of all ages at that inpatient unit. There were males and females from all types of ethnic backgrounds. For some reason, I was shocked to see a young Asian adult there. He looked quite comfortable, and was probably a long-term patient. Perhaps these feelings emerged because I had someone to relate with, inside of that psychiatric ward. Throughout my entire stay there, though, I never did find out his name.

Soon nightfall came, and it was time to sleep. At 10:00 pm, all of the patients would brush their teeth and prepare for bedtime. The administration of our medicines came soon after. Another nurse came to my room to deliver Dr. Lupton's prescription. At 11:00 pm, all of the lights must be turned off. That was a difficult experience for me. The bed I was in felt much stiffer than my bed at home. I stayed awake for some time, and I was scared to fall asleep. It took me about an hour and a half to fall asleep that night.

The nurse's wakeup call came at 7:00 am the next morning. At 7:30 am, breakfast was served within the main cafeteria. There was an assortment of events planned every morning and afternoon. I did not participate though, and since the weather was nice, I decided to explore the rest of the property. The area outside of the main facility had a feeling of openness and it was a very peaceful environment. A couple of days later, I was released from that psychiatric ward and I returned home.

When I came home, I was not troubled by any forms of stress, and I continued to feel quite relaxed. This feeling, however, would soon pose as a problem for me. After a week of taking my prescribed medications, I started to doubt Dr. Lupton's diagnosis. I felt healthy, and at that time, my mind was free from any major delusional states. I probably still suffered from some minor bouts of paranoia, though at that time, I would usually forget about these experiences. In addition, I somehow came to the belief that my previous paranoid thoughts and delusions were normal, and not the symptoms of any illness.

At that time, the paranoid thoughts that I had previously experienced somehow became more regular in my mind. I recalled the fact that I experienced paranoid thoughts throughout my entire lifetime. Therefore, I somehow reasoned that my problems with paranoia were natural to being human. On the surface, this type of reasoning may seem irrational, when analyzed through a mentally healthy person's frame of mind. However, most patients with a mental illness will lack the ability to perceive the world through a rational frame of mind. I probably would have found other reasons to dismiss Dr. Lupton's diagnosis. At that time, I found it difficult to accept the possibility that I may be ill. I also believed that it was in my best interests to doubt Dr. Lupton's diagnosis. Nonetheless, I never came up with any sound reasons to justify this belief. I just assumed it to be true.

In retrospect, this belief may have been generated through another paranoid thought. Basically, I ended up believing that everyone within my social environment was mistaken about my diagnosis, and that I was the only one who could see this. These thoughts gave me enough reasons to stop taking my prescribed medications.

A state of extreme paranoia would eventually retake control over my mind. Indeed, my condition worsened in a progressive fashion. After some time, I rationalized the thought that there was some sort of conspiracy created against me. I believed that I was healthy, and that these medications were prescribed for some ulterior motive which had escaped my grasp. However, because of my paranoia, I believed that this conspiracy was big enough to involve a group of strangers who were previously unknown to me. I then entered into a highly suspicious state, for no real reason. After some more time, I came to believe in the notion that people were feeding me drugs, to keep me from discovering the true reasons behind this conspiracy.

After several more days, my daily functioning was so poor that I rarely left my bedroom. I was eating only one meal a day, though through my recollection, I was never really hungry. I also experienced bouts of insomnia. In time, my mother and sister took me to the emergency room of a local hospital. The hospital lacked empty bedrooms at that time, so the nurses there gave me a bed located within the hallway. A couple of hours passed, and I eventually became drowsy. Another nurse then came over and asked if I would take off my shoes. I was really too tired to think, and I complied with her request. Later on, I discovered that this was a precautionary measure. It prevented me from fleeing the hospital. After another couple of hours, they put me in a square room with a locking door. There was a toilet, and a mattress on the floor. This room resembled a jail cell over anything else.

I fell asleep quickly that night. The next day, a nurse locked the door and I felt alone and secluded. That room was quite large and mainly empty. After a few hours, I decided that I would exercise to pass the time. I started to do some push-ups and sit-ups. I also started to do some stretching. After some time, I was bored and decided to review and practise the martial arts training that I had received as a child. After doing some kicking and punching exercises, the door abruptly opened. Four or five of the hospital staff entered the room and held me down. They injected a needle into my arm and then left hastily. At first, I felt perplexed. I also felt insulted by the manner in which they had treated me. In an angry tone, I shouted, "I am not a criminal" to the hospital staff as they left. They then slammed the door shut.

The hospital staff spoke to my mother the next day. It turns out that they were watching me shadow box via a closed-circuit camera located inside my room. Through their observations, they believed that I could be a danger to either myself or another person. Perhaps they also believed that I would not cooperate with any of the hospital staff. However, today, I believe that the hospital staff had acted this way in order to try to convince me that I was truly suffering from a mental disorder.

That day, the hospital staff opened the door to my room for the duration of my stay there. They also stationed a permanent security guard outside my room. Later on, I began to feel some painful side effects from the drug that they had injected into me. The medicine was loxapine, which was what Dr. Lupton had prescribed for me. The dosage was too high though, and I suffered from painful muscle stiffness as a direct result.

After about six days, I was transferred by an ambulance to the inpatient unit. It was now October, one month after Dr. Lupton's original diagnosis. She lowered my prescription of loxapine from 12.5 milligrams to 10 milligrams, because of my experience with painful side effects. During random points in the day, I felt a sharp pain in my jaw. That pain eventually became so intense that the only way to alleviate it was to keep my jaw fully open. Dr. Lupton soon prescribed 1 milligram of cogentin, to counteract these side effects. I left the psychiatric unit approximately one week later.

After another week, I decided to stop my antipsychotic treatments again, because of my experience with painful side effects. I was then re-admitted back into the inpatient unit, and Dr. Lupton decided to change my prescription. I was now ordered to take 2 milligrams of risperidone during the morning, and 3 milligrams at bedtime. She divided my prescription into two daily doses to address any possible problems with ill side effects. I also took 1 milligram of cogentin, twice daily. On some occasions, I took a small dosage of ativan to help me sleep at night.

Scheduled activities would now become a part of my regular day. During the weekday mornings after breakfast, a gym class would be available at 9:30 am. I especially looked forward to attending gym class, because of my love for exercise and athletics. During the first 20 minutes, we would do some stretching and aerobics. Afterwards, we would play some type of sport for the last 40 minutes. Sometimes I would return to the gym during the afternoons, when I was bored and had nothing to do. The gym was closed during the day but the man in charge of the facility let me know that I could practise there whenever I liked. The compassion he showed me that day helped me to re-consider the possibility that I may be ill.

Once a week, a games night would be available for patients, after dinner at 6:15 pm. There was a pool table, ping-pong table, shuffleboard, dartboard, card table, lounge area, several board games and a stereo in that room. We were free to choose our own activities. At times, I wanted to stay there over the scheduled hour. This is when I started to bond with other patients at that hospital.

Every weeknight at 7:30 pm, a social meeting would take place in the common area. Patients were free to talk about any subject. All of the patients had an equal opportunity to speak. Most of the patients talked about their daily activities. The nurses also asked each patient about anything special that may have happened during that particular day. Some patients would ramble on about issues that nobody else could comprehend. At other times, patients would be overly aggressive and the nurses would moderate their time to speak. We also talked about possible improvements within the ward. However, the main objective in those meetings was to provide the patients with an opportunity to vent their feelings, to someone who would actually listen. Hearing my peers speak also provided me with a better understanding of my illness.

In the beginning, I was quite shy and I never really participated in these social meetings. None of the hospital staff minded, and likewise, no one was ever forced to speak. After about a week or two, my insecurities lessened, and I felt a sense of belonging within that group. I participated whenever I had something to say, though on some occasions, I had nothing to say. Those meetings always lasted for an hour and a half.

The weekends at the unit were mainly informal. There were no scheduled events, except for our meals. If the weather was good, I would usually take a walk around the facilities. There was much parkland to explore, and at times, other patients would be feeding the birds out front. Watching television was also an option. If the room was empty, I could watch whatever I liked. In most cases though, there was someone already present inside that room. I also kept some reading materials in my bedroom. My favourite things to read at that time were car magazines. I also read newspapers and other genres of magazines. Visiting hours were longer on the weekends as well. During the weekdays, visiting hours started after 7 pm, though for the most part, no restrictions were ever enforced.

My hospital stay lasted for about six weeks this time. It was a lengthy stay for one main reason. For the first two weeks, I did not comply with my treatments, and I secretly spit out my medications after they were administered. Dr. Lupton eventually realized this, and soon after, a nurse personally monitored the dispensing of my medicines. After several weeks, my health had improved and I decided to fully comply with Dr. Lupton's treatment plan.

In late November, I was released from the inpatient unit. At that time, Dr. Lupton trusted that I would take my daily medications. However, I also experienced painful side effects from the risperidone treatments. This time, I would experience a differing sharp pain within my mouth. I discovered that if I made a chewing motion, the pain would lessen to some degree. After a while, though, the pain began to increase in severity. I then made an immediate trip to the inpatient unit. When I got there, the nurse in charge told me to wait in a bedroom. After about 20 minutes, she came in and injected another medicine into my backside. I still felt a sharp pain in my mouth for approximately 30 minutes more. I then began to feel drowsy and I fell asleep.

In terms of pain, loxapine was worse than risperidone. Yet, in terms of overall dissatisfaction, risperidone had much more of a negative effect on me. This medicine interrupted my ability to sleep at night. After some time, it caused me to become extremely agitated every night after I prepared to sleep.

I believe that I also had an allergic reaction to risperidone. Whenever I took that medicine, I would soon experience excessive nasal congestion. This problem also interfered with my ability to fall asleep. However, the worst side effect caused severe feelings of anxiety within me. Whenever I tried to fall asleep, I would soon become extremely restless. Frequently, I would need to shake my legs or move around in my bed to relieve this feeling. The anxiety that I felt was just as intolerable as any of the physical pains that I had previously endured. It produced a feeling of extreme uneasiness in me, and this impacted my ability to fall asleep. In due course, I began to loathe my nightly risperidone treatments. In addition, there were no medicines available to counteract my problems with nasal congestion or restlessness. The impact of that medicine on my ability to fall sleep finally became too unbearable. I could not tolerate my nightly problems with sleeplessness, and this negatively influenced my confidence in psychiatric medications as a whole.

I reported these side effects to Dr. Lupton, and about three weeks into December, she changed my prescription to 4.5 milligrams of risperidone. Four days later, she further adjusted the dosage to 4 milligrams, along with 0.5 to 1 milligram of cogentin on an as needed basis. Even so, my problems with nighttime breathing and restlessness persisted.

Finally, in June of the next year, Dr. Lupton changed my prescription to 2.5 milligrams of a newer and a more promising antipsychotic, known as olanzapine. My problems with sleep and restlessness had profound effects on my overall lifestyle. After experiencing seven months of uneasiness and frustration, I lost faith in my society's mental health care system. I was tired of the ill side effects from both my risperidone and loxapine treatments, and I was not looking forward to experiencing any more negative side effects from olanzapine. At that point, I was probably suffering from symptoms of psychosis as well.

That prescription was too low to be effective, though Dr. Lupton prescribed a low dosage on purpose. Increasing the dosage of a medication incrementally is a method used by psychiatrists, which decreases the possible occurrence of any ill side effects. However, my frustration, along with my paranoid thoughts had taken control over my mind again. This and my progressive lack of faith in my community's mental health system gave me a new reason to stop taking my medications for the third time.

Of course, this lack of faith was fundamentally due to my highly irrational frame of mind. I did notice some positive benefits from the risperidone treatments, and the paranoia that I experienced was under some level of control. Yet, I disregarded these positive benefits because of the intolerable side effects. My mental health would diminish as a consequence.

I then began to experience delusions of paranoia and grandeur once more. Whenever I watched television or listened to the radio, I would start to believe that persons within the media were speaking to me. I even believed that the commercials were talking about some aspect of my life. Thus, the severity of my delusions also increased. My delusions were bothering me to the point where I would lie in my bed for the entire day. In addition, on many nights, I had problems while trying to fall sleep. On some occasions, I stayed continuously awake for a period as long as three to four days.

During that time in my life, I also remember experiencing an extreme delusion of grandeur, while I was taking my car out for a drive. I believed in the notion that I was God, and that I was responsible for much of the pain in our world. In particular, I was thinking about some of the tragic events that have occurred both in my personal life, and on a global scale. I believed that, as God, I failed to help these persons. This filled me with much rage and anger. I then got into a minor car accident and called home for help. My sister and mother came to pick me up, though they also called the police. When the police officer came, he asked if I was carrying any sharp objects. In all probability, he knew that I was a schizophrenia patient. I then replied "no" and he frisked me. Afterwards, I told the officer that I was angry with my family, and he politely asked if he could take me to another destination. At that point, though, I recognized that I had nowhere else to go.

That police officer's courtesy also helped to reinforce my trust in Dr. Lupton's professional diagnosis. His demeanour reminded me that no human being is perfect. Memories such as these began to outweigh my paranoid thoughts, and subsequently, I had more reasons to have faith in my society's mental health care system.

I remember that on some occasions, I would travel to a specific house located within my downtown neighbourhood. Every time I went there, I knocked on the door and asked to see an old friend of mine from high school. For some reason, my schizophrenic delusions generated the belief that this person was residing within that home. In fact, I did not know the true owners of that residence. The housekeeper that answered the door always told me that my friend never resided there. She may have also been a bit frightened of me. I recall that when I went there for the third time, she answered the door with a couple of large dogs on leashes. Her reaction was the only reason why I stopped visiting that neighbourhood. At that time, even though I was extremely delusional, I was still able to comprehend the notion that some of my personal beliefs may be wrong.

My delusions did not stop though. One day while lying on my couch, I came to believe that someone was controlling the ticking movement of a clock in the living room of my home. I focused on the ticking sound of the clock and falsely perceived that these movements were not synchronous. This perception then led me to believe that someone was controlling that ticking motion, and that there were persons who were continually watching me within my home. I then concluded that these beliefs would only make sense if was Jesus Christ. My delusions further spiralled to the belief that there were people in the world who were planning to kill me. This succession of rapid thoughts caused me to live in a state of constant fear, for a period of over two weeks.

This delusion of grandeur also forced me to re-examine the idea that I had the power to stop many tragedies within our world. The extreme symptoms of my illness had returned, and I lost all ability to critically examine any of these delusions. Full of rage, I ended up punching a large hole in my bedroom wall. I was angry because I believed that I could have done more to end much of the suffering in our world. My delusions soon became exceptionally problematic. I then decided to ask my mother for help. She told me to take my medications, but I would not listen to her. My mother then took it upon herself to become responsible for my mental health.

During mid June, my mother dialled 911 and a police officer came to my home. This was not the first time that she had called for help. I remember that on one occasion, an ambulance also came to my home. The medics came into my room to see how I was doing, but I refused treatment. On two other occasions, several police officers had also come to my home to check up on me. Again, I refused to be treated. This time, though, I complied with the police officer, and he drove me to the inpatient unit. At that time, I was in a state of confusion and I remember that I was quite scared when I entered the police cruiser. My mother entered the cruiser with me, and we travelled to the inpatient facility together.

My stay at the inpatient unit lasted for approximately one year this time. During the first few weeks, the nurses administered an antipsychotic in liquid form. Dr. Lupton knew that, in my history, I sometimes did not comply with the hospital staff and that I would occasionally spit out my medications. The administration of a medicine in liquid form is much easier to monitor.

I knew most of the hospital staff this time around. In fact, during my first day there, one nurse saw me and asked why I was back. Another staff member wanted me to wear a set of the inpatient unit pyjamas. In the beginning, they put me in a two bed room, but after a month I was transferred into a room with four beds. Trying to fall asleep in a room with a stranger can be difficult. I found it even more difficult to fall asleep in a room with three other strangers. I did not know any of my roommates, and because of my paranoia, I did not trust any of them. My new room was also slightly noisier and this kept me awake on several nights.

One roommate that I particularly remember was of African descent. He was approximately 25 to 30 years old. He also looked quite scared, in my opinion. For the first few days, he would be sitting upright on his bed and he never left the bedroom. After a few days, I realized that he was probably quite ill and extremely delusional. I noticed that he had spent most of the day staring at the wall, on the other side of the room. He was also receiving his meals in the kitchen area of the ward. Only patients who are very ill, or those who are unable to travel to the cafeteria will receive this service. In fact, he only left the bedroom to eat, and he spent the rest of the day looking like he was in some type of hypnotic trance.

After a couple of days, I decided that I would try to talk to him, but I did not know what to say. I noticed that he had not been showering. Subsequently, I shouted at him and told him to go and take a shower. He did not react and I left the room several minutes later. The next day, I remember that he was much more in touch with the world and he seemed to be less restrained. He also started to take care of his personal hygiene that day. I am not sure if what I said had hurt his feelings, but I do know that I somehow reached him in his sickened state. From my personal experience, I knew that this was a major achievement.

I also made a friend at the inpatient unit. His name was Cam and he told me that he had schizophrenia. Cam was an immigrant from China. His English was not perfect, and we spoke in Cantonese on some occasions. Very few patients conversed with each other at that ward, and at times, I would just be sitting in the living room by myself. Cam would sometimes join me, and we mostly sat together without saying a word.

In one respect, I feel that I was a bad influence on Cam. I like to smoke cigarettes and he also picked up this habit. Actually, he preferred to smoke cigars. In any case, we both enjoyed smoking, and we established a connection because of this. At times, I would see him smoking outside on the deck, by himself. At other times, we would go outside and have a smoke together. He would usually give me a cigar, and I would give him one of my cigarettes in return. The fact that we enjoyed each other's company enabled us both to establish a sense of inner peace. Having a friend while extremely ill should have a positive impact on any schizophrenia patient.

At times, I felt quite lonely while residing within that hospital. I do not think that I could have had a deep conversation with any other patient there. Similarly, any relationships with the hospital workers would be strictly on a professional basis. On the other hand, I had a close relationship with Cam, and we probably could have had a meaningful conversation on almost any subject. This never happened though. We were able to sense each other's feelings, and realized that we were both troubled by an element of discomfort. We also held a mutual respect for each other as peers, and this concept was new to the both of us.

I also remember interacting with the Asian male who had previously stolen my shoes while I was asleep. One day, he was sitting in the living room, resting his elbow on the arm of a chair. For some reason, I was in a good mood that day, and I sat in a chair next to him. He did not move, and he was staring straight ahead with a pale look on his face. I then nudged his arm, in an effort to strike a conversation with him. This was a big mistake. From my observations, he believed that I was acting aggressively, and he stared quite angrily at me. I did not expect this reaction, and I stared back at him. After a lengthy moment, he returned to his original position and stared across the room in the same pallid manner. At that point, I realized how ill I must have been when I was first diagnosed with schizophrenia. I also became aware of the amount of progress that I had made since that day.

After some time, I was moved back into the more private two person bedroom. One of my roommates there was a married Caucasian male. The man was around 35 to 40 years old, and he had two daughters. He posted artwork that his daughters had made for him on his side of the bedroom. On the weekends, he would often go out on day trips with his family. I remember seeing his wife come to the unit and pick him up every Saturday morning. It was at this point when I recognized the fact that mental illnesses affect a much broader range of individuals than I had previously thought. I also realized that the patient's family will also struggle, when trying to come to grips with a mental illness.

One weekend I ran out of cigarettes, and thus, I did another very stupid thing. When my roommate went out on his day trips, he left a box of tobacco, some cigarette papers, and a rolling machine inside our room. Instead of buying a pack, I wanted to try his machine. Actually, I could have asked someone in my family to bring me some cigarettes, but I did not think that he would notice if I rolled one for myself. The main problem centred on the fact that I did not know how to use a rolling machine. After about 10 failed attempts, I was finally able to make one. However, after making this cigarette, I essentially compressed a large amount of tobacco into a smaller size. When my roommate returned, he believed that I smoked over half a box of his tobacco. Naturally, he was quite angry. I felt bad about this and I immediately went to the corner store to buy him a new pack.

Throughout my entire life, I remember doing similar things that I would feel bad about at a later time. I know that everyone makes mistakes, and that holding regrets is a very common feeling. However, many of my regrets are in relation to my disease. Whenever I experienced an extreme delusion, I would usually end up making many stupid choices as a direct result. Accordingly, at times, I would purposely act in a manner that I knew was wrong, because of my delusions. In fact, many of the poor choices that I have made in my past were mistakes that I had made on purpose. I remember following my impulses, while making choices that I knew were wrong. In essence, I used the reactions of other persons to my poor choices as a reality check, and this would sometimes enable me to redirect my focus out of a delusional state, back onto the real world.

Hence, making mistakes on purpose would serve as a checkpoint for me. When I intentionally made a choice that I knew was morally wrong, I usually did this in the hope that I would receive some type of negative response. If this was the case, and persons had responded negatively to my actions, I would then conclude that my current perception was focused on the actual world. Conversely, if no persons had reacted to my behaviour, it may be possible that my thought was a delusion, and thus not a real world perception. Therefore, in a way, I was trying to test the integrity and validity of my thoughts, through deliberate action.

If I were to act in a way that I knew was wrong and if I did not receive any forms of negative reinforcement, I would occasionally be able to conclude that my current thought was in fact a delusion that only made sense to me. This personal reality check of mine did not always work though, and at many times, I would subsequently enter into a state of confusion. Furthermore, while in a full-blown paranoid state, I would lack the ability to analyze any of these check points, and I would then remain in a delusional state.

I was also lucky enough to make a female friend, during my stay at the inpatient unit. Her name was Karin. She was approximately 20 years old and she suffered from bipolar disorder. The first time I saw her in the ward, she was lying on the floor in her bedroom. A couple of nurses were in her room, trying to help her onto the bed. She put up quite a struggle though. During the first days of her stay, a nurse was stationed outside of her room for the entire day. This was not common for most patients, and I have only witnessed this on a few occasions.

When she was feeling better, she left her room and became socially active. I was then able to build a bond with her. Everyone in the ward was ill, but I noticed that there was a big difference in her composure, after she received treatment. When my mother came to visit me, she usually brought an assortment of food for me. At that time, I disliked eating fruit, so I decided to give it away and put it into Karin's room every morning.

Many patients in the ward had no visitors. She was one of them, and I am sure that she had appreciated my thoughts. I became her friend, and we enjoyed each other's company. After I met her, I decided that I would try to focus more on what I had in life, as opposed to what I did not have in life.

I remember having contact with another female at the inpatient unit, before I met Karin. During one social meeting, she told the group that her favourite song was Building a Mystery, by Sarah Mclachlan. At that time, I was quite ill, and I believed that this song was written about me. In fact, I took this latter experience to be further proof that I was God. I also believed that Mclachlan's song was recording my use of supernatural powers, to build a greater civilization. This demonstrates the random nature of a schizophrenic delusion. Patients in a state of psychosis can arbitrarily misinterpret real world experiences and form radical beliefs based on these misinterpretations.

The last patient in the unit, that I made a connection with, was a 20-year-old male who was diagnosed with bipolar disorder. I first met him in the television room. When I entered, he wanted to have an arm wrestle with me. We bonded together probably because we were both mentally tough individuals. At that time, the two of us were also determined to improve our mental health, and re-enter our social spheres.

I remember going on several day trips with him. We would often go to the corner store together. He would buy some snacks, while I went shopping for magazines. Another time, we took a taxi ride together and travelled to my city's west end. I was delusional at that time, and neither of us had any money to pay for that taxi ride. I also believed that I had a friend who lived in the area. We got out of the taxi and he became angry when I told him that I could not pay the driver. It was my idea to take this trip, and he assumed that I would have enough money to pay for our outing.

After we stepped out of the taxi, he shoved me and told me not to follow him. That was a very surreal moment for me. I then started to believe that everyone in the area was focusing on me. A few moments later, I was suddenly all alone in an area that was unfamiliar to me. I saw a man that was eating in a nearby restaurant, and believed that he was shaking his head at me. After walking around the area for a little while, I bumped into an elderly male who was jogging on the street. I asked if I could use his home phone and he told me to use a pay phone. I walked a little while longer and found a mini plaza. I first entered a pizzeria there, and asked if I could use their phone. They also told me to use a pay phone. Then I went to a dentist's office in the same plaza and spoke to the receptionist. She called a taxi company for me with no hesitation. The taxi driver then took me home, and I told him that I had no cash on me. When we reached my home, I told him that my mother would reimburse him for his services. He asked me to leave my sweater as collateral, but I told him to come along with me to my home instead. He came with me, and my mother paid him at our front door.

At home, I decided to take a long shower and a nap. It felt good to be at home. The shower was more refreshing and my bed was more comfortable. A couple of hours later, my sister drove me back to the inpatient unit. I saw my day-trip acquaintance in the television room and we did not speak to each other.

The experience of being in a strange area, with no money, was also a frightening experience for me. I thought about exactly what I had done to get myself into that situation, and how I handled myself. After a couple of days, I came to realize that I have no survival skills when I am in a sickened state. I cannot physically care for myself when delusional, and I will most certainly be dependent on third party for help. While in a delusional state, I do not even ponder thoughts related to living and survival. As a result, I eventually realized that living an independent lifestyle may be difficult to achieve, and that any independence that I have enjoyed in the past may be possibly lost for the rest of my life.

Dr. Lupton eventually increased my prescription to 15 milligrams of olanzapine. I took these pills at bedtime, because its major side effect was fatigue. After a couple of months, I also noticed that I was gaining excessive weight. I weighed about 125 pounds before taking olanzapine. Approximately six months later, my weight fluctuated at around 150 to 155 pounds. Dr. Lupton continued to monitor my condition, and she eventually decreased my prescription to 10 milligrams of olanzapine.

Soon enough, I went home after my mental health had stabilized. The side effects of olanzapine were in fact tolerable, but this mode of treatment also had its costs. Upon returning home, I discovered that I would constantly feel drowsy throughout the entire day. My main concern, in this respect, was based on the possibility that I may live the rest of my life in my bedroom, while in a state of deep slumber. Dr. Lupton listened to my problem, and she decreased my prescription to 7.5 milligrams of olanzapine.

Four months later, Dr. Lupton decided to stop practicing psychiatry. She wanted to go back to school and learn more about mental diseases. Dr. Forbes took her place in October, and he then became my psychiatrist.

Dr. Forbes mainly knew me through the notes that were taken by Dr. Lupton and Sharon. I told him about my problems with fatigue and he decided to lower my prescription to 5 milligrams of olanzapine. He then decreased my prescription to 2.5 milligrams of olanzapine, two months later in December.

This dosage turned out to be too low however, and I started to experience some problematic symptoms again. More specifically, at times I would enter into a confused state and experience problems with concentration. In January, Dr. Forbes re-adjusted my prescription back to 5 milligrams, and then after one month he raised my prescription back up to 7.5 milligrams of olanzapine. By this time, though, the medicine's efficacy had dissipated.

All antipsychotic medications require a specified amount of time to become effective. Thus, most patients will need to take a medicine for some time, before they gain any positive benefits. This was the same for me. After Dr. Forbes re-adjusted my prescription, the medication was almost entirely flushed out of my system. As a result, I also began to feel less fatigued throughout the day. Dr. Forbes then prescribed 1 milligram of ativan to help me sleep at night.

In March, my prescription was adjusted again. I started to re-experience problems with fatigue, so Dr. Forbes decided to prescribe a new medication. I discontinued my olanzapine treatments, and started to take 25 milligrams of quetiapine twice daily. In the beginning, I felt much more refreshed in the morning while taking this new medicine. However, after some time, I began to experience additional side effects. This drug also caused problems with extreme nasal congestion at night, and this would disrupt my sleep patterns again. After a month, I decided that excessive fatigue was more bearable than problems with sleep. Dr. Forbes then changed my prescription back to 7.5 milligrams of olanzapine.

On another note, around that time, I also needed to sell the car that I was financing since I was nineteen years old. In fact, I was unemployed for several years due to my illness. Eventually, my sister took it upon herself to sell my car for me.

After I lost my car, I began to think about things that I had lost in life, due to my illness. I also believed in the impression that it would be difficult to regain everything that I lost, after Dr. Lupton diagnosed me with schizophrenia.

In June however, I received a call from an employer who acquired my resume during my first semesters at college. I decided that being employed would give me an opportunity to assess my mental faculties, before I return to any post-secondary studies. The work was in the field of computer technology. I never experienced problems with concentration at that time, and I made few mistakes. After some time and after my responsibilities were increased, I was quite happy to be functioning at such a high level. This work experience gave me confidence in my mental abilities, and I then realized that it was entirely possible to treat my illness.

I was 23 years old when I returned to college, during the following September. The side effects of fatigue and drowsiness still affected me though. In order to counteract these effects, I decided to become a dedicated coffee drinker. Actually, I had been drinking coffee for some time now. I started to drink coffee soon after I left the inpatient unit for the final time. When I returned to my studies, I drank coffee not for leisure purposes, but out of sheer necessity. On most occasions, I could not feel refreshed and start my day in the morning without having a cup of coffee. Before experiencing any major problems with delusions, I would have little trouble waking up in the morning. I also never had to depend on coffee. Today, I feel that I am as addicted to coffee as I am to cigarettes.

When I first registered for my college classes, I had an administrative problem to deal with. During my previous semesters at college, I was delusional and I withdrew from all of my classes. However, the formal procedure that I should have taken was to drop my classes instead. This way there would not be a W noted on my permanent transcript. Yet, at that time, I was too ill to know the difference.

A W on a college transcript usually suggests that the student had attended his class for the entire semester, but then decided to drop it before taking the final exam. Students with unsatisfactory marks on assignments, or those who are too lazy to study for the final exam usually use this method to ensure that their grade point average does not decline. Therefore, the recorded W's on my transcript seemed to imply the possibility that I dropped my courses not for personal reasons, but for reasons associated with poor academic standing.

When I withdrew from my classes, I experienced extreme problems with paranoia. I remember that I was staring at many of my professors, and that I was not particularly friendly with them. Thus, my behaviour, during that period, was not typical of an academically inclined student. The fact that I could not stop laughing at my professor that day in my past also probably reflected negatively upon my character. Under these circumstances, I do not blame any of my professors if they ever perceived me to be a lazy or unmotivated student.

I only realized these latter thoughts upon my return to college. My college record seemed to reflect on the possibility that I was not a serious student, and accordingly, I had problems while trying to enrol in one of my classes that semester. My troubles during the registration phase forced me to speak with my computer science professor in person. Dr. Carter wanted to know why there were so many W's noted on my transcript. At that point, I knew that my academic record was less than satisfactory. Thus, I decided to tell Dr. Carter the truth. I told him that I withdrew from my classes because I was suffering from schizophrenia. He then respectfully asked if I could prove this. I replied that I could. After showing Dr. Carter a note from my psychiatrist, he immediately signed my enrolment form, and I was free to continue with my studies.

I also re-joined the college badminton team that semester. I was a member of the team three years back, before I became severely ill. However, when I withdrew from my college studies, I also stopped attending the team's weekly practices. My former coach never knew that I had schizophrenia, and he assumed that I had just quit playing for the team.

Hence, I faced similar administration problems while trying to re-join the college badminton team. We had a new coach that year. The new badminton coach and the athletic supervisor were both hesitant to let me rejoin the team. I spoke to my badminton coach and told him that I withdrew from the team due to medical reasons. After I proved this with a doctor's note, I was permitted to re-join team. I learned many new skills that year, and this had a positive impact on my self-esteem.

At first, I experienced problems with concentration upon my return to college. In time, my ability to concentrate improved and I performed well academically. I was also laid off from my job in October of that year. My return to college lasted for three semesters and I graduated with an Associate of Arts degree.

The Associate's degree that I completed enabled me to enter into studies at the university level. In college, I achieved a 2.9 grade point average, which was also good enough to gain entry into most universities in Canada. University life was different from life in college. The campus was bigger, the population was greater, and the students were busier. The college that I went to had a relaxed, yet academic atmosphere. The university environment, on the other hand, was more scholarly and achievement oriented.

I always loved to attend class, especially during my college years. It would essentially be the highlight of my day. Academically, university students are graded on a much higher scale, in comparison to college. Likewise, in both institutions, students are granted more academic freedoms when compared to high school. However, university life is complicated and highly structured. In college, students decide their own course load, and the professors there emphasize understanding and knowledge. In university, students are essentially choosing their future and the professors there emphasize self-learning and independence. This increase in student liberties, across the entire academic system, guides the individual into becoming a more responsible adult.

In hindsight, my first year of university studies was quite difficult. University professors expect much more from their students. According to some persons, the average student will notice a third of a grade drop in grade point average, after transferring from college to university studies. I was 24 years old, and my grade point average soon enough dropped an entire letter grade. Another problem that I faced related to my chosen major or specialization. At that point, I did not declare a particular field of specialization, and I foolishly chose an industry based on job availability and monetary compensation. My marks in computer science at the college level were decent, and I believed that I could do equally well in this field at the university level.

During my first two semesters at the university, I enrolled in classes that were prerequisites for a degree in computing science. However, my mathematical skills and short-term memory had degraded significantly since my high school years. During my first year at high school, I scored quite high academically in the subject of math, and I was chosen to represent my school in a nationwide mathematical competition. I always achieved high grades in the subject of mathematics, even during my elementary school years. Nevertheless, due to my disease, I lost the ability to comprehend complex mathematics during my university years. The main mistake that I made was based on the expectation that I would have all of the intellectual faculties that I possessed during my youth, before I was diagnosed with schizophrenia. My expectations were too great though, and I struggled to achieve a passing grade throughout my entire course load.

In time, I feared the prospect that I may be suspended from my studies, because of my low grade point average. In the past, if I scored low grades, this would motivate me to work harder. However, pure motivation would not improve my academic standing at this point in my life. I experienced problems with memory and logic. As a result, I finally had proof that I may have permanently lost some intellectual capabilities, due to my disease.

For some reason, this problem did not affect my studies at the college level. My success in both college, and the work force gave me enough reasons to believe that a university degree was still within my reach.

I always wanted to complete a university degree, even as a child. Yet, at this point, I knew that it would be highly difficult to complete a degree in computing science. I then had to reanalyze my goals and carefully consider another field of specialization. I looked at my college transcript and discovered that I had a keen interest in the subject of philosophy. Moreover, I also held a personal interest in the areas of ethics and human morality. Therefore, I took a chance and declared philosophy as my major at the university level.

After some time, I took advantage of another employment opportunity and worked for my cousin within the computing industry. I was a technician, and my tasks required some computer savvy. My responsibilities included working on both computer hardware and computer software. Some of my other responsibilities were research based, and I was able to work at home. This job also boosted my self-confidence and it enabled me to establish a greater sense of belonging within my community as a whole.

My third semester at the university level was an entirely different experience for me. I was actually interested in the subject matter, and my grades showed improvement. This time I decided to take two courses, instead of three. This reduced the demands that I had put on myself, and it gave me more time to complete my assignments. For the first time during my university studies, I actually enjoyed the experience. The change of my specialization from the sciences to the arts also better suited my aptitudes at this stage in my life. Although my mathematical capabilities have declined due to my illness, I feel that the range of my abstract thoughts has subsequently increased. I scored above average grades that semester.

Also during that semester, I volunteered to act as an executive at the university's badminton club. From my first days at university, I played badminton both at club events and during the intramural sessions. When compared to most of the other students, I was one of the more skilful players. Many of the students who played were new to the sport of badminton.

Engaging in social events will give the individual a chance to meet his peers and make new friends. University clubs make it even easier for students to meet and socialize with each other. As an executive, I was both a leader and a regular player. However, the pressures associated with achieving high grades eventually had its impact on me, and this limited the time that I had allotted for recreation. After some time, the demands of the club had interfered with my studies. Consequently, I resigned from my executive position after one year, and then focused entirely on my studies.

In May of that year, Dr. Forbes also decided to return to school, so that he could learn more about mental illnesses. His replacement, Dr. Freedman, still currently treats me. I told Dr. Freedman about my problems with fatigue and drowsiness. In response, he wanted to retry the antipsychotic quetiapine. Dr. Freedman's knowledge of me was also based on notes that were taken by my previous mental health care team.

I was then prescribed 12.5 milligrams of quetiapine, and this dosage was gradually increased to 100 milligrams by the following November. My fatigue was alleviated by this change in medication, but the side effect of nasal congestion, again, had too much of a negative impact on my sleeping habits. Dr. Freedman then prescribed a suitable dose of olanzapine to stabilize my mental health, then later prescribed a newer antipsychotic known as clozapine.

When taking clozapine, I will need to monitor several possible health risks that have been associated with this medication, through bi-weekly blood tests. Dr. Freedman ended up using a different psychiatric method than Dr. Forbes. He prescribed 7.5 milligrams of olanzapine, in addition to a small dosage of clozapine. This mode of psychiatric treatment is known as tapering. It is a method that is used to change the patient's prescribed medication, while simultaneously treating the symptoms of his illness. Dr. Freedman wanted to ensure that I would not become ill during this change in my prescription, and I was able to maintain my studies without disruption. The dosage of olanzapine was then gradually reduced, in conjunction with a gradual increase in dosage of clozapine. Eventually, I would be taking 275 milligrams of clozapine on a daily basis.

I ended up taking one course during the following spring semester. My plan was to enrol in a light course load, so that I could learn to better cope with the stresses connected to university life. I still had problems with concentration though, and I experienced difficulties while trying to read my assigned texts. I also remember experiencing some mild states of paranoia. In class, I would experience problems while trying to focus on my professors' lectures. Perhaps the changes in my prescription had negative effects on my cognition in some way. That semester my grades dropped to an average standing.

During the next semester, in May, I decided to take three philosophy courses. I experienced great difficulties with one course, which was in the field of mathematical logic. The other two courses focused on abstract philosophical theories. Personally, I felt that my concentration had improved that semester. However, I scored poorly during my midterm exams. I also experienced difficulties with my weekly assignments, and I began to feel the pressures associated with university life again.

I may have been a bit delusional also that semester, and it is possible that I was experiencing paranoid thoughts in one of my classes. That specific class centred on philosophical theory, and I remember seeing my professor stick out his tongue for a period of approximately 10 to 15 seconds. I then experienced a paranoid delusion. At that moment, I concluded that the entire class was focusing on me, and that my professor had acted this way for some reason in relation to this paranoid belief. Today, because of the nature of this memory, I am not even certain if it was a hallucination or if it really did happen. I feel this way about many other strange memories of mine. During that class, I realized that it was highly possible that my symptoms may have returned, and this caused me to experience more undue stress. I also started to experience surreal-like mental states again.

At the same time though, I still possessed the ability to conceive abstract thoughts. Yet, I had problems with my short-term memory and concentration. This was the main reason why I failed a kinesiology course during my first semester at the university. I then decided to consult with Dr. Freedman about my current situation. It was then when I determined that my mental health was failing and that I, therefore, could not continue on with my studies. The decision to take a break from my studies was difficult. I did not know if I would ever return to my studies, and I had to seriously consider the possibility that I may never become mentally healthy again.

Low levels of self-esteem, and an increase in dosage of my antipsychotic treatments gave me two more reasons to take the next fall semester off as well. The fatigue that I experienced also affected my ability to study. In the mornings, I would drink several cups of coffee, and in the afternoon,

I would often need to take a nap. I also often wondered about my future and what I was going to do next with my life. In order to achieve a high academic standing at the university level, students must devote their entire lives to their studies. I realized that even if I had committed enough time for my studies, my problems with concentration and memory could still pose as a difficulty for me. Yet, the time that I took off away from school made me realize how much I wanted to complete a university degree. This gave me the drive and motivation to finish my university studies.

In order to qualify for a full-time status, students must enrol in three to five courses per semester. Alternatively, students with a disability will qualify for a full-time status when enrolled in two courses per semester. A full or part-time status mainly affects the student financially. In my nation, students must enrol in a full-time course load to extend the duration of their student loans.

Other forms of accommodations are also available for students with disabilities. For instance, special needs such as a private room for exams, assistance with note taking, specialized equipment, and several government grants are available for students with all forms of disabilities. I have personally received several bursaries and a few government grants, which have helped to pay off a large portion of my student loans.

I decided to return to school during the next spring semester, when I was 26 years old. I enrolled in two courses that semester, to keep my stress levels low and improve my grade point average. At that time, my academic credits included two years of transferable college credits, and more than fifteen credits of university level courses. To complete a Bachelor's degree, I would need to complete 45 more credits, in both pre-requisite and elective courses.

My grades eventually improved back to an above average standing. I felt healthy enough to take three courses during the following summer semester. In time, I started to feel more comfortable within the university environment, and I had more confidence when completing assignments and taking exams. I managed to improve my grades to a good standing, which was an entire letter grade higher than the majority of my previous semesters at the university level.

My next semester turned out to be a relative success. I was feeling healthy and I held more confidence in my mental capacities. I registered for three courses again, during the following spring semester. However, I would eventually end up withdrawing from my classes again. My ability to concentrate was fine. The problem I faced was based on a relapse of my paranoid delusions.

One delusion that I remember occurred while I was writing a midterm exam. I began to believe that all of my classmates were focusing on me. Perhaps the stressors that come along with university life had finally caught up with me mentally. Well into that midterm, one of my classmates stood up from his seat, stretched his arms, and yawned in a disruptive fashion. At that moment, I believed that he was purposely trying to disrupt my concentration. I looked up at my professor, and he in turn looked back at me. His facial expression seemed to exhibit some form of concern. It was then when I knew that my paranoid thoughts had returned.

I went to see Dr. Freedman and told him about this experience. I also told him that my energy levels were low. After I finished that midterm, I felt tired mentally. I then contemplated about taking a break from my studies again. I felt that I had neither the energy, nor the motivation to complete that semester of studies. Nevertheless, Dr. Freedman wanted to prescribe one more medication before I made any final decisions. That February, he prescribed a low dose of the stimulant dexedrine, to counteract my problems with energy.

Two weeks later, I felt no improvements with my mental health, so I went to see Dr. Freedman again. We talked about my current condition, and I was convinced that I could not complete my courses with a passing grade. He wrote a note, and I dropped my classes the next day.

I took a break from my university studies for an entire year. Drinking coffee in the morning, and having a couple of more cups later on during the day became a regular habit. I also took up a new sport. On a sunny day, I would usually practise at the local driving range, as a daily form of exercise. From watching this sport on television, I knew that I could probably play golf throughout my senior years. I then decided to invest in a set of expensive golf clubs and follow a regular exercise routine. My paranoid thoughts still returned, though, even while I was practising at the range. On some occasions, I believed that other golfers were synchronizing their golf swing with my own. The severity of these delusions was minor though, and I was able to forget about them after I left the range.

I continued to play golf, despite my negative experiences with paranoid thoughts. I decided to concentrate on learning the sport of golf, and if I accomplished this, I knew that a return to my university studies might be possible. In time, I improved my golf stroke, and this bolstered my self-confidence. I knew that, at the very least, the disease had not affected any abilities related to my hand-eye coordination.

In March, Dr. Freedman stopped prescribing dexedrine, because there were no evident positive effects. Instead, he prescribed the anti-depressant celexa, in conjunction with my clozapine treatments. In order to lessen the possible occurrence of any negative side effects, he increased the dosage in a gradual fashion up to 60 milligrams per day. Dr. Freedman did not prescribe this medicine to treat any symptoms related to depression. He believed that I would benefit from its insomnia-like side effects.

Problems with fatigue still affected my everyday functioning though. I felt quite frustrated, because I needed to take a three hour nap on a daily basis. Eventually, the side effects of celexa did help me somewhat, and I noticed a slight improvement in my energy levels. Yet, I still felt drowsy during the day, and I continued to take a nap every afternoon.

I returned to my university studies during the following spring semester. At that time, I was 28 years old. The average student completes a Bachelor's degree in approximately five years. If he entered into university immediately after graduating from high school, he would be around 23 years old by the time that he completes this degree. I still needed 20 credits to complete a Bachelor's degree. It was possible to complete these credits during the next two semesters. However, if I chose this option, I would have to enrol in two full-time course loads. I eventually decided to take my time and spread these academic credits across three semesters. I believed that this was necessary to reduce my exposure to external stressors, which would then reduce any chance of relapse.

That semester I took two courses in the area of philosophical theory. I began to love my commute to campus every day. In between classes, I would often go to the cafe and work on class readings or assignments. I also made a new friend up on campus that semester. His name was Tom, and he was approximately 50 years old. Tom always made good comments during class, and it seemed like he loved to study the subject of philosophy. This is probably what drew me closer to him. At times, his comments during class were equally as conscientious as the professor's comments. When I spoke to him, he told me that his studies were interrupted due to a personal disability. I felt a stronger connection with him because of this. After I met him, I knew that I had peers, like me, who were also in the process of recovering from a major illness.

The government grant that I received included a mobile computer laptop. This enabled me to work on my assignments in private, and during times when I was less fatigued. After going home from class, I would occasionally take a two hour nap. I then ate dinner and returned to my studies. This was the first time when I truly felt good about my life, since Dr. Lupton diagnosed me with schizophrenia. My concentration was clear and I seldom experienced any dreamlike surreal states. My grades also had a good standing, and I was finally pleased with my efforts at the university level.

Dr. Freedman added wellbutrin to my prescription that May. This drug is an antidepressant, but it can also help an individual with his smoking habit. In my case, Dr. Freedman prescribed this drug to treat my low energy levels and fatigue. On the plus side, it does, somewhat, alleviate my addiction to nicotine. I used to smoke about half a pack of full strength cigarettes per day, before taking this medicine. Now I smoke a slightly lesser amount of lower strength cigarettes. Dr. Freedman soon increased my prescription of wellbutrin to two doses of 150 milligrams per day.

During the next semester, I took two more courses. One of my courses was in the subject area of the humanities, and the other course was in the field of philosophy. I particularly enjoyed going to classes during the summer semesters. The university that I attended is located on top of a mountain, and the view is quite serene. My health was also very good at that time, and I was free from most external stressors. I scored slightly higher than above average grades, and I was satisfied with my efforts.

That summer, Dr. Freedman increased my dosage of clozapine to 300 milligrams per day to counteract the insomnia-like side effects of wellbutrin. Personally, I felt that my mental health was good. The last time I felt this good was during a short period of time when Dr. Forbes first started my quetiapine treatments. Dr. Freedman finally found the most effective treatment option for me that summer. I was 28 years old at that time.

The following fall semester was my final semester of studies at the university. I took three courses, all of which were based on philosophical theory. I finally earned a Bachelor's degree, which was one of the main goals that I had set out for myself as a youth. During my graduation, I remember thinking about all of my former professors at both the college and university levels, and the continual support that they gave to me. At that time, my concentration was good, and my short-term memory was probably as good as it will ever be. Of course, I still had to work hard to achieve good grades that term. However, it was less difficult to achieve a good standing during this stage of my academic life. It felt good to complete a university degree. Intrinsically, I felt that I had conquered my disability, and that I had redefined my personal identity as a direct result.

4

Reflections and After Thoughts

I was first diagnosed with schizophrenia when I was 20 years old. It took eight more years to find the right combination of medicines that would both effectively treat my illness, and enable me to function constructively within my society. Nonetheless, Dr. Freedman has recently increased the dosage of my clozapine treatments, to address problems related to motivation. He has also increased the dosage of my wellbutrin treatments, to address problems with an increase in fatigue. Today, I take 400 milligrams of clozapine, 60 milligrams of celexa, and 400 milligrams of wellbutrin per day. This change took place when I was 31 years of age.

At heart, I believe that some of my mental faculties can still improve. This is based on the fact that I still feel fatigued and drowsy throughout the day. If my energy levels improve, I believe that my everyday functioning will also improve. On a positive note, at present times, I still possess the ability to concentrate at an extremely high level.

Even so, my ability to concentrate was at a much higher level during my youth, before my fifteenth birthday. I also remember experiencing fluctuations in my ability to concentrate, when I stopped taking olanzapine and took clozapine instead. My current prescription consists of one antipsychotic and two antidepressants. It is not a perfect cure, but it is good enough to make me feel well and live a fairly normal life.

Permanent memory loss is problem that I have recognized in myself today. My short-term memory is exponentially worse today, when compared to my years at elementary school. Memory is an important element in many technical courses, including courses in the sciences. When I took courses in the sciences at university, I had very little aptitude and struggled greatly during those classes. On the other hand, when I had applied myself as a youth, my short-term memory was good enough to score excellent grades in almost any subject matter. Today, during any random situation, my short-term memory can fail me. Perhaps the problem may be based on a chemical imbalance in an area of my brain that is associated with memory. Through my personal experiences, I speculate that this problem may also be due to a form of permanent brain damage that has been inflicted on me, through the illness itself.

In contrast, my problems with long-term memory are less severe. I can still recall many important events in my life, without too much difficulty. The speed at which I access these memories, though, seems to be slower. I have noticed a decrease in speed when accessing both my long and short-term memories, and this is also probably due to my illness.

I have also noticed that a few of my other thought processes may work quicker than they had during my youth. From my estimation, I believe that I am able to focus on and envision abstract thoughts at a faster pace today. Persons who suffer from schizophrenia will usually experience symptoms related to random and rapid thought processes. Incidentally, I believe that my experiences with this latter symptom may be correlated to an increase in speed in my creative thought processes.

Likewise, I also feel that my imagination has improved. When I was younger, my thought processes were, for the most part, quite logical and methodical. Today, I notice an increase in the range of my imagined thoughts. At the same time, however, I have noticed a decrease in the range of my calculated or logical thoughts. For example, I used to be an excellent chess player during my youth, but now I possess very little competence to perform well in that game. I also used to be an average athlete during my youth, but today, I can learn new sports with relative quickness and ease. In my mind, my aptitude in the human arts may have increased, while my aptitude in the sciences may have decreased, all due to my illness.

Additionally, my personal academic interests have also shifted from subjects based on logic and mathematics, to subjects based on social principles and morality. I believe that my experience with schizophrenia may be responsible for this shift, possibly through an alteration of some physical or chemical properties within my brain.

Today, I also hold many regrets with respect to my lack of cooperation with Dr. Lupton, during the early stages of my diagnosis. I speculate that if I had complied with her from the very beginning, it may be possible that I would have no permanent brain damage today. In fact, much research indicates that there is greater brain damage in patients who experience long, untreated psychotic episodes compared to those who experience shorter, more efficiently treated episodes (Kirby and Keon, 2004). I firmly believe that I would have spent less time in a state of psychosis, had I complied with my antipsychotic treatments at that time. Thus, I may have also lost several years of my life while phasing in and out of a state of psychosis. Likewise, it is possible that my illness would have had a lesser impact on my life today, if I had complied with earlier forms of treatment.

From the best of my memories, I do not recall experiencing any noticeable problems with my memory or concentration, when I first took the antipsychotic loxapine. Gaps in my overall awareness only started to occur after I took risperidone. If my memories are accurate in this respect, then it is possible that an illness like schizophrenia could cause permanent brain damage in a period of less than three months.

I also believe that I would have found the most effective combination of medicines to treat my illness, within two years. If this occurred, then I probably would have also completed my university studies at a much younger age. The time I spent at home struggling with my illness and my lengthy stays within an inpatient facility are parts of my life that I can never take back. I have also lost some social ties as a direct result.

On the other hand, I wonder if it is possible for an individual to deal with a mental illness in any other way. Patients with a mental illness will lack the intellectual faculties that are necessary to understand and have insight, regarding the true nature of their condition. This will clearly interfere with their treatment and recovery process.

Schizophrenia is a debilitating disease that separates the individual from the actual world. A new world, based on fiction, replaces any previous knowledge gained through sound logic and reason. Therefore, because of his delusional state, the patient may also lack an ability to act in his own best interests. It is only possible to treat an illness, when the individual actually accepts the fact that he is ill. If I had accepted Dr. Lupton's professional diagnosis from the very beginning, it is highly likely that the progression of my disease would have been much more manageable.

The first moment when I was certain that something could be wrong with me occurred that day in college, when I could not stop laughing in class. This loss of control over my mental faculties should have made me clearly aware of the fact that I was ill. However, as the severity of my delusions increased, my ability to use reason would steadily decrease. I also came to believe that life in the actual world was somewhat less promising than life in my delusional world. In the real world, I was just an average human being. In contrast, I was a supernatural saviour within my delusional frame of mind. This idea further affected my ability to accept the fact that I was ill. As a result, my choice to believe in a delusional world also affected the treatment of my illness.

In my estimation, it is possible that I could have returned to my college studies, within one year after I was first diagnosed with schizophrenia. It actually took three years and it took five more years to find the most effective combination of medicines for my body type. Yet, it may have been impossible to accept Dr. Lupton's original diagnosis, because my mind was in an exceedingly fragmented and irrational state. In addition, because I did not personally know Dr. Lupton, there was no sense of trust established between the two of us. I hardly trusted my family members at that time as well.

I was paranoid. At that time, my paranoid state caused me to believe that everyone in the world was out to get me in some way. If I accepted Dr. Lupton's diagnosis that day, I would have had to disregard all of my personal beliefs and redirect this trust in a total stranger. In other words, I would have had to have faith in Dr. Lupton's beliefs, while simultaneously dismissing my own.

This concept of trust is the first and most essential step of the schizophrenia patient's treatment process. In my case, I irrationally trusted my own beliefs over anyone else's. This reveals the possibility that my mind may have been in a paradoxical state, at that point in time. I did realize that some of my thoughts were strange, and accordingly, I asked for help. However, when I finally received the help that I asked for, in the end, I fundamentally refused this help.

In time, I had to basically doubt my personal beliefs, and accept another person's counsel. This was not an easy task for me. My immediate family could be described as a dysfunctional family, over anything else. My mother and father seldom spoke to each other, and they slept in different bedrooms for many years before they divorced. Equally, my sisters' relationships with each other were based more on animosity than any forms of unconditional love. My relationships with my immediate family members also declined as my illness progressed. Therefore, I never really established a true sense of trust in any of my immediate family members.

It was quite difficult to let my mother take full responsibility over my mental health. A loss of independence became increasingly more difficult to accept. I also realized that there were still many other battles to face, after I reach a state of good mental health.

Accordingly, another significant battle that I faced, at that time, was my struggle for dignity. At its peak, the disease had taken away many of my mental faculties. When extremely ill, I cannot truly survive on my own and I will most likely depend on other persons to take care of me. Once I had retaken control over my mind, these previous dependencies caused me to lose a sense of pride. It takes a real level of maturity to be able to ask for someone else's help, during times of need. When I understood more about the inner workings of my society in general, I started to regain the pride that I had previously lost. Achieving this level of self-respect is the next element in the schizophrenia patient's recovery process. The respect that I had for myself as an imperfect human being enabled me to transcend many fears associated with societal stigmas and discrimination. After some time, I came to the understanding that no patient should ever feel shame when asking for another person's help.

Accepting the fact that I suffer from a disease was always difficult for me. Whenever I tried to acknowledge this fact, I would often enter into a state of mild shock. Basically, I had to come to terms with the fact that a mental illness will affect me for the remainder of my life. This is another essential element in the individual's recovery process. In my case, the journey towards accepting my illness took many years. Primarily, I needed to establish a sense of trust between Dr. Lupton and myself. Likewise, I also needed to realize the fact that illness is a natural element in human life.

This latter concept may seem rudimentary at first. Still, when an individual suffers from an illness like schizophrenia, he loses pieces of knowledge that he has gained throughout his entire lifetime. In my case, I had troubles differentiating real world experiences from my delusions and hallucinations. I also had to accept the possibility that I will continue to suffer from schizophrenic delusions and hallucinations, for the rest of my life. Therefore, in the journey towards a recovery from a mental illness, the patient must build a new life, one step at a time.

My rehabilitation process could only really begin once I accepted the fact that I suffer from schizophrenia. Dr. Freedman told me that my illness would be chronic. Thus, I knew that I would be taking antipsychotic medications for my entire life. This would be a substantial change in any person's lifestyle. First, I would have to remember to take my medications on a daily basis. I then had to recognize the possibility that my schizophrenic symptoms will return, if I failed to do this. I fear this possibility even to this day. If for some reason, like a natural disaster, I were unable to acquire my medications, it is possible that I will re-enter into a state of psychosis and lose the progress that I have achieved thus far. As a protective measure against this circumstance, I have extra doses of medications stored for times of emergency.

When I take my clozapine treatments every night, I will usually fall into a deep sleep in less than one hour. The medicine olanzapine had a similar effect on me and once I become drowsy, I will find it extremely difficult to wake up and be refreshed for another eight to ten hours. Under these circumstances, it would be very dangerous for me to, for example, drive a car after I have taken these medications. Other patients who experience problematic side effects should also exercise similar forms of discretion. Schizophrenia patients must take proactive measures like these, when dealing with the potential side effects of their prescribed medication.

Regarding the dosage of my prescription, one may ask why I would need such a high dose of clozapine, when such a low dose of olanzapine has worked for me in the past. Actually, the effective dosage really depends on each individual antipsychotic. For my body type, 300 milligrams of clozapine will have a similar therapeutic effect as 7.5 milligrams of olanzapine. For another individual, whose biological makeup differs from mine, a different dosage of a different medicine may be required for a similar therapeutic effect.

Another significant detail about mental disease has to do with the proper procedure for diagnosing a potentially ill patient. When Dr. Lupton first met me, she observed symptoms that are commonly observed in schizophrenia. However, at that time, her diagnosis was provisional. According to the mental health standards in my country, persons who exhibit psychotic symptoms must suffer from these symptoms for a period of at least six months, before they are formally diagnosed with schizophrenia. This length of time is necessary, because it is possible that the individual may exhibit these symptoms temporarily. In addition, it is possible that the individual's symptoms could be due to stress, the use of a narcotic, or other pertinent factors. Therefore, a period of six months is necessary to determine that the patient's symptoms are exclusively due to a brain disorder.

A further psychiatric policy relates to the kinds of medicines that are made available for schizophrenia patients. Dr. Lupton prescribed loxapine as my first mode of treatment. Through a mental health policy, she was only permitted to change this prescription if I experienced intolerable side effects. In fact, it is widely known that muscle pain and stiffness is a possible side effect of loxapine.

Most experienced psychiatrists know that there are newer and more improved medicines that are currently available for schizophrenia patients. Olanzapine is one of these medications. However, Dr. Lupton was obligated by mental health policies to prescribe loxapine as my initial mode of treatment. From my understanding, the policy of prescribing medicines with potentially painful side effects is based on economic reasons. Dr. Lupton was only permitted to prescribe the higher priced medicine olanzapine, after I had tried and rejected two relatively inexpensive forms of antipsychotics.

Therefore, treatments through olanzapine or clozapine are more monetarily expensive in comparison to treatments through either loxapine or risperidone. As a patient, I have a problem with this mental health policy. I believe that my negative experiences with these older medicines were unnecessary and entirely avoidable. In addition, I would not want anyone else to experience the painful side effects that I had to endure. At that time, I was battling problems with denial, and my experience with these substandard medicines served to complicate this issue. The painful side effects that I experienced fundamentally acted as another source of stress. Moreover, the experiencing of painful side effects is a common reason why many patients stop taking their medications. As a result, due to this mental health policy, schizophrenia patients must battle further difficulties associated with inferior medicines. I believe that prescribing the best medicine available will increase every patient's chance to fully recover from his debilitating condition.

Concerning the inpatient unit that I stayed at, that facility was much nicer than I had expected. My only knowledge of mental health wards came from the movie One Flew over the Cuckoo's Nest. In that movie, patients were confined to a particular wing of a hospital, and they slept together in a single room. The only forms of recreation available were a television, a card table, and an outdoor basketball court. However, the most disturbing aspect of that movie was its portrayal of psychiatric nurses. In essence, these workers failed to address the needs of the patients, they lacked compassion, and they also seemed to behave more like prison guards as opposed to mental health nurses.

The head nurse, known as nurse Ratched, appeared particularly menacing in that film. She seemed to control the ward in a dictator-like fashion. She also enforced a set of stringent rules, which restricted the personal liberties of every patient who resided there. Furthermore, many of those patients were not even aware of the fact that they were denied many basic liberties, and this is very troubling. Nurse Ratched enforced a systematic program that seemed to dehumanize most of the patients in that ward. She acted mainly out of pragmatics over empathy. In the end, the majority of the patients in that ward gained a higher degree of sentience, exclusively through the benevolence of a mentally healthy third party.

To be fair, this movie was based in a time when psychiatric medications were less than effective, in comparison to the medications that are available today. All of the patients in that ward took medications, but only one character, the Chief, ever benefited from those treatments.

After watching this movie, I held the impression that all psychiatric facilities would resemble prisons over general hospitals. However, my personal experiences are not consistent with this impression. It is true that some of my freedoms were restricted, while I was residing within an inpatient unit. Yet, as my health improved, my personal liberties also increased. Leaving the hospital, and going on day trips are two privileges that are granted to patients with good mental health. In time, the only restriction imposed on me was a universal curfew.

In addition, the nurses at the inpatient unit were not authoritative, and they acted with compassion. No patients were ever dehumanized, nor were they treated like prisoners. Patients who were severely ill had their basic needs taken care of, and more importantly, all of the mental health workers treated these persons with respect. From my observations, all of the members of the inpatient staff had a genuine interest to help persons with a mental illness, and likewise, they always acted in a professional manner.

The movie One Flew over the Cuckoo's Nest also portrayed electroconvulsive therapy (ECT) as a potentially dangerous method of treatment. In reality, ECT is a safe form of treatment, though permanent memory loss may be a possible side effect. In contrast, the most serious side effects associated with antipsychotic medications are extrapyramidal symptoms, which are distressing acute and delayed movement disorders.

From a critical point of view, I remember a couple of instances when I personally felt annoyed with the inpatient nurses. As a regular duty, one of the nurses would check on every patient, in every bedroom at around midnight. For one week, I remember that a particular nurse would direct his flashlight into my eyes and wake me up purposely. I have witnessed this action before, but I did not understand why the hospital staff had acted in this manner. During that period, I was battling insomnia and the nurse's nightly routine tended to cause feelings of frustration in me.

On the other hand, most of the nursing staff knew that I would sometimes smoke a cigarette out of my bedroom window, whenever I could not fall asleep. During those times, I was still in the process of metabolizing a new prescription. Actually, I knew that it was against the rules to smoke in the building, but feelings of anxiety grew increasingly difficult to bear. Smoking cigarettes had always helped with my anxiety in the past. Therefore, it is possible that this nurse may have been checking up on me, to make sure that I was not smoking in my bedroom.

Another vivid memory of mine occurred when I experienced extreme nasal congestion, due to my risperidone treatments. I had to additionally battle extreme feelings of anxiety while taking that medication, and this had a massive impact on my ability to fall sleep. One night, I went to the public bathroom to blow my nose. After a couple of minutes, my ability to breathe had improved somewhat, and I was ready to return to my bedroom. At that moment though, I suddenly became overwhelmingly dizzy. I then lost my balance, and my head hit the washroom mirror. I had to pause for a few moments to regain my balance. Then, while I was on my way to my bedroom, I began to experience more problems with nasal congestion. Still in a somewhat drowsy state, I was trying to make my way back to the bathroom, when a nurse saw me in the hallway. I think she believed that I was wandering aimlessly throughout the unit, and she forced me back into my bedroom.

That nurse ignored my reason for going to the bathroom, and that made me angry. In fact, she would not even listen to my complaints. I could not sleep because I could not breathe through my nose. I was trying to actively address my problems with insomnia, but from my point of view, that nurse would not permit this.

I would experience sleep problems for the entire period when I was treated with risperidone. I could not breathe properly, and extreme feelings of restlessness had affected my comfort levels. These effects probably lasted for about two and a half hours, before I would eventually fall into a deep sleep. In my opinion, the side effect of restlessness during bedtime was worse than the painful side effects from my loxapine treatments. My experiences with both of these medicines gave me a solid reason to detest psychiatric treatment.

My state of mind had continued to fluctuate, between a somewhat healthy to an extreme delusional state, until I found the right combination of medicines for my body type. There were only two medicines that I could tolerate, which also effectively treated my illness. I was healthy for a long period of time while taking 7.5 milligrams of olanzapine. Three hundred milligrams of clozapine was another effective prescription. In all other cases, either the medicine was ineffectual or its side effects were too intolerable.

A third memory of mine within the inpatient unit occurred when I was exceedingly ill. On one particular day, I had asked to see my cousin Ray. Ray passed away in a car accident when I was twelve years old. At that time, however, I was severely delusional and I believed that he was still alive. My paranoid state of mind produced the belief that my family had purposely lied to me about his death. Yet, due to my rapid thoughts and fragmented state of mind, I never came up with any reason why they would do this to me.

The radical nature of this delusion further demonstrates how disordered a schizophrenia patient may be, during the peak of his illness. In essence, my experiences with paranoid thoughts had altered my sense of the real world and replaced it with a new reality based on fictitious elements. On many occasions, I believed in my radical delusions over anything else.

During the peak of my illness, I was also too sick to recognize the fact that I was suffering from one major symptom of schizophrenia. When I saw

Dr. Freedman during my regular check-ups, he would continue to ask if I ever heard any voices. At first, I told him that I never experienced that symptom. After a few sessions, though, I went home and started to notice that I did hear imaginary voices speaking to me. Strangely, I only started to become aware of this symptom after Dr. Freedman had brought it to my attention. In fact, I remember hearing voices speak to me during moments from as early as my teenage years, but I was only able to realize this after I met Dr. Freedman. The imaginary voices that I heard throughout my life were essentially intrinsic parts of my mind, and I was not able to recognize otherwise.

For some reason, Dr. Freedman also helped me to recognize other things that I had failed to understand about my disease. Perhaps, at this time, my health had improved. Thus, I may have been more in touch with the real world. My failure to recognize the symptom of imaginary voices should reveal the fact that extremely ill patients will lack a degree of personal awareness and insight into their illness. My prior states of denial were also due to a lack of insight, and an inability to utilize sound reason and logic. At times, when I was clearly delusional, I would be unable to distinguish these perceptions from any of my regular thoughts. As a result, a lack of awareness may be a common reason why many severely ill patients will deny the possibility that they are suffering from a mental illness.

In fact, entering into a state of denial may be a common experience among many individuals who develop schizophrenia. An inability to recognize the true nature of one's paranoid delusions and hallucinations may contribute towards this denial. Hence, schizophrenia patients may also refuse medical treatment due to a decreased degree of self-awareness.

A good question now would be to ask how one could convince a schizophrenia patient to break out of his state of denial. Undeniably, the treatment process cannot truly begin until the patient actually accepts the fact that he is suffering from an illness. In Canada, every individual is entitled to civil liberties, and among these fundamental liberties includes a right to refuse medical treatment. Therefore, an extremely sick individual has the right refuse medical treatment, even when there is no logical reason behind this choice.

Trying to reason with the patient could solve this problem. In my case, the delusional state that I entered into during my college studies, and the paranoid beliefs that I held with respect to media personalities should have provided me with enough evidence that would have enabled me to realize that I was suffering from some form of psychological disturbance. I should have also been deeply concerned with my decreased intellectual functioning, especially in the areas of concentration, attention, and working memory. These were problems that I had reported to Dr. Lupton. However, after some time, I was able to normalize and come to terms with my schizophrenic delusions, because of my impaired frame of mind. A snowball effect then occurred, as I became increasingly more ill.

If reason does not reach the individual when he is in a state of denial, a second alternative may be to use an authority figure. An authority figure should be someone whose opinion is highly respected by the patient. The patient's family doctor could be one possible authority figure. An immediate family member, an extended family member, or even a close friend could also serve as a potential authority figure. When my mother's reasoning no longer had any influence over me, she needed to find someone else who could convince me to accept the fact that I was ill.

Authority figures must have an objective point of view, with respect to any given situation. This is due to a possible conflict of interest. I respected the police officers who came to my home, because I knew that they would have nothing to gain by confirming the fact that I was ill. Likewise, for some reason, I did not experience any paranoid thoughts in relation to these officers. As a result, since I had no reason to deny their authority, I also had no choice but to comply with their orders. The use of an authority figure may be necessary to break the deadlock in a psychological conflict that cannot be resolved through discussion or reason.

An objective standpoint is the most essential characteristic of an authority figure. This is necessary to ensure that a lack of perspective does not occur. For example, a lack of perspective can occur when a doctor treats either a family member or friend. When this occurs, the treatment process may be at risk. This is due to possible emotional responses, which could end up affecting the doctor's judgment or point of view. From my perspective, an emotional response from an authority figure may have a seemingly negative effect, which could ultimately de-legitimize his influence over the patient.

5

The Split Mind

Translated from Greek, the word schizophrenia literally means split mind. However, contrary to what some people may believe, schizophrenia is not a multiple personality disorder. In 1911, Eugen Bleuler coined the term based on the fragmentation of thought that is commonly observed in the patient (Weiten, 1995). Patients with schizophrenia can also experience symptoms similar to those observed in severe mood disorders. Nevertheless, their disturbed emotion usually comes about as a by -product of disturbed thought. As a result, schizophrenia is defined as an illness that affects normal human thought processes, and it is totally separate from other forms of mental illnesses, like multiple personality disorder or bipolar disorder.

Multiple personality disorder was renamed to dissociative identity disorder (DID) in 1994, to reflect changes in the scientific understanding of this disorder. DID is a disorder where two or more distinct identities, or personality states, are present in and alternately take control of an individual. Patients suffering from DID are believed to lack a unity of consciousness, with respect to their self-identity. In some cases, individuals with DID can possess over 100 different identities. However, 50% of documented cases involve patients with 10 or fewer identities (Psychology Today, 2008).

Patients suffering from DID will fail to integrate elements such as identity, memory, and consciousness into a single and multidimensional self. Each personality state, or alter, will demonstrate distinct personal histories, forms of behaviours, and physical characteristics. Alters can also differ with respect to age, gender, sexual orientation, and forms of existence. On average, the development of an alter takes six years (MedicineNet.com, 2008).

In many cases, the individual's given name is passive, guilty, dependent and depressed. Passive identities tend to have more limited memories in comparison to hostile, controlling, or more protective identities. A single alter can also possess forms of knowledge held by other alters. Specific alters may additionally deny knowledge of, be critical of, and conflict with other alters (PsychologyToday, 2008).

The symptoms of DID will vary in each case. It is possible that the patient will experience differing symptoms, over an extended period of time. The switching of a personality occurs when an alter takes executive control over the individual's body. In some cases, the individual experiences no loss of continuous memory (Vernon, Kallio and Wilcox, 1990). In other cases, episodes of amnesia may be prevalent. The average mentally healthy person will usually be unable to recall events during his first three to five years of life. However, patients with DID can experience problems while trying to recall memories during their first six to eleven years of life (Merck, 2008). Other symptoms include blackouts, or an experience of time loss where the patient lacks a period of consciousness.

Some patients may also talk, cry, or act like a young child subconsciously. Other patients may find pieces of writing or artwork that were created during a subconscious state. Patients may also discover forgotten material objects in their possession, or they can lose objects without any sense of awareness. Familiar places may also suddenly seem strange to the patient. In other cases, the individual may lack memories of any previous actions or events (Vernon, Kallio and Wilcox, 1990).

Patients with DID can also hear lucid voices or possess thoughts that can be conversed with. Feelings of detachment from the body, or depersonalization, and the feeling that one is not alone within one's body are further symptoms. Derealization occurs when a patient perceives objects, within his physical environment, as distorted and unreal (MayoClinic.com, 2008). Some DID patients may even fail to recognize their close friends and relatives (HealthAtoZ.com, 2008).

Physical pain, with no physiological reason, or a lack of pain, are also symptoms in DID. The patient may have thoughts, feelings or pieces of knowledge, which according to him, belong to someone else. This, in turn, will result in a varying ability to perform familiar skills. Some patients may further refer to themselves from a third person's perspective, or call themselves by different names. Other patients have reported that they do not recognize themselves when looking in a mirror (Vernon, Kallio and Wilcox, 1990).

Additional symptoms can include problems with detailed or sequential memory, especially during highly emotional situations. The individual may also possess strong emotions with no evident origin, or exhibit radical changes in opinion or attitude within similar situations. The patient may further constantly lose his train of thought, change the subject during a conversation, or repeatedly ask the same questions with no awareness. Other patients may produce unexpected intuitive solutions to problems, in areas like mathematics for example (Vernon, Kallio and Wilcox, 1990).

Psychosocial stress also plays a significant role in DID. Patients who develop this illness frequently report that they are the victims of severe physical and sexual abuse, especially during childhood. The transition of identities in the patient is also often triggered by psychosocial stress (Psychology Today, 2008). Some individuals with DID will further suffer from post-traumatic symptoms or post-traumatic stress disorder (PTSD).

In many cases, individuals who develop DID do so as a response to a traumatic experience (PsychNet-UK, 2008). When the patient has no means of escape, he may resort to some form of mental escape, as a way to deal with his physical or mental pains. An anticipation of such pains can also severely affect the individual. The dissociative process essentially separates the individual's thoughts, feelings, memories, perceptions and identity from a conscious awareness, and this allows him to function as if the traumatic experience has never occurred (PsychNet-UK, 2008). Chronic dissociation can lead to a form of psychological dysfunction, while repeated dissociation can lead to a series of separate entities, or mental states, which eventually take on identities of their own.

Patients who develop DID usually dissociate their mental and psychological components during childhood. Nevertheless, not every child who suffers from a traumatic experience will have a capacity to develop multiple identities. Similarly, vulnerable children may not develop the disorder because they are sufficiently protected and soothed by adults (Merck, 2008). As a result, most children who do develop DID are living within a stressful or dysfunctional environment. Accordingly, stress is clearly relevant to the etiology of DID.

The main mode of treatment for DID comes in the form of several years of specialized psychotherapy. Early diagnosis and treatment usually results in a better prognosis. Forms of prevention for DID may require social interventions within abusive families. Treatments through medications are only necessary when the patient's alter suffers from other conditions, like an anxiety disorder or depression.

Several symptoms in DID that are commonly observed among other forms of mental illness include visual or auditory hallucinations, depression, and anxiety. When a patient reports the hearing of alters in his head, DID can sometimes be misdiagnosed as schizophrenia. DID can also be misdiagnosed as a form of depression, in cases where the patient's core personality is subdued or withdrawn (HealthAtoZ.com, 2008).

In fact, my experience with schizophrenia could be, somewhat, comparable to what a DID patient experiences. An identity, or personality state, is essentially an enduring pattern of perceiving, relating to, and thinking about the environment and oneself (MedicineNet.com, 2008). Thus, in my opinion, the belief that I was God could be comparable to a switch in personality states. If I am right, there may be similar physical brain deficiencies common among both disorders.

Dissociative amnesia is another form of dissociative disorder. Patients suffering from this disorder will experience a sudden loss of memory, with respect to important personal information, that is more extensive than standard or regular forgetfulness (Weiten, 1995). Memory loss usually occurs around a single traumatic event, or for a period of time surrounding this event. This disorder is also typically caused by a traumatic or stressful event. In terms of treatment, therapy can help the individual with coping skills, and memory typically returns after some time.

As a closely related disorder, dissociative fugue occurs when the patient has memory loss that encompasses his entire life and personal identity. The patient may forget his name, family, and mode of employment. Travel away from one's home or place of employment may then occur. Other patients can adopt a partial or completely new identity (AllPsychONLINE, 2008). However, most patients do seem to remember things unrelated to personal identity, including how to drive. Extreme stress usually triggers this disorder. On average, the symptoms of this disorder will usually dissipate within one month's time (AllPsychONLINE, 2008).

Schizophrenia is not a mood disorder either. A mood disorder is an illness that is marked by emotional disturbances, which disrupt the individual's physical, perceptual, social, and thought processes. Depression is a unipolar disorder that causes the individual to experience persistent feelings of sadness and despair. Patients who suffer from depression will often lose interest in any previous sources of pleasure (Weiten, 1995).

Approximately 10% of persons in the general population will develop a depressive disorder within their lifetime (MedicineNet.com, 2008). Three main criteria are critical for a diagnosis of depression. Feelings of sadness must last for most of the day, for a period of more than two weeks, and these feelings must both interfere with daily life and impair normal functioning (National Institute of Mental Health, 2008). Besides feelings of hopelessness and despair, other symptoms include feelings of uselessness, helplessness, worthlessness, emptiness, excessive guilt, pessimism, and a preoccupation with failures or inadequacies. The individual may also exhibit fatigue, decreased energy, changes in appetite and weight, or recurrent suicidal thoughts. Individuals with depression can lack all forms of emotion, they may cry very easily, or they may be unable to cry when experiencing feelings of sadness (Centre for Addiction and Mental Health, 2008).

On a further note, depression affects more women than men. Researchers theorize that differences in biology, life cycle, hormones, and psychological factors may be relevant to this statistic. Men are more likely to report symptoms of fatigue, irritability and a loss of interest in pleasurable activities, while women more frequently report feelings of sadness, worthlessness and excessive guilt (National Institute of Mental Health, 2008). In the United States of America, more female patients will attempt to commit suicide, but more male patients will actually die by way of suicide.

Scientists theorize that the etiological factors behind depression include a combination of genetic, biochemical, environmental and psychological factors (National Institute of Mental Health, 2008). It is hypothesized to be a brain disorder because the brains of persons with depression look physically different, when compared to the brains of persons without depression. More specifically, areas of the brain responsible for mood, sleep, thinking, appetite and behaviour appear to function abnormally in depression. Researchers also believe that levels of serotonin and norepinephrine are lower in depression patients (MedicineNet.com, 2008). This chemical imbalance and a genetic predisposition seem to be the most significant elements linked to the cause of depression (National Institute of Mental Health, 2008). Some common triggers of depression include the loss of a loved one, a traumatic experience, or other forms of stressful situations.

Even in the most severe cases, depression is a highly treatable disorder. Clinical depression is rarely permanent, and it can sometimes end naturally without any forms of medical intervention. Nonetheless, the individual's period of depression may end more swiftly with medical treatment (Health Canada, 2008).

Antidepressant medications and professional psychotherapy are the main modes of treatment for depression. Medicines that alter levels of norepinephrine or serotonin can also alleviate some symptoms (MedicineNet.com, 2008). However, as with all medicines, antidepressants may cause side effects. The most common side effects include headache, nausea, fatigue, insomnia, agitation, nervousness, and other problems related to sexual dysfunction (National Institute of Mental Health, 2008).

Selective serotonin reuptake inhibitors (SSRIs), and serotonin and norepinephrine reuptake inhibitors (SNRIs) are the latest forms of antidepressants. The older forms, known as tricyclics and monoamine oxidase inhibitors, are also effective modes of treatment. However, a study conducted in 2004, on over 4000 children and adolescents, reveals the possibility that antidepressants could invoke suicidal thoughts. Researchers have discovered that 4% of subjects in this study thought about or attempted suicide. In comparison, only 2% of subjects taking a placebo thought about or attempted suicide (National Institute of Mental Health, 2008).

Nonetheless, a review of pediatric trials conducted between 1988 and 2006 indicates that the benefits of antidepressant medications likely outweigh their risks, concerning the treatment of children and adolescents who suffer from major depression or an anxiety disorder. As a precautionary measure, children and adolescents who are taking antidepressants should be closely monitored for any irregular side effects, including suicidal ideations or behaviours (National Institute of Mental Health, 2008).

Psychotherapy is another treatment option for patients with depression. Cognitive behavioural therapy (CBT) and interpersonal therapy (IPT) are two forms of psychotherapy. CBT teaches patients how to think and behave, while IPT helps patients with knowledge, understanding and social relationships. In cases of mild to moderate forms of depression, psychotherapy may be effective as a single mode of treatment (National Institute of Mental Health, 2008).

In cases where medications or psychotherapy fail, electroconvulsive therapy (ECT) may be used. The side effects of ECT include confusion, disorientation, and memory loss. However, these side effects are only temporary, and after some time, patients usually do not suffer from any adverse cognitive deficits (National Institute of Mental Health, 2008).

Some common symptoms observed in depression and other forms of mental illness include social withdrawal, irritability, insomnia, oversleeping, and a loss of touch with reality in the form of hallucinations or delusions (Centre for Addiction and Mental Health, 2008). Other common symptoms include restlessness, persistent bodily aches and pains, and difficulties with concentration, memory and decision-making (National Institute of Mental Health, 2008). Patients with depression may also neglect their personal hygiene and suffer from periods of anxiety (Depression Canada, 2008).

Bipolar disorder is a mood disorder where the patient experiences periods of serious depression and episodes of elevated emotional highs. Previously known as manic-depressive illness, this disorder affects approximately three to four percent of the world's population (IsItBipolar, 2008). Some manic symptoms include feelings of euphoria, increased energy levels, extreme optimism, frenzied action, rapid and unpredictable changes in emotion, and a decreased need for sleep (Health Canada, 2008). Extreme manic episodes can also cause an increased level of self-confidence, which may lead to aggressive, reckless, or risk-taking behaviours (emedicinehealth, 2008).

Patients with bipolar disorder will experience extreme manic or depressive states in cycles. In view of that, patients may function normally in between these mood cycles. Researchers have also discovered that the patient's mood swings tend to become closer temporally with age (emedicinehealth, 2008). Patients can further experience a mixed state where the symptoms of depression and mania occur at the same time. Hence, the individual may, for example, think and speak rapidly while experiencing feelings related to anxiety or suicide (Centre for Addiction and Mental Health, 2008).

The cause of bipolar disorder remains unknown. Researchers do know that the majority of all bipolar diagnoses affect individuals during their teenage to young adult years. They have also discovered that certain areas of the brain, in bipolar patients, are physically different, with respect to size and shape. A genetic mechanism, a chemical imbalance, environmental factors, and disrupted hormone levels may be relevant etiological factors in this illness (Bipolar Disorder, 2008).

Although the triggers of a bipolar episode will vary on an individual basis, there are universal stressors that may be common among many patients. For example, an irregular sleep schedule, or the abuse of a substance can trigger a bipolar mood swing. The use of medications for depression or other medical conditions, like a thyroid problem, are other possible triggers. Highly stressful social events like a marriage, a new job, or a disagreement among family members or friends can also trigger a bipolar episode. Likewise, simple environmental elements such as a change in season or a holiday may become bipolar stressors. In other cases, patients can experience mood swings with no obvious trigger (Bipolar Disorder, 2008).

Methods of treatment for bipolar disorder include medicines and psychotherapy. Educating patients in the area of self-insight may also be effective. Treatment through medications, in the majority of cases, is lifelong. Types of medicines for bipolar disorder include mood stabilizers, anti-seizure medications, antidepressants, antipsychotics, and other adjunct medications that address problems with sleep or anxiety. Depending on the specific medication, side effects can include weight gain, nausea, anxiety, tremors, movement problems, dry mouth, hair loss, and a reduction in sexual functioning (National Institute of Mental Health, 2008). ECT may be considered when the patient does not respond to conventional medicines. Modes of psychotherapy can include sessions with a professional counsellor, group therapy, CBT, psychoeducation, and specialized support groups which objectively focus on the individual's mood and personal relationships (Bipolar Disorder, 2008).

Common symptoms observed in bipolar disorder and other forms of mental illness include racing thoughts, rapid speech, extreme irritability, and impulsive behaviours (Health Canada, 2008). Patients may also be easily distracted, exhibit poorer judgment, and suffer from delusions or hallucinations (Centre for Addiction and Mental Health, 2008). Overreactions to stimuli, the misinterpretation of events, and a state of denial are other symptoms (National Institute of Mental Health, 2008). Bipolar patients can also exhibit cognitive profiles that are similar to the profiles of schizophrenia patients, though schizophrenia patients have more severe and widespread impairments (Pradhan *et al*, 2008).

Other complications can arise in cases where a sick individual is not formally diagnosed with bipolar disorder. Firstly, the individual may be prone to abuse alcohol or other substances. He may also develop an eating disorder, like anorexia or bulimia. The development of attention deficit hyperactivity disorder, a panic disorder, or a social phobia is also possible (Bipolar Disorder, 2008). Subsequently, individuals with bipolar disorder are at some risk of developing other forms of mental illness.

Schizophrenia is not an anxiety disorder either. Excessive and unrealistic worries or fears, irritability, and avoidance are the general symptoms of an anxiety disorder. Similar to sadness and depression, most individuals will experience feelings of anxiety at some point in their lifetime. However, also similar to depression, an anxiety disorder is more extreme in nature. An anxiety disorder will sometimes cause the individual to respond inappropriately within a given situation, or it can cause him to lose control over such responses (WebMD, 2008). This type of disorder will also affect the individual's social relationships, social activities, academic pursuits and field of employment (Public Health Agency of Canada, 2008). Specific anxiety disorders include generalized anxiety disorder, a phobic disorder, panic attacks, obsessive-compulsive disorder, and PTSD (Mental Illness Awareness Week, 2008). Approximately 12% of the Canadian population will develop an anxiety disorder. As a result, anxiety disorders are the most predominant form of mental illness in Canada (Mood Disorders Society of Canada, 2008).

Generalized anxiety disorder is characterized by a chronically high level of anxiety that is not tied to any specific threat (Weiten, 1995). Patients may constantly worry about previous mistakes or potential problems. However, most of their troubles are minor in significance. The symptoms of generalized anxiety disorder can include trembling, muscle tension, nausea, dizziness, headache, and a frequent need to go to the bathroom (Health Canada, 2008).

Symptoms of a panic attack can include a rapid heartbeat, excessive sweating, and a fear of death. A panic attack usually occurs without warning, and at times in conjunction with feelings of terror. Persons who experience a panic attack are subject to intense, prolonged feelings of fright and distress, for no obvious reason. A panic attack can also cause other physical symptoms like chest pains, heart palpitations, dizziness, abdominal discomfort, and shortness of breath (Health Canada, 2008). Patients who suffer from panic attacks can sometimes enter into a mental state of unreality where nothing in their environment seems real, or they may be entirely focused on possible looming dangers (Health Canada, 2008). Some patients additionally fear the possibility that they will suffer from a panic attack while in public. This sometimes leads to the development of agoraphobia, which is a fear of going out to public places (Weiten, 1995).

A phobia is a strong and irrational fear associated with an object, experience, or other phenomenon, that presents no realistic danger (Weiten, 1995). For instance, a social phobia can cause the individual to avoid social situations. The patient may be prone to social withdrawal, confusion, a state of extreme self-consciousness, and he may fear the possibility that other persons will observe him while acting inappropriately. For the most part, experiences with fear are common to the average person. However, a phobic disorder necessarily interferes with the individual's daily life and behaviour. Some specific phobias include fears related to heights, bridges, large crowds, public speaking, closed places, and water (Weiten, 1995).

Obsessive-compulsive disorder (OCD) is characterized by the persistent and uncontrollable intrusions of unwanted thoughts, otherwise known as obsessions, and the urge to engage in senseless rituals, which are compulsions (Weiten, 1995). The main symptom in obsessive-compulsive disorder is the repetition of a specific action, due to the belief that this will prevent some feared event or consequence (Mental Illness Awarenes Week, 2008). In OCD, patients may experience general symptoms related to fear and low self-esteem. Most patients experience both obsessions and compulsions, although some patients suffer from only one of these symptoms. A patient's obsession may centre around inflicting harm on other persons, sexual acts, suicide, or personal failures. Constant hand washing or endless and repetitive actions, such as the checking of locks or faucets, are two forms of compulsions. Patients with excessive compulsions may sometimes feel that they have lost a level of control over their mind. By acting through compulsive behaviours, patients will temporarily relieve their personal anxieties (Weiten, 1995).

Patients with obsessive-compulsive disorder have comparable performance profiles with schizophrenia patients. Patients with OCD also have similar, yet less severe impairments in the areas of simple attention and memory. Accordingly, it is possible that a doctor may mistakenly diagnose an OCD patient with a schizophrenia spectrum disorder (Martin *et al*, 2008).

Individuals with post-traumatic stress disorder have usually witnessed or experienced an event where they feared for their life (or another's) and felt they could do nothing to save themselves (or the other person) (Mental Illness Awareness Week, 2008). The symptoms of PTSD include intrusive memories or flashbacks of a traumatic event, the avoidance of anything that may be linked to this event, emotional numbing, and jumpiness (Mental Illness Awareness Week, 2008). Depression, irritability, distress, detachment, isolation, a heightened level of arousal, and feelings of explosive anger are other symptoms. PTSD is largely untreated among adults with a dual-diagnosis. In these cases, the treatment of psychotic symptoms usually takes precedence, and this oversight can lead to complications in the patient's recovery process (Frueh *et al*, 2009).

Researchers theorize that many anxiety disorders are caused by a complex interplay of genetic, developmental, biological, and socio-economic factors, in addition to workplace stress (Public Health Agency of Canada, 2008). The individual may also gradually develop a fear due to the repeated exposure to some embarrassing, abusive, or violent act. A cognitive based theory suggests that the individual will develop an anxiety disorder if he foresees some form of embarrassment or harm. A biological theory focuses on a region of the brain, known as the amygdala, in addition to a genetic cause. Some researchers are further exploring the possibility that an individual may develop an anxiety disorder as a response to parenting practices (Public Health Agency of Canada, 2008).

General modes of treatment for all anxiety disorders include a combination of medicines and CBT. Anti-depressants or anti-anxiety drugs are sometimes used. Support groups can also aid the patient and his family. Under this setting, patients can learn measures that will enable them to minimize and cope with their anxiety related symptoms.

Patients with an anxiety disorder may also experience symptoms that have been observed among other forms of mental disorders. These symptoms include restlessness, difficulties with concentration, fatigue, insomnia, and an unrealistic view of one's problems. Some patients may also suffer from other mental illnesses, like an eating disorder or depression. In general, patients with an anxiety disorder can be easily startled, experience hallucinations, and they may lose interest in any forms of enjoyable activities (WebMD, 2008).

In addition, schizophrenia is not a personality disorder. Some individuals may hold the belief that patients with schizophrenia are prone to criminal behaviour. However, most persons who are prone to criminal behaviour suffer from a personality disorder, and not a schizophrenic disorder. An individual's personality is defined as a complex pattern of deeply imbedded psychological characteristics that are largely non-conscious and not easily altered, which express themselves automatically in almost every area of functioning (Public Health Agency of Canada, 2008). A personality disorder is characterized by extreme and inflexible personality traits, which cause subjective distress or impaired social and occupational functioning (Weiten, 1995). This form of disorder can also be defined as an enduring pattern of inner experience and behavior that deviates markedly from the expectations of the individual's culture (pyschiatryonline, 2008). Persons affected by a personality disorder are usually pervasive, rigid, and self-defeating. Hence, personality disorders are more associated with the individual's temperament and character (Kirby and Keon, 2004).

For a proper diagnosis, the pattern of the individual's personality traits must remain stable over a long duration of time, and its onset will usually be traced back to adolescence or early adulthood (BehaveNet, 2008). A proper diagnosis also requires two symptoms in the areas of emotion, cognition, interpersonal functioning, or impulse control. Nonetheless, many individuals that suffer from a personality disorder are never diagnosed, nor treated (Public Health Agency of Canada, 2008). As a result, the prevalence of personality disorders within the general population is largely unknown.

Scientists have categorized all personality disorders into either an odd-eccentric cluster, a dramatic-impulsive cluster, or an anxious-fearful cluster (Weiten, 1995). Previously known as sociopathic personality disorder, antisocial personality disorder fits into the dramatic-impulsive cluster. Patients with this illness regularly disregard and violate the rights of others. They also reject social norms with respect to ethical principles and moral behaviour. Such individuals can be aggressive, destructive, isolated, and they may disregard established laws and lawful behaviour. They may also be deceitful, manipulative, impulsive, reckless, easily irritated, and they may lack a sense of communal responsibility or common remorse (BehaveNet, 2008). Scientists have further observed that these individuals rarely experience genuine affection for others, and that they will rationalize any forms of pain that they inflict on other persons. Individuals with antisocial personality disorder also pursue immediate forms of gratification or personal profit (Weiten, 1995). They can possess a superficial charm, lack an ability to tolerate boredom, and they may possess a sense of extreme entitlement (MayoClinic.com, 2008).

An inability to feel empathy for other persons often results in antisocial behaviour. Both genetic and environmental factors are theorized to be relevant to the cause of this illness. According to Weiten, biological factors may create a genuine but weak predisposition towards antisocial behaviour. Growing up in a dysfunctional family system has also been correlated to the etiology of this illness. Researchers theorize that the symptoms in this illness will usually emerge throughout childhood or adolescence. Possible warning signs can include difficulties with anger and authority, problems with legal altercations, cruelty to animals, and the setting of fires (AllPsychONLINE, 2008).

Long-term insight oriented therapy is available for patients with this illness. Psychotherapy can also help with the development of appropriate interpersonal skills, which can then instill a moral code (MayoClinic.com, 2008). However, these patients rarely seek treatment for their condition. This is due to the patient's belief that the world itself is primarily responsible for his problems (AllPsychONLINE, 2008). Hence, the individual will usually lack a sense of insight or awareness, with respect to the general symptoms of his disorder.

Patients with antisocial personality disorder are in some danger of developing depression, bipolar disorder, an anxiety disorder, or other forms of personality disorders. This, in turn, puts the patient at increased risk of drug abuse, alcohol abuse, and suicidal behaviour. Early intervention is recommended for the treatment of adolescents who exhibit antisocial behaviour. Modes of prevention can include the establishment of clear rules for conduct and discipline, the teaching of crucial social and interpersonal skills, the application of consistent consequences for maladaptive behaviours, the reduction of punitive methods directed towards the controlling of behaviour, and lessons based on the concept of respect for other individuals within one's community (MayoClinic.com, 2008).

Individuals with narcissistic personality disorder have an inflated sense of their own importance and a deep need for admiration. Even though they hold the belief that they are superior over other persons, their self-esteem is actually quite fragile and vulnerable to the slightest forms of criticism. Other symptoms can include a lack of empathy, and an inability to maintain healthy relationships. Patients with this disorder will often exhibit pervasive patterns of grandiosity, they may hold the belief that they are special, and they may hold the belief that other persons are jealous of them. These individuals may be interpersonally exploitive, they may express disdain against persons who are perceived as inferior, and they can often appear as contemptuous or condescending (MayoClinic.com, 2008). Furthermore, they may believe that they are only understood by persons who are like them, or those who are equally superior in some aspect of life (AllPsychONLINE, 2008).

These patients tend to address an underlying sense of inferiority through a sense of entitlement. When special treatment is denied, the individual can become impatient or extremely angry. He may also envy other persons who have more respect or those who are given more attention (AllPsychONLINE, 2008). In essence, the patient's efforts to belittle other persons are primarily conducted to make himself appear superior, in some other manner.

Theorized causes of narcissistic personality disorder include a dysfunctional childhood with excessive pampering, high expectations, abuse and neglect. Genetics or psychobiological factors may also be important. Short-term lengths of psychotherapy can address issues like substance abuse, depression, and low self-esteem. Long-term insight-oriented therapy can help individuals with the creation of a more realistic self-image. Psychotherapy can also help patients with interpersonal relationships, and with the management of any emotions or motivational factors behind their illness (MayoClinic.com, 2008). However, similar to antisocial personality disorder, patients usually do not seek treatment, due both to a limited amount of insight and the shift of blame or responsibility that they place on their society, with respect to the symptoms of their illness (AllPsychONLINE, 2008).

In histrionic personality disorder, the individual will exhibit a pervasive pattern of excessive emotions and attention seeking behaviours (BehaveNet, 2008). The patient usually expresses emotions that are extremely or inappropriately exaggerated, which can otherwise be viewed as theatrical.

His emotional expressions may also shift in a constant, sudden, or rapid fashion (PSYweb.com, 2008). Other symptoms include an excessive concern with physical appearances, and a false sense of intimacy with other persons (MayoClinic.com, 2008). The individual may be extremely sensitive with respect to the approval of others, he may constantly seek a form of reassurance from other persons, or he may be uncomfortable in situations where he is not the center of attention. In addition, the patient may interact with other persons in a provocative or seductive manner, and he may sometimes utilize an impressionistic style of speech (BehaveNet, 2008).

Borderline personality disorder is a fourth personality disorder. Symptoms in this illness include a pattern of unstable and intense interpersonal relationships, where the patient alternates between feelings of idealization and great admiration, to devaluation and intense dislike. Patients may also possess an insecure self-image marked by impulsivity, rapid changes in mood, self-mutilating behaviours or gestures, chronic feelings of emptiness, inappropriate or intense forms of anger, short episodes of anxiety or depression, and social isolation (BehaveNet, 2008). They may also view themselves as bad or unworthy, or they may feel that they are unfairly mistreated or misunderstood. Patients may exhibit frantic efforts to avoid social isolation, and they may be highly sensitive to rejection with a fear of abandonment (Mymentalhealth.ca, 2008). Accordingly, these patients can also feel helpless, be very needy, and cling to other persons (AllPsychONLINE, 2008).

The etiology of this disorder has been associated with a history of unstable relationships, a dysfunctional family, and childhood neglect. Long-term treatments in the form of insight-oriented therapy can sometimes be helpful (AllPsychONLINE, 2008). Women with borderline personality disorder may also be admitted into a hospital setting, to prevent suicidal forms of behaviour (Public Health Agency of Canada, 2008).

Classified into the anxious-fearful cluster, avoidant personality disorder is marked by an excessive level of sensitivity to potential rejection, humiliation, or shame (Weiten, 1995). Individuals suffering from this disorder may exhibit pervasive patterns of social inhibition, and a hypersensitive response to negative evaluations. These individuals may then purposely avoid occupational activities, and demonstrate restraint in intimate relationships. In new interpersonal situations, the patient may be inhibited by feelings of inadequacy. He may be unwilling to get involved in social situations, unless he is certain that other persons will like him. The patient may also be unusually preoccupied with being criticized or rejected in social situations, and he often views himself as unappealing, socially inept, and inferior to other persons. He can also be reluctant to take risks or engage in activities that could become embarrassing at some future time (BehaveNet, 2008).

Obsessive-compulsive personality disorder involves a preoccupation with rules, schedules, lists, trivial details, and the concept of organization. Patients suffering from this disorder will exhibit extremely conventional, serious, and formal forms of behaviour (Weiten, 1995). Further, they are usually unable to express warm emotions and they may demonstrate a preoccupation with orderliness, perfectionism, and mental and interpersonal control, at the expense of flexibility, openness, and efficiency (BehaveNet, 2008). These preoccupations can also often interfere with both the completion and major point of a given task.

The patient can also be excessively devoted to work and productivity, at the expense of leisure activities and friendships (BehaveNet, 2008). He can be overconscientious and scrupulous in matters related to ethics or morality. In other cases, the patient may be reluctant to delegate tasks to others, unless these persons submit precisely to his way of doing things. This leads to the formation of rigid and stubborn personality traits. Other patients may be unable to discard old objects with little value. They may also view money as something that must be hoarded for future catastrophes (BehaveNet, 2008).

Patients with dependent personality disorder are excessively lacking in self-reliance and self esteem. They may be extremely passive and allow other persons to make their decisions. They may also constantly subordinate their own needs for the needs of other persons (Weiten, 1995). These patients will often experience problems when disagreeing with other persons, due to the fear that they will lose some form of support or approval. They can demonstrate an excessive need to be taken care of, and this often leads to submissive and clinging forms of behaviour, in addition to fears of separation (BehaveNet, 2008).

In some cases, the patient may need excessive amounts of advice or reassurances, or he may need another person to take responsibility over major areas in his personal life. Thus, the patient may go to extreme lengths when acquiring forms of social support from other persons. The patient may also experience difficulties when doing things on his own, and he may feel uncomfortable or helpless when socially isolated. When a close relationship ends, the individual will urgently seek another relationship, and he may hold the relentless fear that he will be left alone to take care of himself, at some future time (BehaveNet, 2008).

Categorized into the odd-eccentric cluster, paranoid personality disorder is marked by a pervasive and unwarranted suspiciousness and mistrust of other people (Weiten, 1995). Another characteristic includes an overly sensitive or hypersensitive attitude, where the individual is liable to take quick offence while in a variety of circumstances. One possible paranoid thought revolves around the belief that a group of persons is plotting to harm the individual in some way. In terms of behaviour, persons suffering from this disorder tend to be argumentative, they may lack a sense of humour, and they may express disdain against other persons who are perceived as weak (Torrey, 1995).

Individuals who are diagnosed with schizoid personality disorder will exhibit a pervasive pattern of detachment from social relationships. The individual will usually lack a desire for or enjoy any forms of close relationships, even with family members. He will often choose solitary activities, and he may have very little interest in sexual relationships. Other symptoms can include an attitude of indifference with respect to the praise or criticism of others, and a restricted range of emotional responses or affectivity (BehaveNet, 2008).

The patient may also be unable to experience pleasure, and he may lack character traits related to motivation and persistence (MayoClinic.com, 2008). He can further experience general feelings related to discomfort or restlessness, similar to the symptoms observed in other mental illnesses. However, the patient must not experience these symptoms during the course of schizophrenia, a mood disorder, or a pervasive developmental disorder to be accurately diagnosed with schizoid personality disorder.

Many complications have been associated with this disorder. Patients may experience troubles when interpreting or responding to social stimuli. They may also have troubles when warding off the predatory behaviour of other persons. Accordingly, they may be more susceptible to victimization, when compared to the average citizen. The patient may then develop a drug or alcohol addiction, as a possible consequence. Patients with this disorder are also at an increased risk of developing schizophrenia, depression, or other forms of mental illness (MayoClinic.com, 2008).

Genetic and environmental factors, during early childhood, are theorized to be etiologically relevant in this disorder. A family history of this illness is also a particular risk factor. Possible modes of treatment include medications, CBT, and group therapy. However, the treatment process can be complicated because some patients will settle into complacency about their emotionally impoverished existence (MayoClinic.com, 2008).

Individuals with schizotypal personality disorder will exhibit social deficits through oddities in thinking, perception, and communication that resemble, but are less intense than, the symptoms observed in schizophrenia (Weiten, 1995). These patients may further experience an acute discomfort or a reduced capacity with respect to the formation of close relationships (MH. com, 2008). Therefore, individuals with this disorder can demonstrate an indifferent or detached attitude towards social relationships, they may experience cognitive or perceptual distortions, and they may also act in an eccentric fashion (PSYweb.com, 2008).

The belief that the media, or other persons, are centring on oneself is a perceptual distortion known as an idea of reference. Persons with schizotypal personality disorder will sometimes experience ideas of reference, and they can hold odd beliefs in the realms of magic, clairvoyance, ESP, telepathy and superstition. Unusual perceptual experiences, like bodily illusions or phantom pains, and suspicious or paranoid thoughts are further symptoms (BehaveNet, 2008).

The patient may also appear, behave, or speak in an odd, eccentric, or peculiar manner. He may exhibit excessive social anxieties because of his paranoid fears, and he may lack close relationships outside of first-degree family members (BehaveNet, 2008). Flat or inappropriate emotional responses are other possible symptoms (MayoClinic.com, 2008).

Scientists theorize that genetics and early life experiences may be relevant to the cause of this disorder. It is further possible that childhood abuse, neglect or stress results in the brain dysfunction that gives rise to schizotypal symptoms (MayoClinc.com, 2008). One major warning sign includes an awareness of everyday executive difficulties. A family history of schizotypal personality disorder increases the individual's risk to develop this illness. Patients are also at an increased risk to develop schizophrenia, major depression, an anxiety disorder, a social phobia, or another personality disorder (MayoClinic.com, 2008).

Treatments for schizotypal personality disorder include medicines that are used to treat anxiety or mood disorders. Psychotherapy, behavioural therapy, cognitive therapy, and family therapy are other modes of treatment (MayoClinic.com, 2008).

In general, researchers hypothesize that genetic factors influence the biological basis of brain function as well as basic personality structure. The personality structure then develops over a period of time, and the individual eventually acquires distinctive ways of feeling, thinking and behaving, in addition to distinctive ways of perceiving the world. As a consequence, the individual's personality structure will influence his response to general life experiences and social interactions (Public Health Agency of Canada, 2008).

The poor regulation of emotional responses, in conjunction with environmental stressors like abuse or neglect, may increase the individual's risk of developing a personality disorder. Developmental challenges during adolescence and early adulthood could also trigger a personality disorder. Thus, the reinforcement of learned responses, modeling, and aversive stimuli may be contributing factors. Personality disorders can also reflect deficiencies in ego and superego development, which may be related to unresponsive, overprotective, or early separation elements amongst mother-child relationships (WD, 2008).

The cultural deviations observed in individuals with a personality disorder are usually mild in terms of severity. Therefore, many patients may not seek treatment because they are able to live normally in other ways, such as maintaining a form of employment. Intense individual and group psychotherapies are the main modes of treatment for most personality disorders, though in some cases, medicines like anti-depressants and mood stabilizers may also have beneficial effects (Mymentalhealth.ca, 2008)). Social support networks within a school or community setting can also help in the development of a stronger sense of self-esteem and more effective coping strategies. Thus, some researchers theorize that a supportive environment may protect the individual from developing a personality disorder (Public Health Agency of Canada, 2008).

These patients may also require treatments for other conditions like alcohol and drug abuse, depression, anxiety, bipolar disorder, obsessive-compulsive disorder, an eating disorder, sexual dysfunction, and suicidal thoughts. Hence, some individuals can suffer from other health conditions in concurrence with a personality disorder (Public Health Agency of Canada, 2008).

A sexual disorder will have profound effects on the individual's sexual performance, desire, and behaviours. As in all other mental disorders, a true sexual disorder will also necessarily interfere with the individual's normal functioning. Paraphilias, in particular, are distressing and repetitive sexual fantasies, urges, or behaviors (AllPsychONLINE, 2008). These symptoms will interfere with satisfactory sexual relations or everyday functioning. The patient may then believe that he is unable to control his symptoms and that these symptoms mainly affect him in a negative manner (AllPsychONLINE, 2008).

Pedophilia is a disorder marked by intense sexually arousing fantasies, urges or behaviors, involving a prepubescent child. The patient must be at least sixteen years of age and five years older than his subject for an appropriate diagnosis.

Sexual sadism involves fantasies and behaviours, which either humiliate or cause physical suffering to another person. Sexual masochism, on the other hand, involves urges and behaviours linked to the personal experience of humiliation, or physical pain.

Sexual fetishism is marked by a fantasy or behaviour that links sex to a nonliving object, situation, or body part. The urge or the act of observing an unsuspected stranger who is naked, disrobing, or engaging in a form of sexual activity is known as voyeurism. In contrast, exhibitionism is characterized by the fantasy or act of exposing one's genitals to an unsuspecting stranger. In transvestic fetishism, the individual experiences sexual urges towards clothing that is typically worn by persons of the opposite gender. In some cases, these patients may experience problems related to gender identity as well.

In general, the causes of most paraphilias mainly involve childhood experiences. Researchers believe that a large majority of pedophiles were sexually abused as a child. However, feelings of inadequacy with same age peers during childhood may also account for the transfer of sexual urges to children. Childhood trauma is theorized to be involved in the etiology of sexual sadism, sexual masochism, sexual fetishism, voyeurism, exhibitionism, and transvestic fetishism (AllPsychONLINE, 2008).

Treatments for most paraphilias typically involve psychotherapy. Such therapies can help the individual recognize and understand any underlying causes behind his behaviour. The prognosis of pedophilia, however, usually declines when the individual is dually diagnosed with antisocial personality disorder. With respect to exhibitionism, some medications are available as a possible mode of treatment.

The categorizing of gender identity disorder as a psychiatric disorder is currently a topic of controversy. In gender identity disorder, individuals will exhibit a strong and persistent identification with the opposite gender. These individuals can feel a sense of discomfort with their physical gender, and they may believe that they were born into the wrong sex. Although gender identity disorder is technically classified as a mental disorder within the Diagnostic and Statistical Manual of Mental Disorders (DSM-IV), it is evident that many persons, who are diagnosed with this condition, function normally in their everyday lives. Consequently, since disability does not necessarily result from the act of identifying oneself as a member of the opposite sex, this phenomenon may not be, in principle, a disorder. In any case, this phenomenon still causes the individual to have a split mind with respect to sex and gender, and accordingly it may have elements in common with other disorders that are classified under the DSM-IV.

Adolescents and adults with gender identity disorder will demonstrate a preoccupation with trying to rid themselves of their primary and secondary sexual characteristics. Individuals within this sub-community may also frequently pass off as a person of the opposite sex, and they may desire to live or be treated as a member of the opposite sex. The individual will also believe that his feelings and reactions are typical of the opposite gender (BehaveNet, 2008).

Children may repeatedly voice that they are, or desire to be, a member of the opposite sex. Boys may believe that their sexual organs are disgusting and that these organs will disappear at some point in the future. Girls may assert that they do not want to grow breasts or menstruate, and they may also believe that they have or will grow a penis. Cross-dressing and preferences for cross-sex roles in make-believe play or persistent fantasies are other symptoms. The child can further demonstrate a strong desire to participate in stereotypical games and pastimes associated with the other sex, or exhibit a strong preference for playmates of the opposite sex (BehaveNet, 2008).

Distress and disability can become potential problems for individuals with this disorder. In young children, distress is manifested by the stated unhappiness about their assigned sex. In adolescents, the failure to develop age-appropriate same sex peer relationships can often lead to isolation and mental hardships. In adults, a preoccupation with the opposite gender can sometimes interfere with regular activities. Furthermore, in all three age groups, relationship difficulties may be common and normal functioning at the school or work environments may be impaired (BehaveNet, 2008).

Parent-child relationships, at an early age, are theorized to be relevant to the cause of gender identity disorder. Difficulties in identifying with a parent of the same sex can be a further etiological factor. Chromosomal anomalies and hormonal imbalances during brain formation in the utero is another possible cause (WD, 2008). Modes of treatment are likely to be long-term, and are manifested in small gains made with respect to any underlying issues involved (AllPsychONLINE, 2008).

Social isolation and low self-esteem, due to stigma and discrimination, are common elements observed in gender identity disorder and other forms of mental disorders. Males may further choose to self-medicate themselves through hormone treatments. Some patients also exhibit depressive symptoms, anxiety, or the general symptoms of transvestic fetishism. Suicidal ideations and attempts are particular risk factors for adolescents with this disorder (Mental Health Sanctuary, 2008).

Individuals with a factitious disorder intentionally produce or feign symptoms, so that they can assume the role as a sick patient. Moreover, some patients will ingest medications or toxins to produce problematic symptoms. The emotional support, pity, and special rights given to sick persons usually serve as a motivational factor (AllPsychONLINE, 2008). Therefore, acts of malingering, where the individual benefits economically, through the avoiding of legal responsibility or unwanted duty, or through an escape from captivity or incarceration are not motivational factors behind this type of illness (BehaveNet, 2008).

Munchausen syndrome is a particular form of factitious disorder where the individual pretends to be sick, or deliberately causes injury, to fulfill deep emotional needs. Patients with this syndrome may make up symptoms, push for risky operations, or try to rig laboratory test results in an effort to win sympathy and concern. These individuals are healthy persons who desire to be physically ill. In Munchausen syndrome by proxy, the patient will make another person ill, to win sympathy for himself (MayoClinic. com, 2008).

Patients with this syndrome can make up dramatic stories, with respect to differing forms of medical conditions. They may be frequently hospitalized, report vague and inconsistent symptoms, seek treatment from many different doctors, or make frequent requests for medications. The patient's medical condition can also get worse for no apparent reason, he may have extensive knowledge of medical terminology, and he may forbid contact between health professionals and his family members or friends (MayoClinic.com, 2008).

Individuals with Munchausen syndrome may further report a false medical history, create self-inflicted wounds, fake their symptoms, or aggravate their current wounds. Some patients will also tamper with medical instruments (MayoClinic.com, 2008). At present, there is no known cause of Munchausen syndrome. Biology, genetics, and life experiences may be relevant. Risk factors for this illness can include a poor sense of identity or self-esteem, poor coping skills, childhood trauma, a serious childhood illness, a seriously ill relative, or the loss of a loved one during childhood.

Although there are no standard modes of treatment for this syndrome, psychotherapy, behavioural counselling and family therapy can sometimes be effective. A nonconfrontational intervention by trained medical staff can also help some individuals (MayoClinic.com, 2008). Medicines used to treat depression or anxiety, and temporary hospitalizations are other modes of treatment.

Somatoform disorders are similar to factitious disorders. Patients suffering from this type of disorder will experience physical ailments, with no medical or biological cause. As a result, their ailments are based solely on psychological factors (Weiten, 1995). Possible ailments can include headaches, nauseas, muscle cramps, pain, numbness, and dizziness. As in all other mental disorders, the symptoms of a somatoform disorder must cause clinically significant distress or impairment in social functioning, occupational functioning, or other areas in life (psychiatryonline, 2008).

Hypochondriasis is a common form of somatoform disorder. Patients with hypochondriasis hold the fear that they have a serious disease, due to the misinterpretation of bodily sensations (AllPsychONLINE, 2008). This preoccupation continually persists in the individual, even when assured by a doctor that no real illness exists. Patients also usually do not recognize that their concerns are excessive or unreasonable (BehaveNet, 2008).

Researchers have not been able to identify a specific cause of this disorder. It usually affects individuals who have had a personal experience with an organic disease, either directly or through a family member. This illness has also been linked with individuals who are affected by everyday stressors (PSYweb.com, 2008).

Psychological therapy is a complicated mode of treatment for hypochondriasis. It is complicated because most persons with this illness do not believe that their symptoms are purely psychological. Stress also increases an individual's risk to develop this disorder (WD, 2008). Accordingly, stress-reduction training may also be effective.

Hypochondriacs are usually sceptical and disbelieving, with respect to their doctor's professional diagnosis. Accordingly, denial is an element in this disease that is common among other forms of mental illness. In fact, most forms of denial may be comparable to a minor paranoid delusion. Hypochondriasis is also frequently diagnosed in conjunction with other mental illnesses, including depression or an anxiety related disorder (Weiten, 1995).

Somatization disorder is marked by a history of diverse physical complaints that appear to be psychological in origin (Weiten, 1995). These symptoms, however, must not be intentionally feigned or produced (BehaveNet, 2008). For a proper diagnosis, the patient's history of somatic complaints must occur prior to the age of 30, and over a span of several years. A significant impairment, or a history of resulting medical treatment is also necessary. Moreover, a physician must lack any forms of explanation for either his patient's reported symptoms or the severity of his patient's complaints (AllPsychONLINE, 2008).

Some evidence exists for both a genetic and an environmental cause of this disorder. In terms of treatment, long-term therapy is usually helpful. Medications can also treat symptoms related to anxiety or depression. In many cases, the patient will have a complicated medical history, from many different doctors (Weiten, 1995). Accordingly, a continuing and supportive relationship with a single health care provider may be crucial. Regularly scheduled appointments, and the development of coping strategies can also be therapeutically effective (WD, 2008).

Patients who are diagnosed with somatization disorder essentially cling to ill health. They may also exhibit symptoms similar to those observed in either an anxiety disorder or depression (PSYweb.com, 2008). In my opinion, the psychological aspects in this illness could be comparable to a state of paranoia observed within the schizophrenia patient.

Conversion disorder is a third kind of somatoform disorder. Patients with this disorder unintentionally lose voluntary motor or sensory functions. Psychological factors are theorized to cause these deficits, because these symptoms are usually initiated or exacerbated by previous conflicts or stressors (BehaveNet, 2008). Unconscious mental conflicts, or disturbances within the patient's central nervous system are other etiological possibilities. Modes of treatment are aimed towards increasing the patient's coping skills. Improvements in interpersonal and social functioning may also be needed (AllPsychONLINE, 2008).

Theoretically, the adaptation of a sick role within one's social network may provide some form of personal benefit. Sick individuals may receive more attention, sympathy, and assistance from other persons. Assuming a sick role can also enable the individual to avoid problems or other challenges in life. Likewise, an illness can provide the individual with an excuse for failures in life, related to self-esteem (Weiten, 1995).

Substance abuse is another form of mental disorder. A substance is defined as anything that is ingested to produce a high, alter one's senses, or otherwise affect functioning. A psychoactive substance is anything that has an effect on the individual's mental state (Kirby and Keon, 2004). These substances can include illicit drugs like marijuana or heroin, alcohol, toxins, medications, caffeine, and nicotine (AllPsychONLINE, 2008).

The individual has a problem with substance abuse in cases where he adopts a patterned use of a substance, despite knowing the negative consequences that may be associated with such use. For a proper diagnosis, the use of a substance must result in significant problems in work, relationships, physical health, financial well being, and other aspects of a person's life (Kirby and Keon, 2004). The use of a substance during hazardous situations, like driving, may be a second criterion. A third criterion is the surfacing of legal problems that directly results from substance abuse. Patients with this disorder will continue to abuse a substance, even when experiencing significant social or interpersonal problems (AllPsychONLINE, 2008).

Substance dependence is another substance related disorder. This illness is based on a loss of control, and a preoccupation with the continued use of a substance. The patient's dependence may involve physical elements, psychological elements, or both. A physical dependence develops through an increased tolerance, where the patient needs greater amounts of a substance to produce the same effect at a lower dosage. A psychological dependence emerges when the individual perceives an intense need to use a substance, to function effectively within a particular situation (Kirby and Keon, 2004).

A high or severe degree of dependence is defined as an addiction. An addiction is an uncontrollable use of one or more substances, associated with discomfort or distress when that use is discontinued or severely reduced. Some behavioural problems, like compulsive or pathological gambling, may also be classified as a form of addiction. According to many researchers, pathological gambling may progress in stages similar to those in alcoholism (Kirby and Keon, 2004).

Patients suffering from substance dependence will have a history of substance abuse. They may also experience withdrawal symptoms when they discontinue their patterned behaviour of substance abuse (AllPsychONLINE, 2008). The consumption of large amounts of a substance, or the consumption of a substance for a longer time period than intended is also a general symptom. The individual may suffer from either a persistent desire for a substance, or an inability to decrease the quantity of a consumed substance. Patients will also spend great lengths of time to acquire their desired substance. In other cases, the individual will miss important social, occupational, or recreational activities due to substance abuse (BehaveNet, 2008). Depression and other mental or physical health conditions may also arise in patients with this disorder (Mymentalhealth. ca, 2008).

Researchers have discovered evidence that associates genetic factors to both substance related disorders. The use of a substance to cover up or get relief from other problems is another etiological factor. However, in the latter case, the act of self-medicating may be a symptom of another mental disorder (AllPsychONLINE, 2008).

Social support is the most effective method of treatment for individuals with substance abuse problems. Detoxification treatments may be necessary to help patients with dangerous withdrawal symptoms. Special organizations, like Alcoholics Anonymous, are also available. However, both disorders are still quite difficult to treat, and many individuals will enter into a cycle of behaviour between abstinence and the continued use of their desired substance (AllPsychONLINE, 2008).

In a similar fashion, patients with an impulse control disorder will exhibit a failure, or extreme difficulty, when trying to control impulsive forms of behaviours, even if they are faced with negative consequences (AllPsychONLINE, 2008). Impulses are impetuous behaviours that may be harmful to either the individual or other persons. Patients who suffer from this type of disorder will experience an increasing sense of tension or arousal before the act is committed. After the act is committed, the patient will experience feelings of pleasure, gratification, or relief (psychiatryonline, 2008). In some cases, the individual can also experience feelings of regret, self-reproach, or guilt after acting impulsively.

Pathological gambling is an impulse control disorder. These patients will exhibit a persistent and maladaptive pattern of gambling that causes difficulties in interpersonal, financial, and vocational functioning (AllPsychONLINE, 2008). The individual usually becomes overly preoccupied with the act of gambling, and he may be largely unsuccessful when trying to control his habit. He may also become restless or irritable when attempting to minimize or stop his gambling habits, and his need to gamble can increase over time.

The individual mainly uses gambling as an escape from other problems in life. Yet, this essentially creates a new problem after he loses large sums of money. The patient may then be compelled to minimize or even out his material loss. Patients with this illness will lie to other persons about their problem, and they may commit crimes to finance their habit. In other cases, the individual may rely on other persons to relieve his often poor and desperate financial situation (BehaveNet, 2008).

The psychological element of risk has been correlated to the cause of pathological gambling, as opposed to financial gain. Individuals with this disorder may be overly concerned with the approval of other persons, they may be highly competitive, and they may be in a position to adopt other addictive behaviours (AllPsychONLINE, 2008). Social groups, similar to Alcoholics Anonymous, are the main mode of treatment.

Kleptomania is another impulse control disorder. Individuals who suffer from kleptomania have an irresistible urge to steal items that they do not need, and which for the most part have little value. Patients usually know that their actions are morally wrong, and they may experience increased feelings of anxiety, tension, or arousal before committing a theft (MayoClinic.com, 2008). During the crime, these feelings tend to lessen and the individual then experiences a form of relief. Most patients who suffer from kleptomania will experience feelings of intense guilt or remorse after they commit a theft. Nonetheless, they will continue to steal when their impulsive urges return.

Individuals with kleptomania may stash away their stolen items, and these items are rarely used. The items may then be donated, given away, or returned to the place from which they were stolen (MayoClinic.com, 2008). Patients with kleptomania are not motivated by either vengeance or psychosis. These elements, though, can be motivational factors behind other cases of shoplifting.

Scientists have linked depression, anxiety, obsessive-compulsive disorder and other addictive disorders to the cause of kleptomania. Further, the brain chemical serotonin has also been implicated in this illness. Stressful events may trigger an episode of kleptomania. Other risk factors include a brain injury, genetics, or a preoccupation with financial success or material gain (MayoClinic.com, 2008).

Treatments for kleptomania typically involve behavior modification. This is successful when the patient gains insight into the nature of his unconscious psychological processes. CBT, medications, and self-help groups can also effectively treat this illness. Nonetheless, many kleptomaniacs never seek treatment, or they may face incarceration after repeated thefts.

Persons suffering from pyromania experience a similar tension or heightened arousal, prior to the act of setting a deliberate fire. They also experience feelings of gratification or relief after the act is completed. Under this circumstance, the act of setting a fire is not an expression of anger, nor is it motivated by psychosis, monetary gain, or personal gain (AllPsychONLINE, 2008). The patient's motivation usually includes a fascination with, interest in, curiosity about, or attraction to fire, in addition to any related situational contexts (BehaveNet, 2008).

Researchers theorize that an environmental component during childhood may be associated to the cause of pyromania. The treatment and prognosis for patients with this disorder is similar to the treatment and prognosis of patients with kleptomania (AllPsychONLINE, 2008).

Trichotillomania is another form of impulse control disorder. The primary symptom in this illness is a recurrent pulling out of one's own hair, which eventually results in significant hair loss (AllPsychONLINE, 2008). Similar to kleptomania and pyromania, the patient will experience an increasing sense of tension before committing the act, and a sense of pleasure or relief after committing the act. Equally, this disturbance must cause clinically significant distress or impairments in social, occupational, or other areas of functioning for a true diagnosis (BehaveNet, 2008).

This disorder usually develops before adulthood. Behaviour modification can be an effective mode of treatment, along with the exploration of any unconscious issues that may be related to this impulsive act (AllPsychONLINE, 2008).

A developmental disorder is another form of mental illness. These disorders are usually first diagnosed during infancy, childhood, or adolescence. In autistic disorder, the child exhibits a substantial delay in the acquisition of communication skills and basic social interactions. Impairments in communication can include a delay or total lack of development of a spoken language, an inability to initiate or sustain a conversation, a stereotyped and repetitive use of language or idiosyncratic language, and a lack of varied or spontaneous make-believe or social imitative play appropriate to the child's developmental level (BehaveNet, 2008). Children with autism may start to talk at a later age, or they may lose the ability to speak previously learned words or sentences. Further, they may fail to make eye contact with other persons, and they may speak with an abnormal rhythm or tone. (MayoClinic.com, 2008).

Social impairments can include a marked impairment in the use of non-verbal behaviours, a failure to develop peer relationships appropriate to the child's developmental level, a lack of social or emotional reciprocity, and a lack of spontaneous motivation to seek enjoyment, share interests, or share achievements with other persons (BehaveNet, 2008). An autistic child may fail to respond to his name, or appear as if he does not hear other persons. He may resist cuddling and he may seem to be unaware of another person's feelings. Autistic children may further prefer to play alone or they may habitually retreat into their own personal world (MayoClinic.com, 2008).

Other symptoms observed in autism include a restricted and repetitive pattern of behaviour, interests, or activities. These symptoms can involve a preoccupation with a pattern of interest that is abnormal in either intensity or focus. Some examples can include an inflexible adherence to a specific and non-functional routine, a stereotyped and repetitive motor mannerism, or a persistent preoccupation with the parts of objects.

Children with autism will display abnormal or delayed social interactions in the areas of language or imaginative play, prior to the age of three (BehaveNet, 2008). They may also become easily disturbed at the slightest change in routine or rituals. They may further move at a constant pace and be sensitive to sensory phenomena, while simultaneously being insensible to pain (MayoClinic.com, 2008).

In general, children with autism usually have difficulties when trying to share their experiences with other persons. They may be slow when acquiring new knowledge or skills, or they may learn quickly while lacking the ability to communicate. Some children possess exceptional skills within a specific subject matter, like mathematics or artistry. These individuals are known as autistic savants. Other patients function at a high level, with their language skills and intelligence intact (Kirby and Keon, 2004).

Genetic errors are theorized to cause problems in brain development, which then results in a susceptibility to develop autism. Accordingly, a combination of many genetic errors may be related to the cause of autism.

Autistic disorder has also been linked to maternal rubella, untreated phenylketonuria, tuberous sclerosis, anoxia during birth, encephalitis, infantile spasms, and fragile X syndrome. Abnormalities within specific neurotransmitters, through increased dopamine and serotonin levels, have also been consistently observed in autism (WD, 2008). Environmental factors like viral infections and air pollutants are other possible causal elements. Problems during maternal labour and delivery, a defect within the immune system, and possible brain damage within the amygdala could also potentially cause autism (MayoClinic.com, 2008).

Early diagnosis is crucial and has been linked with the best chance for significant improvement in autistic children. Behaviour and communication therapies may address problems with social, language or behavioural skills. Patients with autism also often respond to highly structured educational programs. Some forms of medications are available to treat anxiety or severe behavioural problems. Alternative modes of treatment, like art or music therapy, and special diets may also be effective (MayoClinic.com, 2008).

Asperger's syndrome is a condition that may be categorized within the milder end of the autistic spectrum. It is a developmental disorder that affects the patient's ability to socialize and effectively communicate with other persons. Children with this disorder typically exhibit social awkwardness in many different forms. They may engage in one-sided conversations, or demonstrate an intense obsession with a specific or particular subject matter. They may also speak in a monotonous, rigid, or unusual tone of voice. Children with Asperger's syndrome usually appear as if they are unable to understand, empathize with, or be sensitive to another person's feelings. In social situations, they may lack eye contact, exhibit few facial expressions, or use awkward gestures. Patients can also demonstrate poor coordination skills and exhibit an odd posture or a rigid gait (MayoClinic. com, 2008).

Patients with this disorder will also fail to develop peer-to-peer relationships, and they may further lack an ability to share interests or enjoy experiences with other persons. From a viewer's perspective, these patients can often lack social or emotional reciprocity (BehaveNet, 2008).

Asperger's syndrome may be due to genetic elements and structural abnormalities within several regions of the brain. Treatment options include forms of training in the areas of communication and social skills. CBT can also address problems with interpersonal skills. Although there are no medicines which specifically treat Asperger's syndrome, there are medicines available to treat anxiety, depression, and hyperactivity (MayoClinic.com, 2008).

Previously known as attention deficit disorder (ADD), attention deficit hyperactivity disorder (ADHD) is the most common childhood mental disorder. Even though it interferes with the child's learning processes, this disorder is not technically classified as a learning disorder. ADHD essentially hinders the child's attention span, and this impairs function in a variety of settings, including the academic environment.

Children with ADHD may act impulsively or they may demonstrate difficulties when trying to sustain their attention during specific tasks or activities. Patients may also fail to maintain close attention to details, and they may make careless mistakes (Mymentalhealth.ca, 2008). Other children may not appear to be listening when spoken to, and thus, they may fail to follow instructions. The child may also forget things of importance and exhibit forgetfulness during daily activities.

Within the classroom setting, the child may demonstrate problems while waiting for his turn, he may blurt out answers to questions, or he may interrupt or intrude on other children. The patient can also exhibit problems with organization, and he may dislike activities that require a sustained mental effort (BehaveNet, 2008). Accordingly, the patient can also be very easily distracted.

Hyperactive children will fidget and squirm within the classroom setting. The child can also experience restlessness and leave his classroom seat, or he may act excessively in inappropriate situations. He can also talk excessively and lack the ability to participate quietly during leisure activities (BehaveNet, 2008).

In adults, ADHD is marked by the same core symptoms of distractibility, hyperactivity and impulsive behaviours. However, these elements often manifest themselves differently and far more subtly in adults. For example, adults are more likely to be restless and experience problems with relaxation. Problems with concentration and organization may also be prevalent. Impulsivity, mood swings, intense outbursts of anger, an inability to complete tasks, and an inability to deal with stress are other common symptoms in adult ADHD (MayoClinic.com, 2008).

Concerning possible complications, children with ADHD are at risk of developing a learning disability, an anxiety disorder, depression, oppositional defiant disorder, conduct disorder, or Tourette syndrome. ADHD has also been associated with an increased risk for alcohol abuse, drug abuse, and delinquency. Further, patients with ADHD tend to have more accidents and injuries of all kinds, when compared to the average person (MayoClinic. com, 2008).

It is theorized that genetic components may be causal factors behind ADHD. This is due to the observation that neurotransmitters within the brain behave differently in ADHD. Researchers have further observed less activity in the areas of the brain that control activity and attention. Likewise, scientists have observed that the brains of children with ADHD are approximately 4% smaller than the brain volumes of children without ADHD (MayoClinic. com, 2008).

Maternal smoking and drug use is known to increase a child's risk to develop ADHD. Childhood exposure to toxins, like lead or PCBs, is a further risk factor (MayoClinic.com, 2008).

Effective modes of treatment can include psychotherapy, behaviour therapy, family therapy, social skills training, parental skills training, and specialized support groups. Psychiatrists also often prescribe medications, known as psychostimulants. Antidepressants can address problems related to disturbances, or mood instabilities. According to a large-scale study, younger children are more susceptible to the side effects of these medications. Nevertheless, it also reveals the fact that the use of medications for children is both safe and effective (MayoClinic.com, 2008).

Children with separation anxiety disorder display recurrent and excessive forms of distress when away from home or from those to whom they are emotionally attached. They will hold persistent worries about losing a major attachment figure, either through some harm or through some untold event. Patients may also refuse to go to places, such as school, because of their fears. Affected children may fear to be alone and they may be reluctant to go to sleep when they are not near their attachment figure. Other symptoms include the experiencing of repeated nightmares based on the theme of separation, and repeated complaints of physical ailments when the patient is separated from his attachment figure (BehaveNet, 2008).

Repeated involuntary movements and uncontrollable vocal sounds, or tics, are characteristic symptoms of Tourette syndrome (WD, 2008). Tics are usually sudden, brief and repetitive, and they mainly involve a limited number of muscle groups. Alternatively, complex tics are distinct and coordinated patterns of movement that involve several muscle groups (MayoClinic.com, 2008).

Simple motor tics can include acts such as eye blinking and head jerking. Complex motor tics may include the touching of one's nose or the flapping of one's arms. Hiccupping and throat clearing are two forms of simple vocal tics. Complex vocal tics can include the use of different intonations, and the repetition of words or phrases (MayoClinic.com, 2008). Tics will usually vary in type, frequency and severity over time. They can also worsen over periods of intense stress, and appear during the patient's sleep.

Researchers believe that the cause of Tourette syndrome may be due to a combination of genetic and environmental factors. Tics usually develop when the child experiences a period of overwhelming anxiety (WD, 2008). Infections and head trauma may also be significant etiologically. Dopamine and serotonin chemical abnormalities have also been linked to the cause of this disorder (MayoClinic.com, 2008).

Medications like antipsychotics, antidepressants, stimulants, and central adrenergic inhibitors can help to control or minimize tics. Deep brain stimulation is another effective mode of treatment. Psychotherapy can help patients with their emotional problems, obsessions, anxiety, and depression. Other studies indicate that physical activities and hobbies may reduce the frequency and severity of an individual's tics (MayoClinic.com, 2008).

Patients with a learning disorder will exhibit cognitive abilities that are below expected levels, with respect to their age and grade level (BehaveNet, 2008). A learning disorder will usually be linked to a specific academic field, such as reading, mathematics, or written expression.

Genetic defects and perinatal insults have been associated to the cause of a learning disorder. Subtle disturbances in brain structure and function are also believed to have an etiological role. However, other theorists speculate that learning disorders do not stem from a single or specific cause. Rather, individuals suffering from a learning disorder demonstrate difficulties when connecting information among various regions of the brain (WD, 2008). Stimulants have been known to improve cognition, in the areas of attention and concentration. These medicines can also help children with their impulsive or hyperactive behaviour. At present, though, there are no medications available to treat problems with speech, language, or academia (WD, 2008).

Mental retardation is diagnosed in individuals who have a significantly lower than average level of general intellectual functioning (PSYweb. com, 2008). More specifically, the individual must obtain a score of 70 or lower in a standard intelligence quotient test. The patient must also exhibit deficits in the realm of adaptive functioning. Patients may display impairments in the areas of communication, social skills, academic skills, self-care, self-direction, leisure, employment, home living, and health or safety (BehaveNet, 2008). In addition, the onset of illness must occur before the age of 18 to accurately diagnose an individual with this disorder.

Researchers theorize that predisposing factors, such as deficient prenatal or perinatal care, and inadequate nutrition may be involved in the cause of this illness. A poor social environment or poor child-rearing practices may also be relevant. With respect to treatment, prenatal screening for genetic defects, along with special education and training for children during their infancy can be effective (MedlinePlus, 2008).

A cognitive disorder is a clinical deficit where a significant change from a previous level of functioning occurs (psychiatryonline, 2008). Delirium is a cognitive disorder that mainly affects individuals over the age of 65. It is characterized by a decline in attention, awareness and mental clarity (MayoClinic.com, 2008). Patients with delirium will often exhibit a fluctuating level of consciousness (BehaveNet, 2008). Other symptoms include feelings of restlessness, fear, irritation, and anger. Patients may also be constantly shifting their attention, or they may remain in a state of confusion and disorientation. They can also ramble, speak disruptively, or be extremely forgetful (MayoClinic.com, 2008).

There are three subtypes of delirium. Hyperactive delirium is marked by symptoms of agitation, combativeness, and rapid or loud speech. Hypoactive delirium is characterized by drowsiness, apathy, and little speech or movement. Patients with mixed delirium alternate between quiet and restless states (MayoClinic.com, 2008).

Medications are the most common triggers of delirium. Some examples include pain medications, sleep medications, antipsychotics and antidepressants. Sleep deprivation, low levels of oxygen, constipation, changes in bodily chemistry, and metabolic changes due to blood loss, dehydration, or alcohol withdrawal are other known causes. A change in environment, an infection, a physical disease, and head trauma may be other causal elements (MayoClinic.com, 2008).

Addressing the underlying causes of delirium is the main form of treatment. Therefore, stopping a medication, or treating an infection can effectively address the individual's symptoms. Other possible triggers such as the use of restraints, frequent room changes, loud noises, poor lighting, and a lack of natural light can also be addressed. The symptom of disorganized thinking can sometimes be treated through antipsychotic medications. Supportive care within a family or hospital setting may also be necessary (MayoClinic.com, 2008).

Symptoms observed in delirium and other forms of mental illness include disruptions in sleep, anxiety, and the experiencing of hallucinations. A quarter of patients with delirium will also experience problems with memory, attention, and other forms of cognition. The patient's length of delirium can last from several hours to several years. However, scientists have correlated this illness with increasingly poor health and impending death (MayoClinic.com, 2008).

Dementia, on the other hand, is an illness that is characterized by symptoms that are commonly observed in delirium. Delirium can sometimes mark the onset of dementia. Contrarily, two-thirds of persons who develop delirium will already suffer from dementia. These patients will often experience a dramatic drop in their cognitive functioning. Nonetheless, dementia develops more slowly than delirium, and delirium is, for the most part, a temporary condition (MayoClinic.com, 2008).

Dementia involves the deterioration of mental, behavioural and emotional functioning. A loss in mental capacity is usually accompanied by personality or behavioural changes. On a positive note, some forms of dementia are reversible (PSYweb.com, 2008).

Technically classified as a degenerative disorder, Alzheimer's disease is the most common cause of dementia. Patients with this disorder will suffer from a loss of intellectual and social abilities, that are severe enough to interfere with daily functioning. In Alzheimer's disease, the patient's healthy brain tissue will degenerate. A steady decline in memory and other mental capacities will then result. Most patients who suffer from this illness are 65 years of age or older (MayoClinic.com, 2008).

During the preliminary stages, Alzheimer's disease usually causes slight memory loss and a state of confusion. It eventually leads to extensive impairments in the areas of reason, memory, imagination, and learning ability. Patients will usually exhibit increasing and persistent forgetfulness. They may experience difficulties with abstract thinking, and they may enter into a constant state of disorientation. Patients can also experience greater difficulties with acts that require planning, decision-making, or judgment (MayoClinic.com, 2008). Eventually, they will experience difficulties when performing routine or familiar tasks. Communication, reading, and writing skills will further diminish in the patient. In some instances, the patient may exhibit changes in personality, as the disease progresses. These personality changes can take place in the form of a mood swing, stubbornness, mistrust, or social withdrawal.

In Alzheimer's disease, neurons among certain regions of the brain begin to expire. This results in a lower production of neurotransmitters, which eventually leads to signalling problems within the brain. Researchers theorize that alterations within specific proteins, genetic mutations, or an inflammation within the brain may also be linked to the cause of this disorder. Other etiological theories for Alzheimer's disease include a combination of factors like an infection, reduced circulation, and a genetic susceptibility (MayoClinic.com, 2008). Overexposure to toxic substances or a severe physical head injury may also be linked to the cause of this illness.

At present, there is no cure for Alzheimer's disease. Nonetheless, some medications may effectively delay its onset. These medicines work either by improving levels of neurotransmitters within the brain, or by protecting brain cell damage from the chemical messenger glutamate (MayoClinic. com, 2008). Patients with Alzheimer's disease can also suffer from depression, anxiety, and restlessness.

Huntington's disease is another progressive illness that causes certain nerve cells in the brain to waste away. General symptoms usually develop during mid-adulthood, though children can also develop this illness. During the early stages of development, patients with Huntington's disease can exhibit personality changes and a decrease in their cognitive abilities. They can also demonstrate problems when remembering information, answering questions, or in general learning (MayoClinic.com, 2008).

Early physical symptoms in this illness include problems with balance, clumsiness, involuntary facial movements, and seizures. The progressive symptoms of this illness include slurred speech, severe problems with balance and coordination, and sudden, jerky, or involuntary movements. Some patients also exhibit difficulties with swallowing or in the shifting of their gaze (MayoClinic.com, 2008).

An abnormal gene has been linked to the cause of Huntington's disease. Researchers have also discovered that a protein, which is expressed by this gene, may interact with another protein, which thereby disturbs the accumulation of cholesterol within the brain. This then disrupts the individual's motor, cognitive, and language skills. The patient may have inherited this gene from one of his parents, or the gene may have evolved through a genetic mutation. Moreover, every individual who possesses this gene will eventually develop Huntington's disease (MayoClinic.com, 2008).

The symptoms in this illness will continue to develop until death. Patients with this illness can also develop problems with anger, irritability, and depression. Medications cannot stop nor reverse this illness, though they may be effective in controlling symptoms. Speech, physical, and occupational modes of therapy are also available. Regular exercise, and maintaining a proper nutritional diet can also help patients improve both mentally and physically (MayoClinic.com, 2008).

Patients with Parkinson's disease can also develop dementia. Parkinson's disease develops gradually within the patient, usually during middle or late life. It often starts as a minor tremor in one hand. In time, the individual will suffer from muscular rigidity or stiffness, an impaired posture, and a reduced ability to initiate voluntary movements. Patients can also lose automatic movements, such as blinking and smiling. Problems like hesitating before the act of speaking, speaking in a monotone, and the slurring or repetition of words are further symptoms of this disorder (MayoClinic.com, 2008).

Etiological theories for Parkinson's disease include genetic mutations and environmental toxins. Many symptoms in this illness may also be due to a lack of dopamine within the brain (MayoClinic.com, 2008). In fact, abnormal dopamine levels are theorized to be involved in many other mental disorders, including schizophrenia. As a result, patients with Parkinson's disease can develop widespread symptoms like depression, problems with sleep, and sexual dysfunction.

Treatment for Parkinson's disease involves many forms of medications. Levodopa, dopamine agonists, MAO B inhibitors, catechol o-methyltransferase (COMT) inhibitors, anticholinergics, and antivirals are used to control specific symptoms in this illness. Physical therapists can aid patients with their range of motion. Speech therapists, on the other hand, can improve problems with speaking and swallowing. For patients who suffer from an advanced form of this disease, surgery by way of deep brain stimulation is also an available mode of treatment (MayoClinic.com, 2008).

Sleep disorders form another category of mental illness. Dyssomnias are related to the amount, quality or timing of sleep. Parasomnias are related to the abnormal behaviours, or physiological events that occur during the sleep process or during sleep-wake transitions (AllPsychONLINE, 2008).

Approximately 10% of adults and 25% of elderly persons suffer from primary insomnia (AllPsychONLINE, 2008). Difficulties with falling asleep and maintaining restorative sleep are the main symptoms in this illness. Patients will face these problems on a regular or frequent basis, and for no apparent reason (MayoClinic.com, 2008). The individual may also experience symptoms of daytime fatigue or irritability due to a lack of sleep. Fatigue can further lead to a diminished mental alertness and poor concentration. Likewise, a lack of sleep can have negative effects on the individual's mood and immune system.

Possible causes of insomnia can include anxiety, depression, the use of stimulants, or the long-term use of sleep medications. Stress, changes in one's environment or work schedule, and painful medical conditions may also be causal factors. Individuals that worry, or those who try too hard to fall asleep can also experience bouts of insomnia. A form of conditioning can further affect individuals who find it difficult to sleep within their bedrooms (AllPsychONLINE, 2008). In other cases, individuals who eat too much, or those who eat too late in the evening may suffer from insomnia. In elderly patients, changes in sleep patterns, daily activities, or their physical health can also cause insomnia (MayoClinic.com, 2008).

Treatments for insomnia include behavioural therapies, and sleep medications. Self-help techniques like exercise, avoiding caffeine, limiting naps, eating healthy foods, keeping a predetermined sleep cycle, and the act of resetting one's bodily clock may also be effective (MayoClinic.com, 2008).

Patients who suffer from chronic insomnia are at risk to develop other psychiatric illnesses, like depression or an anxiety disorder. Long-term sleep deprivation can further increase the severity of other conditions, like diabetes or high blood pressure. Thus, insomnia is often an etiological factor in other illnesses (MayoClinic.com, 2008).

On the other side of the spectrum, primary hypersomnia is diagnosed when the patient experiences excessive sleepiness, either during the night or during the day. In some cases, the patient may need daytime naps even after having completed 12 hours of uninterrupted sleep. In addition, individuals with hypersomnia may enter into a state of confusion when awakened (WD, 2008). In order to be diagnosed with hypersomnia, these symptoms must persist for a period of at least one month, and they must cause significant distress in the individual's life. Up to 5% of the population will suffer from hypersomnia at some point in their life (AllPsychONLINE, 2008).

Although there are many causes of hypersomnia, sleep disruptions during the night that cause a reduction in rapid eye movement (REM) sleep may be most significant. Periodic limb movements and restless leg syndrome are other possible causes (WD, 2008). Modes of treatment can include medicines, exercise, and a change in one's diet. When the symptoms of this illness are linked with other medical conditions, like depression, they will often dissipate when the associated illness improves (AllPsychONLINE, 2008).

Narcolepsy is a sleep disorder that affects the individual's control over sleep and wakefulness. Patients can become extremely drowsy during the day and fall into a deep sleep, even when they have completed an adequate period of nighttime sleep. Accordingly, individuals with narcolepsy experience REM intrusions while awake, which results in half-sleep dreams or temporary paralysis.

After the individual takes a nap, his feelings of drowsiness will usually return and another cycle of REM intrusion may reoccur. Narcolepsy can also cause fragmented or frequent awakenings during nighttime sleep (WD, 2008). A brief episode of a sudden bilateral loss of muscle tone, known as cataplexy, or an REM intrusion must occur in a wakened individual to correctly diagnose him with this illness (BehaveNet, 2008).

The true cause of narcolepsy is currently unknown. A malfunction in the individual's immune system may be a possible cause. Genetics may also be relevant. Modes of treatment can include medications like central nervous system stimulants and amphetamines (WD, 2008).

Sleep apnea is a disorder where the patient suffers from a temporary cessation of breathing during sleep (WD, 2008). Actually, many individuals are unaware of the fact that they suffer from sleep apnea. Obstructive apnea and central sleep apnea are the main forms of this disorder. In obstructive sleep apnea, the individual's throat muscles will shift into a relaxed state. In central sleep apnea, the individual's brain will fail to send signals to the specific muscles that control breathing. Complex sleep apnea is a combination of obstructive and central sleep apnea (MayoClinic.com, 2008).

Common symptoms in sleep apnea include hypersomnia, insomnia and loud snoring. Abrupt awakenings with dry mouth, sore throat, shortness of breath, or morning headaches are other symptoms (MayoClinic.com, 2008).

Upper airway obstructions can cause obstructive sleep apnea. Risk factors include obesity, a large neck circumference, a narrowed airway, and hypertension. A family history of obstructive sleep apnea, the use of alcohol or sedatives, and smoking are further risk factors (MayoClinic.com, 2008). Heart disease and strokes are theorized to be both causes of and risk factors for central sleep apnea.

Treatments for obstructive sleep apnea include the use of machines, which aids the patient with nighttime breathing. Continuous positive airway pressure therapy, or the use of adjustable airway pressure devices or oral appliances are other modes of treatment. Surgery can further remove any excess tissue that blocks the upper air passages within the patient's nose and throat (MayoClinic.com, 2008).

Special devices are also used in the treatment of central and complex sleep apnea. The addition of supplemental oxygen during sleep, and medical care for any associated health problems are other forms of treatment. Self-care strategies, like sleeping on one's side or abdomen, and the use of nasal sprays can also effectively treat central sleep apnea (MayoClinic.com, 2008).

Sleepwalking disorder, or somnambulism, is classified under the parasomnia subgroup. This illness is characterized by the repeated episodes of rising from bed during sleep, where the individual ends up walking about. During a sleepwalk, the individual will usually have a blank or staring face, and he will be relatively unresponsive to other persons. When the patient awakens, he can experience a short period of confusion or disorientation, and in some cases, he may retain no memory of his sleepwalking episode (BehaveNet, 2008).

Individuals who sleepwalk can roam within their entire house, while opening and closing doors, or turning lights on and off. They may also perform routine activities, like getting dressed or making a snack. Patients may further move or speak in a clumsy manner (MayoClinic.com, 2008). Some sleepwalking episodes last for a few seconds, while other instances can last for over 30 minutes.

Factors like fatigue, stress, anxiety and fever may be related to the cause of sleepwalking. Health conditions like abnormal heart rhythms, gastroesophageal reflux, seizures, sleep apnea, panic attacks, and post-traumatic stress disorder can also cause sleepwalking. The use of alcohol or medicines like antibiotics, sedatives, or sleeping pills can also trigger a sleepwalking episode (MayoClinic.com, 2008).

The act of sleepwalking is not necessarily a serious concern, from a medical standpoint. However, this act can become dangerous if the sleepwalker goes outdoors and performs actions like driving a car. Prolonged sleep disruptions, caused by sleepwalking, can also lead to daytime sleepiness and impairments in social or other areas of functioning (BehaveNet, 2008).

Treatments can include the short-term use of benzodiazepines or antidepressants (MayoClinic.com, 2008). Engaging in relaxing activities before bedtime, or getting more sleep can also help patients with this disorder.

In nightmare disorder, the individual will experience repeated awakenings from long periods of sleep or naps, due to exceedingly frightening dreams. He usually wakes with a detailed recollection of his nightmare, which typically involves threats to his survival, security, or self-esteem (BehaveNet, 2008). A single nightmare may also repeat on multiple nights. After awakening from a nightmare, the individual will usually be rapidly oriented and alert.

Many factors can trigger nightmares. Stress, illness or a traumatic event are some causes. Viewing scary works of art like books or movies, eating bedtime snacks, and some forms of medications can also trigger a nightmare (MayoClinic.com, 2008). The individual should seek treatment when his nightmares become frequent and disrupt his sleep patterns on a regular basis. Nightmares that lead to dangerous behaviours are further symptoms in this disorder.

Treatments for nightmare disorder are usually focused on the underlying causes of the individual's nightmare, such as stress or anxiety. Though rarely used, medications that suppress or reduce REM sleep are also available under some circumstances (MayoClinic.com, 2008).

On a general note, the individual's sleep disturbance must not be due to the direct physiological effects of a substance, like a narcotic or medication, or some form of medical condition (BehaveNet, 2008). Many patients with schizophrenia or depression will suffer from bouts of insomnia. However, the individual must suffer from a sleep disruption exclusively, and not during the course of another disorder, to be properly diagnosed with a sleep disorder.

An eating disorder is another class of mental illness. Affecting mostly women, an eating disorder is marked by extreme emotions, attitudes and behaviours involving weight and food (WebMD, 2008). Approximately ten to twenty percent of patients will die from the effects of an eating disorder. Accordingly, this is the highest mortality rate among all forms of mental illness. In Canada, 3% of women and 0.3% of men will suffer from some form of eating disorder within their lifetime (Mood Disorders Society of Canada, 2008).

Anorexia nervosa is an eating disorder where drastic weight loss occurs through fasting, and in some cases, excessive exercise. Intense fears related to gaining weight or becoming fat are the underlying issues behind this illness. Patients suffering from anorexia nervosa will have a body weight that is typically less than 85% of the healthy expected average weight, based on the age and height of the individual. In some instances, the individual may view himself to be overweight, even when he is actually dangerously underweight and grossly thin. In other cases, the individual may acknowledge that he is underweight, while denying the seriousness of his problem.

Patients with this illness are extremely unhappy with their body weight and shape, and they tend to evaluate themselves solely through these characteristics (Kirby and Keon, 2004). As a consequence, the patient will adopt strange eating habits to control his weight, like eating in small quantities or avoiding meals (Mymentalhealth.ca, 2008). In the end, persistent starvation can have vast effects on organ function, which could ultimately lead to death (Mental Illness Awareness Week, 2008). Ailments like kidney failure, an electrolyte imbalance, and problematic heart conditions can also arise in patients with this eating disorder (Public Health Agency of Canada, 2008). Other symptoms due to malnutrition include dehydration, a decreased metabolic rate, an irregular heartbeat, and shortness of breath.

According to some researchers, patients with anorexia feel powerful and in control when losing weight. When the individual wants to block out troubling feelings or emotions, weight loss is often viewed as the easiest method to accomplish this task. Patients for the most part have low self-esteem, and they may hold the belief that they do not deserve to eat. Some patients may frequently check their body weight, and strongly deny that they are ever hungry. Likewise, many patients resist therapy because they view these interventions solely as measures that will force them to eat.

Bulimia nervosa is an illness where the individual repeatedly engages in the act of binge eating, while subsequently utilizing compensatory methods to prevent weight gain. These compensatory methods can include self-induced vomiting, fasting, an extreme exercise program, laxative abuse, and the use of diuretics or diet pills (Eating Disorders, 2008). As in anorexia nervosa, patients with bulimia nervosa place excessive importance on their body shape and weight. However, most bulimia patients are healthy, in terms of body weight.

Bulimia patients also have problems with self-esteem and self worth. They may strive towards the approval of others, and they may view food as their only source of comfort. Other symptoms can include weight fluctuations at an average of 15 pounds, mood swings, severe self-criticism, the avoidance of social events, and the fear that one cannot stop eating voluntarily. Health complications can include malnutrition, and damage to the esophagus, mouth, and teeth due to the repeated exposure to acidic vomit (Mental Illness Awareness Week, 2008). Additionally, most bulimia patients realize that they are suffering from an eating disorder (Eating Disorders, 2008).

Binge eating disorder (BED) is characterized by the episodic uncontrolled consumption of food, without the compensatory activities observed in bulimia nervosa (Kirby and Keon, 2004). The act of overeating often takes place in secret and is usually carried out as a means of deriving comfort. The eating of excessive amounts of food, and a lack of control during this act typically marks an episode of binge eating.

Patients suffering from BED are compelled to eat more rapidly than normal, eat until uncomfortably full, eat large amounts of food when not hungry, and eat in isolation to avoid feelings of embarrassment. Feelings of shame, disgust, depression, and guilt after episodes of overeating are other diagnostic criteria (Mymentalhealth.ca, 2008). Further symptoms can include low self-esteem, anxiety, fluctuations in weight gain, and the active avoidance of social situations where food will be present (Eating Disorders, 2008). Patients may also suffer from a form of marked distress related to their eating behaviours, and they may be obese or overweight.

With respect to the causes of binge eating, patients may essentially use food as a way of blocking out troubling feelings or emotions. Excessive eating can also be used as a means to numb oneself, fill a personal void, or as a way to cope with daily stressors. The health complications associated with binge eating include obesity, diabetes, high blood pressure, high cholesterol, osteoarthritis, cardiac arrest, decreased mobility, heart disease, and liver or kidney problems (Eating Disorders, 2008).

Eating disorders, in general, are theorized to be caused by biological elements, personal factors, and the promotion of a thin body image within the individual's society. With respect to the latter two factors, eating disorders can sometimes be adopted to cope with problems in life (Mymentalhealth. ca, 2008). Researchers believe that most eating disorders will begin as unhealthy eating patterns, that later develop into compulsive actions and behaviours (Public Health Agency of Canada, 2008).

Nutritional stabilization is the primary mode of treatment for all eating disorders. When the patient regains a healthy lifestyle, psychotherapy can serve as a further mode of treatment. Family counselling, education, body image therapy and CBT are some common forms of psychotherapy. Antidepressants have been effective in the treatment of bulimia nervosa, and likewise, other medicines have been useful in treating BED. Hospitalization for patients with anorexia nervosa may be necessary, to treat metabolic complications (Public Health Agency of Canada, 2008).

From my point of view, the principle of denial that most anorexics have, with respect to the seriousness of their disease, could be comparable to the state of denial that I entered into when Dr. Lupton first diagnosed me with schizophrenia. Likewise, the compensatory methods utilized by patients with bulimia could be comparable to my experiences with social withdrawal. Furthermore, the marked distress, exhibited by patients with binge eating disorder, could be comparable to the feelings of anxiety experienced by patients with other forms of mental disorders. The fact that all eating disorders arise as a coping strategy to deal with psychological problems may also be similar to the act of self-medicating oneself. Low self-esteem, depression, fatigue, insomnia and irritability are also common symptoms observed in eating disorders and other forms of mental illness.

Elements such as our society's definition of beauty, and the individual's consequent negative self-image, are significant etiological factors in most eating disorders. In my opinion, it is possible that similar variable psychosocial elements may also be etiologically significant in other mental disorders. In fact, psychosocial elements, like our society's definition of beauty, are liable to change. This demonstrates the possibility that we can effectively address deep psychological problems through changes in our society. The cultural stigmas that exist against mental illnesses can also vary and be subject to change. Accordingly, if certain psychosocial elements in our society were to be addressed, this could directly minimize many of the psychological problems that surface in patients with mental illness. Therefore, a further possible mode of treatment can transpire when every individual in our society realizes the values of acceptance, tolerance and diversity.

Now that we know what schizophrenia is not, let us examine its true effects on the individual's mental processes. Schizophrenia is a thought disorder. Individuals that suffer from a thought disorder will experience distortions in their awareness and thinking. Moreover, rational thinking and judgment may be severely impaired. Delusions and hallucinations are the most prevalent symptoms observed in schizophrenia and other thought disorders.

Schizophreniform disorder has a diagnostically similar criterion to schizophrenia. However, patients who suffer from this disorder will experience schizophrenic symptoms for a period of less than six months. Patients who exhibit these symptoms, for a period of less than one month, are technically diagnosed with brief psychotic disorder (Torrey, 1995).

Biological components are theorized to be relevant etiological factors in schizophreniform disorder. Medications are available to treat both psychotic and affective symptoms. Psychotherapy can also improve the patient's well-being (AllPsychONLINE, 2008).

Individuals suffering from delusional disorder exhibit non-bizarre delusions that could be true, even though they are greatly exaggerated. For example, the individual may believe that he is being followed, conspired against, or loved by someone at a great distance (AllPsychONLINE, 2008). Delusional disorder can be further classified into six subtypes. The erotomanic subtype is based on the delusion that some one of a higher status is in love with him. Patients who are diagnosed with the grandiose subtype have delusions of inflated self worth, power or identity. The delusion that one's sexual partner is unfaithful may be categorized into the jealous subtype. In the persecutory subtype, the patient believes that either he or a loved one is being oppressed in some manner. The somatic subtype involves the false delusion that one is suffering from some type of medical condition. Lastly, the mixed subtype is characterized by more than one of the previous subtypes, with no predominant theme (BehaveNet, 2008).

Some researchers theorize that the cause of delusional disorder may be due to a combination of biological and hereditary factors. Severe stress and childhood experiences within an authoritarian family structure are other possible etiological factors. Medical conditions such as a head injury or chronic alcoholism, in conjunction with aging, may also increase the individual's risk to develop delusional disorder. Predisposing factors linked to aging can include isolation, a lack of stimulating interpersonal relationships, a physical illness, and impaired hearing or vision (WD, 2008).

Medications are the main mode of treatment for delusional disorder. However, many patients will refuse treatment because they believe that they are functioning normally in all other respects. The patient's belief that his delusions are real can also affect his compliance during the treatment process (AllPsychONLINE, 2008).

In shared psychotic disorder, the individual develops a delusion that is similar in content to that of another person, who already has the established delusion. The patient will usually have a close relationship with this other person (BehaveNet, 2008). At present, the cause of this disorder is not well understood. Researchers theorize that the best mode of treatment may take form in a separation from the other individual (AllPsychONLINE, 2008).

From my perspective, the term split mind can equally describe other mental disorders beyond schizophrenia. All mental disorders involve an alteration in the individual's thinking, mood, or behaviour. The fact that many mental disorders share common symptoms seems to imply the possibility that they may be caused by similar physical defects within the brain. By definition, a mental illness will impair the individual's ability to function in areas of everyday life. As a result, the mind of any individual who develops a mental disorder may be disunited in one respect or another.

Approximately 20% of the Canadian population will directly suffer from a mental disease, during the course of their lifetime. An exponentially larger portion of the population will have an indirect experience with a mental illness, either through a family member, friend, or associate. It is common sense that mental disorders, and every other form of illness for that matter, may be diagnosed in persons of all ages, ethnicities, and income levels. Mental disorders are generally caused through a complex combination of genetic, biological, personality, and environmental elements (Public Health Agency of Canada, 2008).

Equally, every mentally healthy individual will experience feelings of isolation, loneliness, and emotional distress. Patients who are diagnosed with a mental disorder are different in that they suffer from a more radical form of these psychological problems. Subsequently, mental disorders may be more natural than many persons are willing to accept.

Mental health has also been scientifically correlated to physical health. For example, persons suffering from a mental illness can experience problems with heart disease, biochemical imbalances, reductions in immune system efficiency, gastrointestinal problems, and weight gain or loss (Health Canada, 2008). In contrast, persons with physical health problems can develop a form of anxiety or depression. In Canada, mental illnesses account for approximately 40% of all forms of disability. Therefore, the rate of mental disabilities may be more or less equivalent to the rate of physical disabilities in my nation.

In addition, some individuals who are affected by a mental illness may go on to develop another form of mental illness. For instance, a patient suffering from depression may go on to develop an anxiety disorder because of his mood. Likewise, an individual that suffers from schizophrenia may develop a substance abuse disorder because of his delusional frame of mind (Public Health Agency of Canada, 2008). This would seem to indicate that there may be a causal relationship between some mental disorders. It could also imply the possibility that some mental disorders may share similar etiological components. Hence, it is possible that a single mechanism within the brain may produce symptoms that are consistently observed among several different categories of mental disorders.

Problems with substance abuse may pose a significant problem for many individuals who are later diagnosed with a mental disorder. Likewise, there is also a considerable risk of suicide among individuals that suffer from a mental illness. However, both problems essentially stem through societal stigmas. It is true that all persons who suffer from a mental illness will face an uncertain future, with respect to their health and quality of life. They may also believe that they are, or will become, a burden to either their family or community at large. In my opinion, this feeling of burden is due directly to social stigmas. If we are able to eliminate this concept of burden, many patients will have less reason to abuse a substance or contemplate suicide. Likewise, patients should be able to better focus on improving their mental health as a direct result.

Educating the public on the subject of mental illnesses should eventually solve the problem of societal stigmas. Stigmas usually arise through old belief systems, a lack of knowledge and empathy, superstition, and the tendency to fear and exclude persons who are perceived as different (Public Health Agency of Canada, 2008). Patients will react to societal stigmas through feelings of fear, embarrassment, anger, or avoidance. The patient may also consequently enter into a state of denial. Patients then become isolated from the rest of their community, and this further complicates their treatment process.

Government interventions can help address the problem of societal stigmas. Personally, I have faced discrimination during my search for employment. For one thing, I did not disclose the fact that I suffer from a mental illness to any potential employers, because of the existence of social stigmas. This, in turn, affected my ability to be fully honest during the interview stage. Likewise, I was ill for a period of over three years, and was therefore unable to account for this period on my resume. While applying for employment within the public sector, I was also subject to both direct and indirect discrimination due to my illness. I was directly dismissed as a possible applicant at least on one occasion, and I have been dismissed indirectly on other occasions, because of problems with my illness.

The fact that I need to lie about my mental health seems to imply the notion that at least some form of intolerance against mental illness exists, within my community. In addition, the high standards associated with gaining competitive employment may exclude most patients from the interview process, if they were to reveal the true nature of their mental health. The low employment rate of persons with schizophrenia also seems to indicate that some form of discrimination exists within my society. According to Statistics Canada, in 2006, the employment rate for persons with disabilities was at 53.5%, while the employment rate for persons without a disability was at 75.1% (Statistics Canada, 2008).

Persons who are employed may also face workplace discrimination, if they are later diagnosed with a mental disorder. If the individual's employer subscribes to societal stigmas, then acts of prejudice will most likely result. It is possible that the individual will be disregarded for possible promotions, face a demotion, lose desirable working- shifts, or even be fired due to his mental health. Therefore, I believe that societal stigmas will provide some employers with a justifiable reason to discriminate against any individuals that suffer from a mental illness.

In Canada, every person is equal under the rule of law. Therefore, the schizophrenia patient's basic right for equality is violated when he is not granted an equal opportunity, with respect to gaining potential forms of employment. However, the solution to this problem may be quite complex. Governmental institutions cannot obligate individuals, within the private sector, to obey principles based on an equal opportunity. Laws of this nature would be difficult to enforce. Yet, I believe that a responsible government can address and eliminate much of the discrimination that exists against the mentally sick.

To accomplish this, a nation's governing body itself should not endorse any forms of special treatment. From my experience, persons with a mental disability are not treated equally on a universal basis. Some patients are granted financial support to continue their education, while others are not. Furthermore, some forms of employment within the public sector only consider individuals who are members of a visible minority group. Thus, the governing body in my nation is utilizing the principle of affirmative action to address social inequality. However, the principle of affirmative action is essentially a form of reverse discrimination (Stanford University, 2008). In effect, by utilizing this principle, my government is discriminating against persons who are not members of a visible minority. Accordingly, while a just government may believe that it is addressing the problem of discrimination through affirmative action, it may be reinforcing the concept of discrimination as a secondary effect.

On the contrary, I do not hold the belief that any employer should hire persons that are unqualified, with respect to an available employment opportunity. What I am saying is that some patients with a mental illness are not considered for positions, even when they are fully qualified. An individual should not be dismissed as a possible applicant, solely because he suffers from schizophrenia. To solve this problem, a top-down basis of reform, with respect to the implementation of ethical social principles, must be endorsed, and this will ultimately build a non-discriminating society. I believe that the onus is on governmental bodies across the world to ensure that all of its citizens are given a fair and equal opportunity, whether they are affected by a mental illness, a physical illness, or if they have perfect health.

Not all persons, who suffer from a mental illness, will qualify for a government grant to complete their education. This is a form of discrimination in itself. I do appreciate the governmental aid that helped me to complete my university studies. Nonetheless, other schizophrenia patients in my nation will not be approved for a similar mode of support, and this troubles me. A society can only properly address the element of discrimination, if its governing body treats every citizen on an equal basis. Therefore, from my perspective, government aid for post-secondary studies should be available for all persons with a disability, whether it is mental or physical. The fact that I was given special treatment reflects on a form of injustice based on the absence of an equal opportunity, which is a fundamental principle among all democratic nations. A form of negative precedence may then be set. In my opinion, this inequity essentially legitimizes the act of discriminating against persons who may be less functional comparatively.

Lower levels of formal education have been positively associated with low socio-economic status. Poverty has also been correlated to unemployment and mental illness, and it further increases the individual's risk of exposure to chronic or traumatic stress. Thus, mental illness seems to be a barrier that prevents the patient from succeeding in a complex post-industrial society (Public Health Agency of Canada, 2008). As a consequence, many individuals that are diagnosed with a mental illness will be stuck in an endless cycle of poverty both prior to, and after their diagnosis.

Suicide is another significant social problem associated with mental illness. In Canada, 40% of schizophrenia patients will attempt to commit suicide, and 25% of these individuals will actually succeed (schizophrenia. com, 2008). Patients who consider suicide will experience feelings of extreme hopelessness, helplessness, and desperation. These symptoms are habitually observed in depression. Primarily, the patient may believe that he has lost the ability to live an independent way of life, due to his illness. He may also believe that he will become fully dependent on a third party, for his everyday living. Many individuals would find this loss in personal autonomy extremely difficult to accept.

When an individual loses his independence, feelings of hopelessness and desperation may then arise. The patient may suffer from further depressive symptoms like sleeplessness, social withdrawal, or a loss of appetite. The patient can also lose interest in any enjoyable activities, or he may act recklessly. In some cases, the patient will express feelings related to death or dying to another person. Sudden plans or preparations for death, like the act of applying for life insurance, are other possible warning signs (Mymentalhealth.ca, 2008).

The specific factors related to suicide will vary among differing subgroups within a mixed society. For example, men usually express their despair through fatal acts, like the use of a firearm or through hanging. In contrast, women will usually choose less lethal acts, like a drug overdose, where their resuscitation is possible (Public Health Agency of Canada, 2008). Youth suicides are usually impulsive and revolve around developmental stress. Problematic issues within social or educational spheres, in conjunction with a particular vulnerability to commit suicide may contribute towards a higher risk of suicide within this subgroup. A loss of social relationships increases the risk of suicide among seniors. Death and mortality associated with themselves, or their loved ones can cause suicidal thoughts within this subgroup as well.

The reasons behind suicidal behaviour can be complex. Predisposing factors may create a vulnerability to commit suicide within an individual. Examples of these factors include a mental illness, abuse, or the loss of a loved one. Precipitating factors are crises in life such as interpersonal conflicts, financial difficulties, and social rejection. Contributing factors, moreover, increases the exposure of the individual to either predisposing or precipitating factors. Such factors can include a physical illness, isolation, or substance abuse. In contrast, protective factors may decrease the individual's risk to commit suicide. Personal resilience, adaptive coping skills, and a positive attitude can sometimes counteract suicidal ideations (Public Health Agency of Canada, 2008). In some cases, an attempt to commit suicide may be mediated by a combination of elements among all four subcategories.

At times, the causal elements behind the act of suicide may be common among the subject's peers. Therefore, many persons who do not attempt to commit suicide may experience similar and equally distressing social problems. Accordingly, we should examine what differentiates a suicidal individual from his non-suicidal peer. The answer to this question may surface in differences among the individual's predisposing, precipitating, contributing, and protective factors.

Actually, most persons have thought about the concept of suicide, at one point in their lives. Similarly, when an individual commits suicide, this is rarely a sudden event. It usually results after a process of reckless deliberation.

Individuals, who are diagnosed with a mental disorder, will develop predisposing factors, in relation to suicide, throughout their entire lifetime. Likewise, because of their illness, they may also lack an ability to develop protective factors. Conversely, their mentally healthy peer will never face this predisposition. Similarly, a mentally healthy peer should also have a greater ability to build protective factors, during the course of his lifetime.

Individuals will usually have no power over any forms of predisposing factors. These elements occur beyond the individual's realm of control. Accordingly, one solution to the problem of suicide may be found in the development of protective factors. Providing mentally ill persons hope for a prosperous future should be effective on a universal basis. Educational or employment options can provide the patient with this form of hope. Reducing the patient's personal stressors, related to daily living, can be a further effective measure. The patient will be able to adopt a more positive lifestyle, if he does not have to worry about everyday problems like food, shelter, or poverty.

Research indicates that 90% of suicide victims have a diagnosable mental illness or substance use disorder (Kirby and Keon, 2004). Nevertheless, this figure does not include sick individuals who never sought medical attention for their psychological problems. This latter group of individuals may be in the developmental stages of a mental illness, and accordingly, they may be exhibiting a milder form of symptoms. If this is true, perhaps an even higher percentage of suicide victims are persons who suffer from some type of mental disorder.

According to the World Health Organization, suicide is the leading cause of violent deaths worldwide, over homicide and war-related deaths (Kirby and Keon, 2004). Subsequently, much of the world's population may underestimate the impact of mental illnesses on their society.

In many cases, the patient will not seek medical help when he first experiences problematic symptoms. Therefore, a third party's ability to recognize the warning signs of a mental illness can aid in the patient's preliminary treatment process. Educating the public on the subject of mental illness warning signs is necessary for this to occur. Likewise, alleviating any fears in relation to discrimination, or negative stereotyping can also motivate the individual to seek immediate help when he first experiences questionable symptoms. These are examples of some of the actions that an entire community can undertake, which will further facilitate the modes of treatment that mentally ill persons desperately need.

In summation, the term split mind may be a bit misleading for any individuals who lack knowledge of mental illnesses in general. A good question would be to ask if the term Split mind truly describes what we know about schizophrenia, as a disease itself. I would have to answer yes. Schizophrenia causes the individual to have a divided perception of the actual world.

Nevertheless, the term split mind could also potentially describe many other forms of mental illness. Patients who suffer from dissociative identity disorder will demonstrate characteristics belonging to more than one identity. Bipolar disorder causes the individual to experience extremes on both ends of the emotional spectrum. Individuals that suffer from anorexia nervosa will hold an extremely distorted self-perception. In a factitious disorder, the patient will seek help that he truly does not need. Researchers have also recently drawn a relation between autism and schizophrenia, in that both illnesses are polar opposites of one another (Meadahl, 2009). Therefore, different forms of mental illnesses may be associated to the concept of a split mind, through many different respects.

6

Diagnosing Schizophrenia

It is estimated that 1% of persons in the world suffer from schizophrenia. However, according to some studies, there is a worldwide variation in the prevalence of schizophrenia. Schizophrenia is mainly divided into categorical subtypes. Patients who fit into different subtypes will experience different classes of symptoms. In recent times, some specialists have asserted that there are no meaningful differences between these subtypes in etiology, prognosis, or response to treatment (Weiten, 1995). Accordingly, the illness of schizophrenia may be better divided into two major subtypes, based on a different grouping of symptoms. The categories of positive and negative symptoms may be more pertinent, for patients and doctors alike.

The differences between positive and negative symptoms are quite significant and they usually result in differing prognoses for each individual patient. Positive symptoms involve behavioural excesses that are not observed in healthy persons (Weiten, 1995). The most common positive symptoms are hallucinations, delusions, unusual thoughts, disorganized speech, and bizarre behaviours. Thus, positive symptoms reflect an excess or distortion of normal functions (schizophrenia.com, 2008). Patients who exhibit positive symptoms are more frequently correlated with a better prognosis and responsiveness to drug treatment, in comparison to patients that exhibit negative symptoms.

Hallucinations are sensory perceptions that occur in the absence of a real, external stimulus (Weiten, 1995). The most common type of hallucination, in schizophrenia, is the hearing of voices. In my case, I heard voices even before I was formally diagnosed with schizophrenia, though I did not realize this until a much later time. During my youth, I would hear voices only for a short duration of time and mainly at random. However, while in a deeply psychotic state, I would hear voices throughout much of the day. These imaginary voices never seemed strange to me, at the time when I was perceiving them. I also mainly experienced these hallucinations when alone.

The voices that I heard would usually be speaking to me, as if I was having a telepathic conversation with them. These voices would sometimes encourage me to believe in certain things, act in a certain way, or perform a specific action. In my mind, I believed that these voices were coming from some friends of mine that I met in high school. After having a conversation with these voices, I would often wonder how these persons were communicating with me. During my youth, I never believed in psychic communication, telepathy, or other forms of supernatural phenomena. Later in life, while severely ill, I eventually concluded that these voices were communicating through a state of the art microchip that was implanted into my head. I probably got this idea from my paranoid state of mind, in combination with something that I may have seen on television or in a movie.

Scientifically, auditory hallucinations are sometimes caused by an abnormal sense of agency (Haggard, 2003). A normal sense of agency is grounded on the belief that one is responsible for his own actions. However, many auditory hallucinations are externalized by the schizophrenia patient. Therefore, the patient will believe that another person is responsible for his auditory hallucinations. The act of externalization has been significantly correlated with the severity of the voice's comments, the delusion of being controlled, and other concepts related to thought insertion (Startup, 2008).

On other occasions, my head, or another body part, would move involuntarily or twitch at random. Whenever I experienced this, I believed that the voices in my head were responsible for these movements, and that they had taken partial control over my body. In time, I started to hear auditory hallucinations in conjunction with these involuntary bodily movements.

The patient can generally view his hallucinations as a positive or a negative experience. When a patient believes that his hallucinations are useful and beneficial, this will usually create a barrier in his treatment process. However, according to one study, the first auditory hallucinations that schizophrenia patients hear are, for the most part, reported as having a negative effect. Positive voices, on the other hand, mainly occur among non-psychotic subjects (Jenner, 2008). Moreover, between forty to sixty percent of the patients in this study heard positive voices for the duration of their entire lifetime. Positive voices are mainly experienced as direct addresses from a second person's point of view. Furthermore, the perceived control of these voices has been highly correlated with the wish to preserve these voices. Therefore, positive hallucinations can be equally as dangerous as negative hallucinations.

Through my experiences, I also wished to preserve my positive auditory hallucinations. The voices that I heard had come from females who, at some point, were romantic interests of mine. Therefore, due to the fact that I was lonely and isolated, I personally felt that I had benefited from my auditory hallucinations. Whenever I heard these voices, I would no longer be alone and I also felt that I was being loved. As a result, the extreme mental states experienced by severely ill patients can sometimes be more preferable than their real life. This provides the patient with another reason to enter into a state of denial and refuse medical treatment.

Persons who experience visual hallucinations will also sense persons or objects that are not truly present within their physical environment. In some cases, the individual may believe that he is having a conversation with an imagined person (National Institute of Mental Health, 2008). Hallucinations can also affect the other human senses. Thus, it is possible that a patient will also feel, smell or taste objects that do not exist (schizophenia.com, 2008).

Delusions are a second positive symptom in schizophrenia. Persons who experience delusions maintain false personal beliefs, even when they are presented with evidence that their beliefs are false or illogical (National Institute of Mental Health, 2008). Therefore, a delusion is a persistently false and radical belief regarding the actual world. Some of my personal delusions may be characterized as extremely severe, when viewed through a healthy and rational frame of mind. For instance, in some of my delusions, I firmly believed that people were speaking to me as if I was God. I maintained this belief even after experiencing other perceptions that would lead me to believe the contrary. During many other occasions, I believed that persons were speaking to me as if I was a mortal human being. Even though I was partially aware of this conflict in identity, I never really acknowledged the fact that they contradicted each other. I knew that some of my perceptions were wrong. However, I lacked an ability to determine which of my perceptions were true and which were false.

When I believed that persons were addressing me as a mortal human being, I would usually evaluate these to be normal perceptions. However, my delusions of grandeur were, perhaps, more vivid or lively within my mind in comparison. As a result, this made me more inclined to believe that my delusions of grandeur were, in fact, true. During some brief moments, I envisioned some form of insight with respect to my condition. At these times, I was able to rationalize the fact that if my delusions of grandeur were false, I would most likely be suffering from some type of illness. Nonetheless, I would usually ignore these deductions, because I feared the shame and stigma that may have been associated with that particular deduction. In fact, I experienced the delusion that I was God throughout much of my adolescence and childhood. From a personal standpoint, this gave me one solid reason to believe that many of my radical thoughts may actually be true.

Another delusion that I experienced was based on the belief that persons within the media were communicating with me. I believed that some personalities on the television and radio were either speaking directly to me or through a code that only I could understand. While severely ill, I held the delusion that every television program and song on the radio was based on my life. During other extreme moments, I held the belief that all of the disc jockeys on the radio were viewing me through a hidden camera in my home, and that the musical artists were performing live on the radio for my personal benefit. This perception was one of my most extreme delusions. After analyzing this delusion, I further reasoned that this type of service would never be carried out for the average human being, and that therefore I was someone of great importance.

This is usually how a schizophrenic delusion forms. A false perception causes a false belief, and the delusion will continue to expand through an irrational frame of mind. In general, a paranoid delusion will usually be based on the belief that a group of persons is focused on the individual. One of my other extreme paranoid delusions was based on the belief that a group of persons in the world wanted to harm me in some way. The most exorbitant delusion that I experienced was based on the belief that I was Jesus Christ. My previous delusions, where I believed that persons were speaking to me as if I was God, together with my Christian background probably gave rise to this belief. This then led to the extreme paranoid delusion that everyone in the world wanted to kill me. Accordingly, a schizophrenic delusion usually snowballs from a misinterpreted perception, into a severely false belief regarding the actual world.

During one of my paranoid episodes, I was extremely frightened at the prospect of leaving my home. However, I also believed that I was not safe, even within my home. Eventually, after some time, my fears were temporarily alleviated when my mother telephoned the police, and a constable came to my home. I felt safe in his presence and trusted him when he stated that he wanted to take me to a psychiatric hospital. Perhaps my paranoid delusions, coincidently, also gave me a reason to cooperate with that police officer. He offered me a sense of security that I needed during that stage in my life.

Patients with schizophrenia can also experience somatic delusions while in a state of psychosis. Individuals with somatic delusions have false beliefs concerning their physical body. Thus, the schizophrenia patient may believe that he is affected by some terrible illness, or he may hold the belief that there are foreign objects within his body (schizophrenia.com, 2008). My somatic delusions stemmed from the paranoid belief that there were persons in the world who were spying on me. I believed that some state of the art technology was embedded within the bodies of these persons, aimed specifically to help them perform this task. Moreover, I also believed that a similar computer chip was installed into my brain, so that these spies could both communicate with me and read my personal thoughts. Therefore, my somatic delusions coincided with, and were directly linked to my auditory hallucinations. In all somatic delusions, the patient is mainly preoccupied with his belief, even when it is extremely irrational.

From a scientific perspective, features characterizing space in a schizophrenic delusion are those of an imaginary space. Therefore, in the patient's mind, internal and external realities are blurred, and subject-object distinctions are ignored. This essentially forms a single perception of reality that dominates all other conflicting perceptions.

The concept of time may also be distorted within the patient's mind. As a result, imaginary causal relationships can often be reversed. In other cases, socially sanctioned landmarks in time may be recognized. Likewise, the dreaming state and a state of delirium may also be confused within the patient's mind. Therefore, fragmented thoughts that create relational deadlocks, a paradoxical state of mind, and a contradiction of perceptions may be the main underlying factors behind psychosis and psychotic thoughts (Gauthier and Widart, 2008).

Disorganized thought is a third kind of positive symptom. Individuals exhibiting this symptom will have unusual or illogical thought processes. Patients may also demonstrate difficulties in the organization of their thoughts (National Institute of Mental Health, 2008). In my case, I experienced racing disorganized thoughts. Racing thoughts can be defined as a large group of random, unrelated thoughts that are connected together through a state of psychosis.

I remember experiencing racing thoughts on many occasions while residing within the inpatient unit. In one instance, I was sitting in my bedroom, and I remained in a trance-like state. For the most part, I would be thinking about past experiences and events within my lifetime. Then, I would somehow link these seemingly distinct and arbitrary thoughts together, as if they were related to each other in some way or another. On one occasion, I remember asking one of the nurses at the inpatient unit about my score in a math competition that I had competed in, during my high school years. These thoughts somehow connected my participation in this math competition to the very reason behind my stay at the inpatient unit. This seemingly illogical conclusion of mine illustrates how racing thoughts can link two random and distinct thoughts, into a single and cohesive conception.

Racing thoughts or the loosening of associations usually occurs during a period of meditation. At some point, seemingly random thoughts become rationalized and united within the mind of the patient. In my case, whenever I turned my attention back onto the real world, my racing thoughts would usually take precedence over any of my regular thoughts.

From the best of my memories, I mainly experienced racing thoughts when severely ill. After my mind returned back into a more natural state, at times, I would hold an awareness of my previous unusual mental states. This awareness, though, gave me no further insight into my condition. During these moments, I was able to recognize that my mind was producing irrational thoughts. However, after I became aware of this fact, I would usually forget this assessment at a later time. Perhaps, the ongoing development of my illness had affected me in this respect. In time, I would lack the ability to analyze or be consciously aware of any of my delusions, hallucinations or racing thoughts. These thoughts would then become fluid and ordinary from my point of view. At this point, I would have lost all ability to use reason and think through a rational frame of mind.

In addition to racing thoughts, schizophrenia patients can also experience interruptions within their functioning mental processes. For example, maintaining cognitive elements like attention and concentration during my high school studies became increasingly difficult, as I grew older during my teenage years. At some points, I would be focused on a single topic, and then my concentration would abruptly diminish. When this occurred, I found it quite difficult to redirect my focus and attention back onto my class work. As the disease progressed, my attention span and concentration would become steadily more difficult to maintain.

Interruptions in my thought processes still occur today, especially during times when I am under a high amount of stress. On some occasions, I may be having a conversation with someone and I will then suddenly lose my entire train of thought. To deal with this problem, I usually try to ignore all forms of external stimuli within my environment. However, I must also try to accept the fact that my concentration and memory may be permanently impaired, because of my illness.

Schizophrenia patients who exhibit disorganized speech patterns will also be affected by disorganized thoughts. They may speak incoherently, or they may lack an ability to effectively communicate at all. Other telltale signs include disjointed or rambling monologues (schizophrenia.com, 2008). Under these circumstances, the patient could be talking to himself, or he may be hallucinating and talking to an imaginary person.

Unusual or bizarre movements and behaviours are further positive symptoms. In some cases, the patient may be moving in an uncoordinated fashion (National Institute of Mental Health, 2008). Patients can also experience involuntary movements. I started to become aware of the fact that some of my body parts were moving involuntarily, after taking clozapine. However, as I recall, I experienced involuntary bodily movements shortly after I met Dr. Lupton. While severely ill, I linked these involuntary movements to my somatic delusions. At times, I viewed these involuntary twitches as positive experiences. I also believed that the main purpose of these bodily twitches was to affirm or deny random thoughts in my head, and that this was essentially a form of communication. On other occasions, I perceived these twitches to be negative. For example, when I suffered from extreme bouts of insomnia, I held the belief that some imagined persons were purposely opening my eyelids, as a form of torture.

Today, I still experience involuntary twitches on occasion. They usually occur while I am watching television. At some point during the day, my finger will move, or one of my other muscles will twitch. Even so, today I view these involuntary movements as random twitches and nothing else. Thus, I do not attribute the cause of these twitches to a microchip within my body. Actually, the twitches that I experience today are fairly equivalent in severity to the twitches that I experienced while extremely ill. However, it is no longer a cause of concern for me, and this could be indicative of my good mental health today.

The repetition of specific movements is another form of unusual behaviour. During my initial stays at the inpatient unit, I was entering into early adulthood and my facial hair started to grow. While in a state of psychosis, this latter experience annoyed me. At that time, I was not taking care of my hygiene on a regular basis, and I did not shave. As my facial hair grew longer, it started to become more of a nuisance to me. To deal with these feelings, I developed the habit of pulling out my facial hairs. I remember that I had continued this repetitive behaviour for an extensive amount of time.

In addition to my moustache and beard, I also began to pluck out my eyebrows. In retrospect, this turned out to be a big problem. While looking at photos that were taken of me at that time, I realize today that I was actually very ill. I remember that I had lost a degree of self-awareness, and that I was repeating this habit at a subconscious level. After being discharged from the inpatient unit and while my mental health was stable, I remember that I still continued this repetitive behaviour, even while in public. I eventually stopped pulling out my facial hairs after my health had improved, when I became fully aware of my behaviour. Essentially, I was able to address this problem after I regained a higher level of consciousness, when I had a better grasp over my self-awareness.

Other forms of strange behaviour can include sudden or irregular forms of anger, agitation, a trivial attitude or carelessness, and social withdrawal. In my case, I started to have problems with anger while in a state of psychosis. The first time I stopped taking my prescribed medicines eventuated due to feelings of anger. My mother insisted that I was ill and she told me to continue my antipsychotic treatments. However, after a week, I personally felt no differences in my state of mind. In fact, my schizophrenic symptoms were in the process of being controlled. I was unaware of this fact though, and I continued to perceive paranoid thoughts.

At this time, I believed that both my family and my doctors were conspiring against me. I further believed that I was being falsely diagnosed with a mental illness. In time, I also came to believe that I was prescribed these medications, so that other persons would have the power to control my thoughts and behaviours. Yet, I could think of no clear reasons why anyone would want to do this. The belief that I was a God-like figure was one distant possibility. In any case, I held feelings of anger directly because of these delusions.

I remember experiencing more problems with anger, after I was stable on clozapine. Things of very little importance started to cause feelings of agitation in me. Even after long periods of intense meditation, I would still experience troubles while trying to calm my demeanour. One common element, though, is based on the fact that my anger was usually directed towards my mother. I never held the same degree of anger towards any other person, even persons who I extremely dislike today. Perhaps there were things in our personal history that sparked my anger. Furthermore, after improving my health, I probably expected that the relationships between my immediate family members would become more functional than they ever were.

In any case, I also believe that the anger that I held towards my mother was also due, in great part, to my brain chemistry. In my heart, I know that I have an extremely quiet and calm temperament. Accordingly, it is possible that my experiences with anger may have been the latest symptoms of my illness, that were not being properly treated. It is further possible that a particular combination of antipsychotic and antidepressant medicines could have invoked this side effect in me. During many moments, my problems with anger were severe and uncontrollable. Participating in athletic hobbies was one method that enabled me to partially cope with these feelings.

Catatonic behaviour is another positive symptom in schizophrenia. Although I have never been in a state of catatonia, I have observed this symptom in other individuals within the inpatient hospital. Persons who are catatonic usually remain in a motionless state. They may be unaware of their surroundings and they may be unresponsive within their physical environment. From my own observations, I believe that catatonic patients also hold an indifferent attitude towards any forms of external stimuli. Catatonic behaviours may also be marked by rigid or bizarre postures, and aimless or excessive motor activity (schizophrenia.com, 2008). Psychomotor slowing, or the slowing of movements, is a further catatonic behaviour (Morrens *et al*, 2008).

I have only witnessed two patients that exhibited catatonic behaviours. Both individuals remained motionless and they seemed to be in a continuous trance or dream-like state. From my perspective, these patients may have been in a state of deep thought or meditation. It also seems to me that catatonic patients will purposely ignore their physical environment. Perhaps they believe that their train of thought is more important than the actual world. I have also held this belief while in a delusional state.

However, it is also possible that their mind may be ostensibly blank, with no particular idea or topic of focus. According to the National Institute of Mental Health, catatonic forms of behaviour were more common when there was no treatment for schizophrenia, and it is rarely observed today because of the progress made within the field of antipsychotic medications (National Institute of Mental Health, 2008).

Additionally, there are other less severe forms of positive symptoms. Some schizophrenia patients may demonstrate inappropriate reactions when exposed to specific situations or stimuli. Unusual pacing or rocking could be a warning sign, though irregular pacing alone does not provide enough cause to diagnose an individual with schizophrenia. Character traits like depersonalization and derealization can also be symptoms in schizophrenia, under some circumstances. However, these symptoms must be observed in conjunction with other symptoms to have any medical significance. Thus, observing one of these symptoms in an individual, exclusively, will not necessarily lead to the diagnosis of schizophrenia.

In contrast, the negative symptoms of schizophrenia are characterized by a loss, or a reduction of normal emotional and behavioural states. The main difference between positive and negative symptoms remains in the fact that positive symptoms are defined as strange or abnormal traits, while negative symptoms encompass significant decreases in normal functioning. Apathy, the flattening of emotions, poverty of speech, a lack of pleasure in life, and difficulties with the persistence of goal-directed behaviours are common negative symptoms (schizophrenia.com, 2008). According to some studies, severe negative symptoms during the early stages of treatment can often indicate a poor prognosis.

Some researchers view diminished expression and amotivation as the key underlying elements behind all negative symptoms. Furthermore, avolition, or a lack of motivation, has been correlated to the patient's functional outcome (Rassovsky *et al*, 2010). However, many persons with good mental health may experience similar problems with motivation. Therefore, it is possible that the patient may be mistakenly perceived as lazy, unmotivated, or depressed when exhibiting this negative symptom.

The flattening of emotions is defined as a reduction in the range and intensity of emotional expression. This reduction will affect the individual's facial expressions, eye contact, tone of voice and body mannerisms (schizophrenia.

com, 2008). In my case, I remember having problems with abnormal eye contact on several occasions. My first memory of this occurred during my teenage years, when I was working in a restaurant. One day, I stepped into the general manager's office for a private meeting. After I sat down, I remember that I had struggled to maintain my eye contact with him. In fact, I experienced problems with concentration and attention, and I was not fully engaged in our conversation that day. I also remember that he had glared at me, with a squint in his eyes. He may have believed that I was staring him down, and I probably was doing this, though at a subconscious level. After I became aware of the intense and glaring look on my face, I tried to maintain my eye contact through a less aggressive manner. That day, I experienced problems with concentration and could not focus on anything besides my eye contact, including the conversation itself.

I also remember experiencing similar problems with eye contact during my university studies. At that time, I was struggling with my grades and I went to discuss this problem with one of my professors. Once I sat down, I would experience problems while trying to maintain my attention on our conversation. The only thing I could really focus on was maintaining my eye contact. My professor recognized this and gave me a look similar to the one my general manager had given to me, that particular day in my past. However, this happened approximately 10 years later.

I had a similar experience with another professor of mine, during the next semester. His reaction to my intrusive and abnormal eye contact was also, for the most part, negative. In every case, I never became truly aware of my menacing stare until after the fact. In retrospect, I believe that this strange behaviour may have been due to a flattened emotional state. I also believe that problems with cognition may have also limited the range of my emotional expression.

In fact, very ill schizophrenia patients will almost always have severe empathic dysfunction. Several researchers have linked deficits in empathy with impairments in other social cognitive tasks. They also found a large discrepancy between the patient's self-assessment and his relative's assessment, with respect to empathic skills. Therefore, very ill patients may be unaware of the fact that they lack important emotional traits, and this element probably provides another basis for societal stigmas and discrimination.

According to another study, higher schizotypy has been associated with a reduction in empathy, an increase in negative affect, and poorer social functioning (Henry *et al*, 2008). These researchers also discovered that affective empathy serves as a partial mediator between negative schizotypy and social functioning. Consequently, an ability to empathize with other persons is a crucial element in healthy social functioning.

In my history, I have possessed a trivial attitude towards the world, while in a state of extreme paranoia. During these episodes, I would stay at home and lie in my bed for the entire day. I left my room only when I wanted to eat or go to the bathroom. I also had troubles with insomnia, and I remained awake during many nights. Further, I did not maintain my personal hygiene, and I had no volition to do anything else during the day.

When my mother called the police for the second time, my emotional state was mostly non-existent. Two police officers came soon after to check on my condition. When they entered my bedroom, I was lying comfortably in my bed and I did not respond to their presence. After initially ignoring the officers, one of the constables then decided to tear off my bed sheets. He wanted to test my aggression to see if I could pose as a potential danger to other persons. In response, I stared at the constable for a few seconds and I then briskly returned to my sleeping position. My attitude then re-entered into a state of indifference. In fact, I remained in this emotional state for a period of over several weeks. This lack of concern for life in general is a common negative symptom observed in schizophrenia.

Social withdrawal is a symptom that, in most cases, results from a trivial attitude towards life. Participation restriction has also been associated with depressive symptoms in the schizophrenia patient (McKibbin *et al*, 2008). I never had any desire to contact my friends, while in a state of psychosis. Even after I became stable on olanzapine, I still experienced problems with social withdrawal. Today, I do go out on occasion, but I see my friends less frequently at this point in my life. This could be due to my disease, though it could also be due to my age as well.

Personal fears could serve as another reason behind my partial withdrawal from society. Even though I was stable on olanzapine for several years, I still feared the possibility that I would suffer from a relapse while in public. Therefore, I feared that I may be stereotyped or discriminated upon because of my illness. When extremely ill, these fears were probably based more on paranoia than anything else. However, even when my health was stable, I still held the same fears. My fears could have evolved through my paranoid thoughts. Perhaps my experiences with paranoia still have some influence over me, even at times when my illness is actually in a state of remission.

Poverty of speech is another negative symptom defined as the lessening of speech fluency and productivity (schizophrenia.com, 2008). I experienced this symptom while severely ill; however, I still experience this symptom today when I am under a state of extreme stress. When Dr. Lupton first came to see me at my home, I remember that I was exceedingly withdrawn. After Dr. Lupton and Dr. Adrian's questions, I would often reply in short or one word answers. At that time, I feared the possibility that I could be severely ill. However, my thoughts were simple, and I found it difficult to elaborate on these thoughts. On some occasions, I would also slur my speech or speak in fragmented sentences. Accordingly, poverty of speech is a symptom where the individual's speech pattern is reduced to a point where he does not speak thoughtfully or coherently. In fact, my public speaking skills had deteriorated in a gradual fashion, throughout most of my teenage years.

A lack of pleasure or interest in life is a further negative symptom. On the surface, any individual who exhibits this symptom may be viewed as a lazy or unmotivated person. On the inside however, these individuals lack an ability to be fully conscious within their environment. This lack of consciousness causes the individual to hold a blunted perspective of life. The patient is not concerned with concepts like survival or independence, because he lacks a higher form of cognition, imagination, and awareness. Scientifically, the symptoms of ambivalence and anhedonia have also been correlated with impairments in both higher-level emotional processes and everyday functioning (Trémeau *et al*, 2009).

Feelings of fatigue, low energy, and depression may also be relevant to the symptom of anhedonia. When I experienced this symptom, I did not necessarily feel sad or depressed, but I did lose many forms of happiness in life. The main problem was based on the fact that I did not appreciate what life had to offer, nor was I happy to be alive. I would describe my level of awareness, at that time, to be comparable to the level of awareness that an average person has when first waking up in the morning. Nevertheless, I felt this way pretty much throughout the entire day. It took much effort, on my part, to be active during the day, even when I was not suffering from any problems with insomnia.

Difficulties with goal-directed behaviours are a fifth negative symptom. Sometimes, the patient will lack the cognitive ability to complete a goal, while at other times the patient will lack the ability to initiate constructive forms of behaviour (National Institute of Mental Health, 2008).

When I suffered from this symptom, I believe that this experience was mainly due to my poor short and long-term memory. Persons suffering from Alzheimer's disease will lack the ability to complete a goal because they experience periods of extreme forgetfulness when engaged in a particular activity. When severely ill, patients suffering from Alzheimer's disease cannot even initiate an activity, because of their impaired memory. I believe that a similar principle applies, with respect to persons with schizophrenia.

I remember experiencing this problem during a family meeting that occurred two months after I was diagnosed with schizophrenia. As the meeting progressed, I suddenly experienced problems while trying to remember why I was engaged in a meeting, at that particular time. Consequently, I lacked an ability to actively participate in that meeting as well.

On another occasion, I was performing usher duties at my cousin's wedding. At times, I would forget my role in that wedding, and I would then stand aimlessly. During those states of confusion, I found it increasingly difficult to be fully aware within my environment. Subsequently, I did not really fulfill my role at that wedding party. From my perspective, a state of confusion will also give rise to this particular inability.

My worst experience with this symptom occurred when I purchased a DVD machine, after I returned home from the inpatient unit for the final time. When healthy, I am quite knowledgeable in the operation of electronics, but problems with memory had impeded my abilities at that time. The main problem was based on the fact that I could not directly connect that DVD player to my television. The television that I had at that time was quite old and it lacked a necessary connection socket. Accordingly, I then tried to connect my DVD player through several other methods. First, I tried to use my VCR as a converter between my DVD player and television. When that failed, I decided to purchase a large combination of wires and converters. I spent more than a month trying to connect that DVD player to my television, utilizing many differing conversion tools with no success. It was only after I purchased a new television when I realized that my efforts were essentially futile, and that it was impossible to connect that DVD player to an older television.

Thus, I spent an entire month trying to accomplish something that was never possible. In fact, I was never truly aware of the amount of time that had passed. Hence, I also lacked a full sense of awareness within my physical environment. My inability, in this respect, was probably mainly due to my poor memory and this lack of self-awareness. These elements, in turn, had diminished my cognitive functioning, which subsequently affected my ability to complete a goal-directed behaviour.

The average person may essentially view this inability as a disability. Accordingly, this may be the most common symptom observed among all persons who suffer from a mental illness. In my case, I still experienced problems with this symptom, even when many of my other symptoms had improved. During this period, I had no interest in any recreational activities. As a result, I slowly came to believe that I was still ill and suffering from other symptoms. Contrarily, however, Dr. Freedman observed that my mental health had improved, and that I was no longer ill. I did not believe him, and this could have been due to problems with motivation or self-esteem. Thus, it is possible that a purely psychological problem may have interfered with my ability to complete a goal-directed behaviour, at this point in my life. Accordingly, a magical pill may not necessarily cure this symptom. Eventually, I realized that I would need to fully apply myself to achieve any goals that I set out to pursue.

Even though I never truly entered into a catatonic state, I have lacked the ability to independently take care of myself. This deterioration could also qualify as a difficulty with a goal-directed behaviour. When I neglected my personal hygiene, I also did not eat on a regular basis. This is probably the most devastating symptom in schizophrenia. Persons who lack the ability to take care of themselves will require many special needs. Third party interventions like government funding and professional nursing services should be readily available to address this specific problem.

Cognition is a third and highly debated category of schizophrenic symptoms. Cognitive, or the disorganized symptoms of schizophrenia, centre on the intellectual faculties of reasoning and concentration. Patients with schizophrenia can often exhibit cognitive problems like poor executive functioning, poor working memory, and difficulties with attention (National Institute of Mental Health, 2008). Large deficits in central executive working memory, phonological functioning, and visuospatial functioning are further symptoms (Forbes *et al*, 2009). Other cognitive problems can include slow thinking, difficulties with understanding, poor concentration, troubles with thought expression, and an inability to integrate thoughts with feelings and behaviours (schizophrenia.com, 2008). Patients who suffer from cognitive symptoms may face difficulties when trying to complete their education or in obtaining a meaningful career. As such, problems with cognition can be a source of frustration for any patients who achieve a state of remission.

Poor executive functioning is defined as an inability to absorb or interpret information, and make decisions based on this knowledge (National Institute of Mental Health, 2008). I experienced poor executive functioning many times while in a state of extreme psychosis. At times, I would be unable to envision and hold two distinct concepts within my mind. Therefore, my cognitive abilities were limited to the point where I could concentrate on only a single topic. When a schizophrenia patient demonstrates signs of decreased executive functioning, he will also lack an ability to complete goal-directed behaviours. Accordingly, reduced executive functioning often severely impacts the patient's ability to live a normal life.

Difficulties with attention and concentration are other forms of cognitive symptoms. When I had problems with concentration during my college years, I focused more on my delusions than the actual world. Furthermore, I had no choice in this matter. Perhaps the chemical imbalance within my brain had gone rampant. At that time, my thoughts were quite fragmented. I was unable to concentrate on my class work, even through my greatest efforts. Subsequently, I would draw a positive correlation between extreme deficiencies in these cognitive functions and full-blown delusional states.

Problems with attention are similar to problems with concentration. However, while the faculty of concentration implies understanding, the faculty of attention implies awareness. In fact, it is possible for a schizophrenia patient to be aware of his surroundings, while lacking an ability to be an active member within that environment. At times, while I was residing within the inpatient unit, I would be consciously aware of the fact that I was present at a psychiatric hospital, but I could not come up with any reasons why I was there. I would then enter into a prolonged state of confusion. Conversely, patients who are able to concentrate, while having problems with attention, may experience rapid or fragmented thought processes.

Poor working memory is a cognitive symptom that I still suffer from today, even though I have reached a state of remission for many years. I still possess the ability to access my long-term memories, but in retrospect, I believe that these processes have also been negatively affected to some degree. Most of my troubles with short-term memory occur when I am in a stressful or demanding situation. At times, I may repeatedly ask similar questions of little importance. At other times, my short-term memory will fail altogether and I will struggle to remember elements while engaged in a conversation.

Working memory is more or less equivalent to short-term memory, based on its primary definition. Patients who experience problems with working memory will lack an ability to recollect recently learned information, and use it in an immediate fashion (National Institute of Mental Health, 2008). Problems with working memory will have an immense impact on both the patient's normal functioning and his ability to live independently.

Confabulation is defined as a fabricated, distorted, or misinterpreted memory of oneself, with no intention to deceive. It sometimes results through a combination of memory deficits and the individual's tendency to fill these lapses in memory. Deficits in self-monitoring and reality monitoring, and the phenomenon of temporal context confusion are other causes of confabulation. Hypothetically, a confabulator will fail to suppress previously activated memory traces or currently irrelevant memory traces. This process will then intrude on his thought processes. Problems with the regulation of autobiographical recollection may also be associated to the act of confabulation. Multiple lesions involving the basal forebrain and the orbitofrontal cortex, including the striatum or the dorsolateral prefrontal cortex have been observed in patients that exhibit severe difficulties with this memory problem (Funayama and Mimura, 2008).

Another cognitive symptom is an inability to express one's thoughts. The individual will generally exhibit lengthy pauses within his verbal mannerisms. Following these pauses, he may offer irrelevant details, or he may cease to elaborate further with respect to a particular topic of conversation. In most cases, the patient's thought processes are not in sync with his attempts to verbalize his thoughts. On other occasions, the patient may be under duress, or he may be pondering thoughts that are irrelevant within his particular situation.

On a further note, mentally healthy persons may also experience troubles with any of the cognitive symptoms that I have previously mentioned. Difficulties with executive functioning, attention, concentration, memory, and thought expression are cognitive obstacles that almost every person has faced at some point in his life. However, schizophrenia patients that suffer from cognitive symptoms will experience these problems more frequently and for an indefinite period of time.

The last cognitive symptom in schizophrenia is the patient's inability to integrate his thoughts with his feelings and behaviours. Under these circumstances, the patient may exhibit confused or illogical mannerisms and behaviours. On one occasion, I remember seeing an elderly male patient that was walking slowly around the inpatient unit, completely naked. When I looked at his face, he had a blank look and seemed to be quite oblivious with respect to his current condition. He did not know either that he was naked, or else he held the belief that he had done nothing wrong by walking around the facility in this fashion. From my point of view, he exhibited thoughts that were inconsistent with his feelings and behaviours. By walking naked in a public area, without showing any signs of awareness or feelings of embarrassment, I observed this man to be quite out of touch with the real world. I believe that his state of confusion essentially stemmed through an inability to integrate his thoughts, feelings, and behaviours into a single and coherent mind-set.

I have also observed this symptom in another patient, when I visited a schizophrenia support group within my neighbourhood. It was the first time that I had attended the weekly meeting there. Support groups, such as these, are available for individuals who no longer require treatment at an inpatient facility. The main purpose of these support groups is to provide schizophrenia patients with an opportunity to meet their peers. That night, a schizophrenia outreach worker was present. His primary job is to aid outpatients with the acquisition of social support mechanisms. During that meeting, a middle-aged woman became increasingly agitated. She based her anger on the fact that there were no professional psychological counsellors present at that meeting. She then began to focus her anger towards that outreach worker, mainly because he was not a medical specialist.

From my point of view, that woman's attitude was unreasonable, and her behaviour was irrational. Firstly, every schizophrenia patient should already have access to a professional counsellor. I continue to see both my psychiatrist and a mental health nurse on a regular basis. Secondly, the main function of that support group is to provide patients with an additional resource, beyond mental health professionals. Therefore, I believe that she behaved irrationally, due to her disorganized and fragmented thought processes.

In fact, I believe that she was able to grasp these foregoing ideas. In my eyes, that woman was expressing her anger at the wrong target. She was essentially blaming that outreach worker for her personal problems. I also observed her thought processes to be quite patchy. Therefore, irrational action will usually follow when the patient is unable to integrate his thoughts with his emotions and behaviours.

I also suffered from this cognitive symptom on one occasion. During my second semester of university studies, I was under an extreme amount of pressure to succeed academically. I took courses in the sciences and in mathematics that semester, and my preliminary grades began to falter.

One school day, I failed to complete an assignment. When I spoke to my professor after class, he told me that he sent an email to every student regarding that assignment. Therefore, the onus is on the student to check his assignments electronically. During that time, I was performing quite poorly during my exams and on my assignments, and I was under some pressure because of this. While experiencing the exceedingly high demands of university life, I snapped at my professor. In my mind, I felt angry that I had not checked my email account, though I also felt frustrated with my poor academic performance. On that day, I blamed my professor for my own mishaps. In essence, I shifted an underlying responsibility to complete that assignment over to my professor. Today, I concede that my behaviour was irrational and wrong. I believe that I had expressed feelings of anger towards my professor, because of my fragmented state of mind. In essence, I failed to integrate my thoughts and emotions with a proper form of behaviour.

Most schizophrenia patients will exhibit a combination of positive and negative symptoms (Weiten, 1995). On the other hand, cognitive symptoms are more subtle and are usually detected after a neuropsychological test is performed (National Institute of Mental Health, 2008). Cognitive symptoms can also reflect an underlying dysfunction common to several psychotic disorders (schizophrenia.com, 2008). Therefore, while positive and negative symptoms typically characterize schizophrenia, cognitive symptoms do not.

The symptoms of schizophrenia have been historically grouped into other subtypes. This was the first method that psychiatrists used when categorizing different forms of schizophrenia. Schizophrenia patients often exhibited a specific grouping of symptoms. In view of that, the main subtypes of schizophrenia were previously known as paranoid schizophrenia, catatonic schizophrenia, disorganized schizophrenia, residual schizophrenia, schizoaffective disorder, and undifferentiated schizophrenia.

Paranoid schizophrenia is the category that best fits my experience with this illness. Delusions of paranoia are the main symptoms in this subtype. The belief that one is being persecuted, or the belief that one has many enemies who are out to get him are common paranoid thoughts.

Delusions of grandeur are also prevalent within this subtype. The act of identifying oneself as an important figure in history, or as someone who is famous, is a common delusion of grandeur. In my case, the delusions that I first experienced led to the belief that everyone was focusing on me. This delusion then increased in terms of severity, and I eventually believed that I must have been somebody important. This, in turn, led me to believe in the delusion that I was God. Strange delusions and hallucinations are the main characteristics of paranoid schizophrenia, along with exceedingly suspicious feelings against a group of persons or the world in general.

Catatonic schizophrenia is marked by striking motor disturbances, ranging from muscular rigidity to random motor activity (Weiten, 1995). In some cases, the patient may enter into a state of catatonic stupor. The patient will then remain motionless and he may seemingly lack an awareness within his physical environment. Patients can also be isolated from their peers, be socially withdrawn, and possess a negative attitude (schizophrenia.com, 2008). A state of catatonic excitement is a further symptom. Individuals who exhibit this symptom will behave in a hyperactive and incoherent manner. In other cases, patients can experience both states in a systematic fashion. At present, very few patients suffer from catatonic schizophrenia, and its prevalence seems to be on the decline (Weiten, 1995).

Disorganized schizophrenia is a subtype where the patient exhibits moods or emotions that are not appropriate within a given circumstance (schizophrenia.com, 2008). The patient is usually verbally incoherent, and he may be actively babbling or giggling. Other symptoms can include emotional indifference and complete social withdrawal. Nonetheless, these patients usually do not suffer from any forms of hallucinations (schizophrenia.com, 2008). I suffered from this form of schizophrenia at the time when Dr. Lupton first diagnosed me with this illness.

In residual schizophrenia, the patient lacks motivation and interest in all daily activities. Patients who fit into this category will not suffer from any delusions or hallucinations, nor will they exhibit any forms of strange or disorganized behaviours. In my case, I suffered from residual schizophrenia while taking antipsychotic medications that both treated my positive symptoms and caused feelings of fatigue in me as a side effect. When I felt tired and drowsy, I often wanted to take long naps, instead of being active during the day. I would also fail to participate in many other forms of activities. After I addressed my problems with fatigue through coffee and prescribed medicines, I began to enjoy life again and I eventually started a daily work out regime. Therefore, in my case, I suffered from residual schizophrenia during the preliminary stages of my treatment process.

Schizoaffective disorder is a special condition where the patient suffers from schizophrenic symptoms, in addition to the symptoms of either major depression or bipolar disorder. In this particular diagnosis, the patient must suffer from schizophrenic symptoms exclusively and without any other forms of symptoms, for a period of two weeks (Torrey, 1995). Currently, there is some debate as to whether schizoaffective disorder should be truly classified as a form of schizophrenia. The latest research indicates that most instances of this illness belong to a broader category of schizophrenia, while a minority of these cases may be associated to bipolar disorder. Furthermore, the treatment of this disorder is nearly identical to the treatment of schizophrenia, and its prognosis has been statistically better when compared to the prognosis of the average schizophrenia patient (Torrey, 1995).

Undifferentiated schizophrenia is a category for patients who do not fit into any of the latter five subtypes. Doctors will diagnose undifferentiated schizophrenia in patients who exhibit symptoms of more than one subtype, with no clear predominance in any single category. Therefore, these patients suffer from idiosyncratic mixtures of schizophrenic symptoms (Weiten, 1995). Generally speaking, this form is quite common.

There are several factors necessary for a proper diagnosis of schizophrenia. The diagnostic and statistical manual of mental disorders (DSM-IV-TR) is a tool that guides psychiatrists into making universally standard diagnoses. According to this manual, the patient must exhibit two or more positive symptoms, for a duration of at least one month, to be properly diagnosed with schizophrenia. In other cases, only a single symptom will be required, if the patient experiences an extremely bizarre delusion or hallucination.

In contrast, negative symptoms are more difficult to recognize, because in some cases, they may not be related to the illness itself. For example, in some instances of early detection and treatment, antipsychotic medications may cause negative symptoms as a side effect. In other cases, persons may develop negative symptoms psychologically. Additionally, some negative symptoms may be too minor in severity to satisfy the diagnostic criteria within the DSM-IV-TR (schizophrenia.com, 2008).

From my own experience, psychiatrists will only diagnose an individual with schizophrenia when that subject exhibits these disturbances for a period of at least six months. Signs of disturbance can include negative symptoms exclusively, or two or more symptoms in an attenuated form (schizophrenia.com, 2008). If the patient experiences symptoms for less than one month, due to successful treatments, then it is also possible to diagnose him with schizophrenia. This period is required because many different forms of mental disorders will share similar symptoms. Therefore, medical professionals require some time to determine the precise cause of their patient's symptoms.

The patient must also demonstrate signs of social dysfunction, for a significant portion of time, since the onset of his illness. Social dysfunction may occur within the academic or occupational environments, within interpersonal relationships, or in daily living. Psychiatrists will also consider sudden dysfunctions in social, academic, or occupational environments, in cases where the onset of illness occurs prior to adulthood, during the individual's adolescence (schizophrenia.com, 2008).

Another condition requires that the cause of a patient's disturbance must not be due to any extrinsic sources. For example, some individuals can experience delusions or hallucinations through illicit drug abuse. Other types of medications, or combination of medicines, can also cause symptoms similar to those observed in schizophrenia. Psychiatrists must also consider other forms of medical conditions to ensure that their patient is indeed suffering from schizophrenia, and not any other illness.

The individual's medical history may also be relevant. The diagnostic process will be more complicated if there are prior cases of developmental disorders in the patient's family history. This is due to the fact that autism is sometimes misdiagnosed as schizophrenia, in children (schizophrenia.com, 2008). Recording a family history of illness can aid medical professionals during the diagnostic stages of their patient's illness.

Hence, psychiatrists must exclude illnesses like schizoaffective disorder, bipolar disorder, and depression from the diagnostic process. If the patient exhibits psychotic and manic symptoms concurrently, he will be suffering from schizoaffective disorder and not schizophrenia. Any problems with mood must also be brief if the patient is strictly suffering from schizophrenia. Other health problems like brain injuries, genetic disorders, or chromosomal disorders can also mimic the symptoms of schizophrenia. Thus, in some cases, a proper diagnosis may face complications.

Mental health professionals, who are responsible for diagnosing illnesses like schizophrenia, have a variety of methods at their disposal. After Dr. Lupton was confident with her diagnosis, she arranged a further magnetic resonance imaging (MRI) brain examination for me. The purpose of this test was to confirm the probability that I possessed brain abnormalities that are similar to the brain abnormalities observed in other patients with schizophrenia. I have also taken several psychological tests, which measured both my cognitive abilities and the severity of my schizophrenic symptoms. Blood tests also have a 95% accuracy rate, and a test for the sense of smell has also been recently developed (schizophrenia.com, 2008).

Electroencephalogram (EEG) testing is another method used for the same purpose. When an EEG test is performed, the average schizophrenia patient will exhibit significantly reduced amplitudes in all analyzed frequency bands, mainly at anterior locations. This activity seems to indicate that there are multiple deficits within the oscillatory networks and this, in turn, indicates a disturbance in the temporal integration and interaction of all frequency components (Basar-Eroglu *et al*, 2009).

To close, the average age of onset in schizophrenia ranges somewhere around the age of 18 years for males, and 25 years for females (schizophrenia.

com, 2008).   Though rare, childhood onset schizophrenia is also possible, and it seems to emerge through a gradual fashion.   Possible warning signs for children include the hearing of conversations within one's head, the hearing of derogatory or imagined voices, the act of talking to oneself, the act of staring at imagined things, and a loss of interest in the development of friendships.   Other symptoms include lags in motor and speech skills, impaired memory, irrational thoughts, flattened emotions, and problems with attention (schizophrenia.com, 2008).   Nonetheless, it is important to note that these symptoms may also be observed in other disorders, like autism.

Late-onset schizophrenia (LOS) is characteristically diagnosed in patients who are over 40 years of age.   While onset during childhood is slightly associated with a male predominance, late-onset schizophrenia may be slightly associated with a female predominance.   Similarly, the general rule that the later the onset of the disease, the better the prognosis does not apply for individuals who are affected by late-onset schizophrenia (Torrey, 1995). On the contrary, patients that are diagnosed with schizophrenia, who are over the age of 40, will usually have a worse than average prognosis.

Patients with very-late-onset schizophrenia-like psychosis (VLOSLP) experience symptoms when they are over the age of 60.   Both LOS and VLOSLP are very rare.   In comparison, LOS patients are more apathetic, and they present more abnormal psychomotor activity than VLOSLP patients (Girard and Simard, 2008).

7

The Science of Schizophrenia

It is widely agreed between doctors and the scientific community that schizophrenia is a disease that affects the human brain. Furthermore, some researchers believe that schizophrenia is a progressive brain disease. Detailed studies seem to indicate that brain maturation, during the third and forth decade of life, is abnormal in schizophrenia patients (van Haren *et al*, 2008).

Nevertheless, the fundamental cause of schizophrenia has still yet to be determined. One theory proposes the possibility that persons who are diagnosed with schizophrenia possess a genetic predisposition to develop this disease. In fact, researchers believe that the brain volume abnormalities observed in schizophrenia patients mainly involve genetic factors (Harms *et al*, 2010). According to this hypothesis, an individual will develop schizophrenia if he possesses a specific group of genes, which act in combination with a set of environmental factors.

Another theory suggests that there is dopamine neurotransmitter dysfunction within the brains of schizophrenia patients. Researchers base this theory on the fact that the major targets of all antipsychotic medicines are dopamine D2 receptors.

A third possibility is the glutamatergic theory of schizophrenia. According to this theory, the abnormal functioning of the individual's glutamate receptors may be associated to the psychotic symptoms observed in schizophrenia.

Recent scientific findings also associate the GABA class of neurotransmitters to the pathology of schizophrenia. GABA interneurons are a major target of dopamine fibres, and accordingly, alterations in the manner in which dopamine regulates these interneurons have been correlated to the cause of schizophrenia.

A final theory associates schizophrenic brain abnormalities to a particular phase in brain development. Therefore, schizophrenia may be a disorder where the individual's brain has, at some point, failed to develop in a regular and normal fashion. These five hypotheses are the most widely recognized etiological theories among the scientific and medical communities at present.

First, let us examine what scientists know about this disease. When compared to a healthy person's brain, the brain of an individual with schizophrenia has notable abnormalities, in terms of volume and structure. In particular, the hippocampus and the prefrontal cortex are two areas of the brain that are important in the pathology of schizophrenia. Both structural and functional abnormalities within the hippocampus are prevalent in schizophrenia. Researchers have further noted a decrease in volume within the hippocampus and fornix, during the early stages of schizophrenia (Kendi *et al*, 2008). Hippocampal formations on the inner, lower margins of the right and left temporal lobes also appear to be typically altered in the schizophrenia patient.

The hippocampus is an area of the brain that has been associated with certain types of memory. Many researchers suspect that it may be involved in the underlying neuropathology of schizophrenia. The prefrontal cortex may have a similar involvement. This region of the brain is crucial for information processing, attention, working memory, and other higher cognitive functions. Much scientific evidence suggests that there are defects in the anatomy, neurochemistry, and functioning of the prefrontal cortex in schizophrenia.

Other studies indicate that there is both activation and deactivation within specific areas of the prefrontal cortex. When compared to control subjects, schizophrenia patients showed reduced activation within the right dorsolateral prefrontal cortex. Pathological dysfunctions may also, theoretically, disrupt the intrinsic circuitry within the dorsolateral prefrontal cortex. Accordingly, there is a significant impairment in functional connectivity between this region and other task-relevant regions of the brain

Greater activation within the anterior cingulate/ventromedial prefrontal cortex has also been observed in schizophrenia. Failures to activate may be associated with an impaired performance in psychological tests, while failures to deactivate may be associated with functions related to maintaining one's sense of self (Pomarol-Clotet *et al*, 2008).

A reduction in size, within the anterior callosal regions connecting the frontal cortex, has also been observed during the onset of schizophrenia (Walterfang *et al*, 2008). Patients may experience impaired cognition as a direct result. Other research implicates a reduction in activity within the prefrontal cortex of patients that exhibit negative symptoms. In addition, abnormal neuronal activity within the prefrontal cortex is theorized to cause attention deficits.

Some researchers have linked both the prefrontal cortex, and the medial temporal lobe to schizophrenic delusions and hallucinations. More specifically, impaired pre-attentive processing of speech in fronto-temporal networks has been correlated to auditory verbal hallucinations (Fisher *et al*, 2008). Other researchers have drawn a relationship between auditory hallucinations and middle-ear disease. This is significant because, historically, psychiatrists believed that an ear disease could cause insanity through an irritation within the brain. Accordingly, current knowledge regarding the role of the temporal lobes, and their proximity to the middle ear seems to support the hypothesis that middle-ear disease may also be involved in the etiology of schizophrenia (Mason *et al*, 2008).

In healthy persons, the left temporal and frontal lobes of the brain are activated when the individual is trying to make sense of language and visual stimuli. However, these brain regions are abnormally structured in the schizophrenia patient. Subsequently, while healthy individuals utilize language functions within the left half of their brain, schizophrenia patients consistently have more language activity within the right half of their brain.

The left temporal lobe of the brain is believed to be responsible for sensory filtering deficits, which has been associated with poor memory performance and planning. Scientists have also correlated abnormal functioning within the medial temporal lobe to problems with declarative memory. Declarative memory is crucial for everyday life experiences. Prospective memory, which is the ability to do something at future times without the use of prompts, is also impaired in patients with chronic schizophrenia. Further, deficiencies in functioning prospective memory have been linked to dysfunctions within the prefrontal lobe (Tirapu-Ustárroz *et al*, 2005). Deficits in speech production also suggest the possibility that schizophrenia patients have impaired relational memory processes (Kircher *et al*, 2008).

In addition to the prefrontal cortex, other forebrain regions that have been linked to schizophrenia include the amygdala, the nucleus accumbens, and the cerebral cortex. With respect to the amygdala, its elevated function is believed to be an underlying cause of the cognitive dysfunction observed in schizophrenia. In fact, a significant dysregulation has been observed between the excitatory (amygdala) and inhibitory (prefrontal) limbic regions in medicated schizophrenia patients. Dysfunctions in specific brain systems like the lateral prefrontal cortex, the midbrain dopamine system, and the anterior cingulate cortex have also been correlated to problems in cognitive control, related to thought and action in a goal-directed manner.

Thus, researchers agree that schizophrenia is a brain disorder that affects several regions of the brain. There are definite impairments observed within the parietal lobe. More specifically, dorsal stream dysfunction is prevalent in schizophrenia. Researchers have also observed dysfunctions within the limbic cortical regions of the brain, like the entorhinal cortex.

According to Oyebode, schizophrenia-like psychosis of epilepsy may be linked to seizures originating within the limbic structures. Reduced seizure frequency, left-sided electrical foci, and neurodevelopmental lesions manifesting as cortical dysgenesis may influence the likelihood of these episodes (Oyebode, 2008).

Furthermore, delusional misidentification syndromes have been associated with impairments in face recognition memory. These syndromes are believed to be linked to the frontal and parietal lobe, in addition to any organic lesions affecting the limbic structures. Other evidence reveals the possibility that right-sided lesions predominate in the aetiology of delusional misidentification syndromes. Visual and auditory hallucinations also seem to arise from functional changes in the same cortical areas subserving the normal physiological functions of vision and audition (Oyebode, 2008). For instance, auditory association cortices responsible for voice recognition may play a role in the perception of auditory hallucinations.

Activation of the lateral occipital complex (LO) is also more widely distributed in schizophrenia. It is theorized that deficits in object-recognition tasks may be mediated by LO activity. In addition, the superior temporal gyrus, located on the lateral side of the brain, is smaller in patients with schizophrenia. This area of the brain is responsible for language and thought processes. Dysfunctions in cortical function, which are mediated by the coordinated actions of excitatory projection neurons and inhibitory interneurons, have also been correlated to schizophrenia.

The insula is also abnormally structured in the brains of schizophrenia patients. This region of the brain has been associated to feelings of mistrust and paranoia, through neuroimaging evidence. Other studies reveal that schizophrenia patients have a significantly smaller right inferior colliculus, in comparison to healthy control subjects (Kang *et al*, 2008). In addition, disturbances within the frontal portion of the cingulate fasciculus have been observed in schizophrenia. This area has been linked with deficits in attention, affect, and motivation.

A defect in brain white matter may also play some type of role in the development of schizophrenia. A decrease in white matter seems to be inversely linked to the progression of illness in many patients (van Haren *et al*, 2007).

In the majority of cases, schizophrenia does not become visible until after puberty. This suggests that biological changes between adolescence and adulthood may also be significant. After puberty, individuals with early lesions within the ventral hippocampus have experienced dopaminergic deficits similar to those observed in the schizophrenia patient.

Changes in brain circuit connectivity could be a defining feature among many mental disorders. Much documented research reveals that neuronal and synaptic circuitry, within the brain, is altered in diseases like schizophrenia and depression. In particular, the cortical-cerebellar-thalamic-cortical brain circuit has been linked to schizophrenia. This circuit facilitates communication between these regions of the brain, and it also temporally coordinates and synchronizes the brain's cognitive, affective and motor processes.

The abnormal functioning of nerve circuits within the outer regions of the brain may also be linked to schizophrenia. One etiological theory is based on the abnormal processes that alter modes of communication among brain cells. Debruille has discovered that N400 brain electrical activity is greater in highly delusional individuals and has linked this element to the patient's integration of delusional knowledge (Debruille, 2008). Neuronal metabolism could also be related to the progression, arrest and reversal of schizophrenia.

However, the most widely accepted causal theory of schizophrenia is based on a genetic vulnerability, as opposed to a dysfunction within specific neurotransmitter systems. Genes are DNA segments that serve as the key functional units in hereditary transmission (Weiten, 1995). An individual possesses a genetic vulnerability, or predisposition, when his genetic makeup makes him susceptible to develop an illness. Hence, persons with a genetic predisposition must also experience certain environmental factors before they develop schizophrenia.

Some scientists theorize that multiple genes will each produce a small effect. Furthermore, complex gene and environmental interactions that involve genomic variations and specific environmental events must necessarily occur (Zhang, 2008). Rare de novo germline mutations and rare genetic lesions at many different loci could also be significant etiological elements (Xu *et al*, 2008). When these factors are combined, the risk to develop schizophrenia increases until a certain threshold is reached. After this point, the disease will then subsequently begin to develop.

Thirty percent of individuals that have 22q11 deletion syndrome will be affected by either schizophrenia or bipolar disorder. One implication from this statistic may be that 70% of persons with this genetic trait will never encounter any environmental stimuli that could trigger a mental instability.

More specifically, the catechol-o-methyltransferase gene (COMT) could play a role in schizophrenia. Scientists have drawn an association between DNA sequence variation at the COMT locus and schizophrenia. This gene is located within the microdeletion region of 22q11.2, and its role is to encode the enzyme that degrades dopamine. This thereby balances dopamine levels within the brain. In fact, an imbalance of dopamine levels within the brain has been linked to the cognitive impairments observed in schizophrenia. The COMT gene has been additionally linked to deficits in sensory processing and cognition. It plays a role in the metabolism of catecholamine neurotransmitters, which are known to modulate several symptoms in schizophrenia.

Proline dehydrogenase (PRODH), and Gnb1L are other schizophrenia susceptibility genes located within the region of chromosome 22q11.2 (Prasad, 2008). This segment also contains the thioredoxin reductase 2 gene (TXNRD2) and the armadillo repeat gene (ARVCF). The latter genes are involved in functions that have been correlated to schizophrenia. The TXNRD2 and ARVCF genes also play a pivotal role amongst cell-to-cell communications and some developmental processes. Abnormalities in these genes are believed to increase the individual's behavioural defects, along with his susceptibility to develop schizophrenia.

Another gene that has been linked to schizophrenia is the PICK 1 gene. Located on chromosome 22q11-13, PICK 1 is considered to be a genetic locus for schizophrenia. The phosphatidyl-inosital-4-kinase-catalytic-alpha gene (PIK4CA) has also been connected to schizophrenia. It is also located in the 22q11.2 region. Some scientists theorize that variation at PIK4CA may be a risk factor for individuals with 22q11 deletion syndrome (Vorstman *et al*, 2009).

Indeed, the chromosomal region 22q11 is an area of interest in schizophrenia research. According to some genetic studies, 22q11 microdeletions represent the highest known genetic risk factor for the development of schizophrenia. This region is a section of DNA that is known to cause neuropsychological and behavioural deficits in children. Moreover, the absence of a small section of DNA on chromosome 22 could further influence proper brain development.

Microdeletions in this section can also lead to the development of velocardiofacial syndrome. This condition increases the individual's chance to develop schizophrenia by a factor of 50 to 100. Contiguous gene syndrome has also been linked to 22q11 microdeletions, which increases the risk to develop an illness when more than one gene is involved.

The neuregulin gene (Nrg) is another schizophrenia susceptibility gene that is located on chromosome 22q11. Nrg is a cell-to-cell signalling molecule that is mutated in some patients. Expressed in the developing forebrain, Nrg is theorized to modulate the differentiation of glial cells and neuronal migration to appropriate locations in the developing cortex.

Neuregulin 1 is a schizophrenia susceptibility gene that affects the expression levels of the Type IV gene. This suggests that some biological pathways involving the isoform may be altered in schizophrenia. Neuregulin 1 is also known to regulate hippocampal synaptic plasticity, short and long-term cognitive functions, and sensorimotor gating behaviours. It is essential for brain development and it can modify glutamatergic transmission by way of regulating the NMDA receptor.

Another major gene implicated in the cause of schizophrenia is the disrupted in schizophrenia gene (DISC1). There is strong evidence which suggests that a mutation in DISC1 may lead to a rare genetic form of schizophrenia (Ross, 2008). More specifically, as a regulator of cortical development, studies have shown that over-expression of mutant DISC1 interferes with neurite outgrowth in neuronal PC 12 cells. This finding indicates a possible role of DISC1 in the developmental defects and pathogenesis of schizophrenia. Researchers have also discovered that a mutant DISC1 gene will fail to associate with nudel, which is a neuronal migration protein. This suggests the possibility that certain proteins may also be involved in the onset of schizophrenia. Researchers theorize that DISC1 may further interact with the brain's glutamate receptors.

Several genes related to mitochondrial function and oxygen metabolism have been connected to schizophrenia, through studies conducted on the post-mortem brains of schizophrenia patients. Altered neural cell adhesion molecule (NCAM) expression has also been discovered within the post-mortem brains and cerebrospinal fluid of some patients. The two main roles of NCAM are to develop nerve cells that recognize and signal to neighbouring cells, in addition to forming a connection between these cells. Subsequently, researchers are studying the gene that encodes NCAM.

Other scientists believe that a combination of multiple genes and an environmental insult during the early stages of development engenders a process capable of causing the disease in a genetically vulnerable individual. They have noted that mutations in several genes, including the alpha 7 acetylcholine receptor gene (CHRNA7), may be further associated with schizophrenia. The CHRNA7 gene, located on chromosome 15, is believed to be involved in a specific defect, which decreases the brain's ability to filter out irrelevant stimuli. Mutations of the NOTCH4 gene have also been correlated to schizophrenia.

Chromosome 8p is suspected to be a locus for both schizophrenia and bipolar disorder. The NRG1 gene maps to this chromosome, and the VMAT1/SLC18A1 gene, which has been linked to both disorders, is also located within this region. Other studies have connected a region on chromosome 5q22-34 to schizophrenia.

The G72 gene, located on chromosome 13q, may be a risk factor for the development of schizophrenia, bipolar disorder, panic disorder and unipolar depression. This seems to suggest that G72 may underly traits common among several different psychiatric phenotypes. G72 is also known to activate the D-Serine oxidase gene, which lowers levels of the D-Serine molecule. D-Serine activates the NMDA neurotransmitter, and researchers theorize that an overactive G72 may cause lower levels of D-Serine. This, in turn, causes an under active NMDA receptor. NMDA glutamate receptors are further believed to be relevant to the etiology of schizophrenia.

Recent studies have identified other genes that may be related to schizophrenia. The methylenetetrahydrofolate reductase gene (MTHFR) may predispose the schizophrenia patient to more severe symptoms. Researchers note that it is important for folic acid metabolism. The 14-3-3 gene family is also a target of further research. Likewise, nicotinic 7 receptors are other candidate genes that may be related to the cause of schizophrenia.

The syntaxin gene (stx-1) could be important as it plays a role in the release of neurotransmitters from synapses, and this is essential for communication between nerve cells. Likewise, the HOPA-12bp gene has been discovered in 5% of subjects who are diagnosed with schizophrenia. This gene has been linked to hypothyroidism, which produces marked cognitive deficits similar to those observed in Alzheimer's disease. RGS4 gene variations have also been implicated in schizophrenia. Early studies indicate that patients with this gene variation will also have reductions in prefrontal grey matter.

Additionally, two protein pathways that have been associated with schizophrenia are known to be regulated by the Egr3 gene. This gene provides a molecular link between the regulation of brain gene expression and environmental events. It also maps to a major schizophrenia locus. In further studies, Egr3 deficient mice have produced schizophrenia-like abnormalities (Gallitano-Mendel et al, 2008).

The imprinted gene LRRTM1, located on human chromosome 2, is also being studied. Imprinted genes can have different roles in brain development, depending on which parent they are inherited from. In actual fact, every individual has an active and inactive copy of LRRTM1 in every cell of his body. Studies have indicated that a region near this gene may be associated to both left-handedness and a susceptibility to develop schizophrenia, when the paternal copy is active. Left-handedness and schizophrenia are two phenomena that have been associated with unusual patterns of brain asymmetry.

Recent research also links genomic copy-number variants (CNVs) to schizophrenia. It has been discovered that recurrent CNVs may disrupt several genes that have been linked to neuronal functioning, including MYT1L, CTNND2, NRXN1, and ASTN2. This may then play a role in the individual's susceptibility to develop schizophrenia (Vrijenhoek *et al*, 2008).

Some of the genes associated with schizophrenia are also variable by nature. Therefore, some candidate genes may be associated to schizophrenia in some populations, but not in others. For example, polymorphisms in the region of the Chitinase 3-Like1 gene (CH3L1) are believed to be schizophrenia predisposing single nucleotide polymorphisms within the Han Chinese population. However, this association was not established among two other ethnically identical Chinese or Japanese samples (Yamada *et al*, 2009). Furthermore, variation within the Epsin 4 gene has been associated to psychotic disorders within the Latin American population. This gene encodes enthoprotin, which suggests that this protein may also be involved in the pathogenesis of schizophrenia (Escamilla *et al*, 2008). Researchers have also discovered a genomewide significant linkage of schizophrenia to 8p23.3 and a second independent susceptibility locus on 8p21.3, among European and African American test subjects (Holliday *et al*, 2008).

The genetic theory of schizophrenia is mainly based on the hereditary factors that have been observed in this disease. Two of the highest known risk factors for the development of schizophrenia includes being the child of two affected parents, or being the monozygotic co-twin of a formally diagnosed patient. Velocardiofacial syndrome and chromosome 22q11 deletions are other high risk factors (Murphy, 2002).

According to Murthy, the complex multigenic nature of schizophrenia implies the possibility that single gene disruptions may lead to compensatory adjustments in the brain, but multiple gene disruptions lead to failure of such compensations (Murthy, 2008). A further theory postulates that the underlying genetics in schizophrenia involve a combination of modest effects, which are essentially caused through several susceptibility genes.

In this hypothesis, environmental elements are also significant to the cause of schizophrenia. Crair asserts, persons with identical predispositions to schizophrenia may not develop the disorder unless they are exposed to appropriate external environmental stimuli. If this is true, then certain environmental factors are also necessary in the development of schizophrenia. He theorizes that sensory experience or abnormal neuronal activity within early development could also be important causal factors.

Hence, the individual must possess particular biological traits and experience specific environmental stimuli to develop schizophrenia. According to some researchers, specific emotional states may lead to sustained changes in the structure of the individual's central nervous system.

Moreover, it is known that stress may cause permanent brain changes through varied neuroendocrine and immunological mechanisms. Observed decreases in hippocampus activity also seem to suggest that posttraumatic stress disorder, and the role of trauma may be relevant to the development of psychosis. This decrease in activity is theorized to be caused by an oversecretion of cortisol within the brain. It has been observed that this stress hormone is dysregulated in patients with schizophrenia, and in individuals who are at a high risk to develop psychosis.

Chronic stress also induces change in biological systems like the GABA-benzodiazepine system. This system has also been linked to schizophrenia. In addition, scientists have associated sensitization, or the repeated exposure to stress or stimulants, with enhanced dopamine release and dysregulation (Benkelfat, 2008). Dopamine is an important neurotransmitter that has been correlated to schizophrenia by many researchers.

Additionally, changes in stress regulating mechanisms and the activation of cooperating neurotransmitters may play a role in the pathogenesis of other mental disorders, beyond schizophrenia (Szubert *et al*, 2008). Stressful stimuli are known to trigger a neuroinflammatory process. This process could contribute towards both functional and structural damage within the brain (García-Bueno and Leza, 2008). Stress, viral exposure, hypoxia and anoxia have also been linked to schizophrenia, because these elements can affect the expression of an underlying genetic predisposition.

Other genetic predispositions may originate through genes that have been linked to the immune system. An altered immune response may predispose for a disturbed defense of viral infections. Therefore, immunological related genes may also be associated to the development of schizophrenia.

Nonetheless, the specific environmental factors relevant to a genetic predisposition, as of yet, have not been established. Scientists have identified some candidate genes though, and it is probable that they will discover further genetic factors. The genetic theory is currently the most widely accepted etiological theory of schizophrenia. A second theory is based on the abnormal functioning of the dopamine neurotransmitter. This theory also has a long chain of evidence, which suggests that dopamine may additionally play some type of role in the cause of schizophrenia.

Researchers base the dopamine (DA) hypothesis of schizophrenia mainly on the therapeutic effectiveness of antipsychotic medications. Proponents of this theory assert that the clinical symptoms in schizophrenia are due to an imbalance within the DA system (Alves *et al*, 2008). Known as D2R antagonists, antipsychotic medicines mainly target and block dopamine D2 receptors. Moreover, the down-regulation of D2R signalling, within the brain, is believed to be partly responsible for some of the symptoms observed in schizophrenia. On a further note, irregular levels of dopamine are also theorized to be involved in other illnesses like depression, attention deficit hyperactivity disorder, and Parkinson's disease.

According to many studies, hypoactivity within the prefrontal cortex has been consistently observed in schizophrenia. Similarly, enhanced prefrontal activity associated with alleviation of negative symptoms and improvement of cognitive functions has been observed following atypical antipsychotic treatments. Atypical antipsychotics are also known to be effective in the regulation of functions within the striatal area of the brain (Alves *et al*, 2008).

There are some notable differences between typical and atypical antipsychotic medications. Research reveals that atypical antipsychotics can markedly increase the release of dopamine within the prefrontal cortex. This has proven to enhance cognition in the schizophrenia patient. Atypical antipsychotic medicines also inhibit D4 receptors. In contrast, typical antipsychotics mainly inhibit D2 receptors.

Other findings indicate that D1/D5 dopamine receptor signalling, within the prefrontal cortex, may be deficient in the schizophrenia patient. This signalling is known to control working memory. The interaction between dopamine and the neurotransmitter norepinephrine may also be linked to the cognitive dysfunctions observed in schizophrenia. Theoretically, the differential regulation of these dopaminergic systems by way of their noradrenergic afferents may provide a means of selectively regulating their activity to offset schizophrenia with minimal side effects.

Research indicates that the dopamine D1 receptor is abnormally regulated within the frontal cortex of the schizophrenia patient. Moreover, D1 agonists, which mimic D1 receptor behaviour, are known to improve cognition in the patient. Dopamine receptor interacting proteins (DRIPs), which partially regulate D1 receptors, are also known to be upregulated in schizophrenia. Likewise, scientists have observed that the interaction between D2 receptors and the dopamine transporter (DAT) is further altered in schizophrenia.

The release of dopamine within the brain is known to be chiefly regulated by way of communication between the prefrontal cortex and striatum. Dopamine release within the prefrontal cortex has been scientifically correlated to working memory, cognitive dysfunction, and the pathogenesis of schizophrenia.

Hippocampal impairment has also been linked to DA dysregulation. The hippocampus is an area of the brain that is responsible for the regulation of independent pathways, which control the population of phasically active DA neurons.

Schizophrenia may further result from the abnormal activity of dopamine neurons within the mesocortical system. The mesocortical dopaminergic neurons of the ventral tegmental area have been linked to the brain functions of voluntary motor movement, working memory, and reward.

Other research reveals the possibility that imbalances in dopaminergic transmission, within the cerebral cortex, may be related to the cognitive and psychotic aspects of schizophrenia. Discoveries like these seem to imply the hypothesis that dopamine dysfunction is the root cause of schizophrenia. This theory is based on the role of dopamine within the brain. Dopamine is a precursor of adrenaline. Increases of dopamine, in some regions of the brain, are known to cause symptoms such as delusions and hallucinations. In the schizophrenia patient, deficits of dopamine have been observed in regions of the brain that are important for cognitive functions and memory.

Dopamine is produced from a collection of cells located within the midbrain. These cells have excitatory inputs responsive to glutamate neurotransmission. When stimulated by the glutamate system, dopamine cells are released from the midbrain. Highly stressful experiences can make dopamine-producing cells significantly more responsive to excitatory stimulation. This would thereby increase dopamine levels within the brain.

Scientists have further correlated dopamine with the cell-signalling molecules Akt and GSK3. Dopamine D2 receptor antagonists and lithium, which may be utilized in the treatment for schizophrenia, can antagonize both molecules. Anandamide, which is a normal substance in the human brain, has also been connected to the D2 receptor. The activation of the D2 receptor has been linked to alterations in the release and receptor signalling of anandamide, which in turn causes alterations in mood, perception, and cognition.

D2 receptors may also be sensitive to amphetamine treatments. According to some researchers, amphetamines may increase dopamine release between nerve cells. On a similar note, the dopamine D2 receptor is known to inhibit N-Type calcium channel activity. In effect, too much calcium can produce highly toxic side effects within an individual's brain.

The role of dopamine has also been connected to the individual's mood, reward system, learning ability, and memory (Seal, 2008). Dopamine containing neurons can be activated directly or indirectly by most drugs of abuse. Subsequently, this could be one reason why many mentally sick persons choose to abuse illicit substances.

Leung further theorizes that the brain's endocannabinoid system may be out of balance in schizophrenia. This hypothesis is based on the higher densities of cannabinoid receptors, and the elevated fatty acid amide (FAA) concentrations observed within the dorsolateral prefrontal cortex. Another study indicates that an endogenous cannabinoid system may be involved in the regulation of striatal dopamine release (Wenger and Fürst, 2004). As a result, the abuse of cannabis may escalate dopamine release within the brain, which could produce a mental state that is similar to a state of psychosis.

According to another study conducted in the Netherlands, cannabis use may be considered as a contributory cause of schizophrenia. Even so, these researchers admit that only a small proportion of cannabis users will go on to develop some form of psychosis. As a result, the risk to develop psychosis may be due to an interaction between cannabis and multiple variations within multiple genes (Henquet et al, 2008).

From my personal experience, I believe that some patients, who possess a high sense of awareness, may wish to compare their experiences with psychosis to the highs that are produced by illicit drugs. Through my clouded frame of mind, I held the naive belief that if my states of psychosis were dissimilar to the mental states produced by illicit drugs, this would give me one reason to assume that my paranoid thoughts were abnormal. I also believed in the notion that if an illicit drug did produce a state of psychosis in me, then it would be possible that someone was purposely poisoning me, which would then account for my experiences with extreme delusions and psychosis.

In fact, this latter belief of mine was actually a paranoid thought. Nonetheless, I believe that many other schizophrenia patients will have had a similar experience with paranoia, before they experimented with any forms of narcotics. Hence, the individual's state of psychosis may have some influence over his choice in this respect. The patient may also experiment with an illicit substance, in an effort to treat the symptoms of his illness. In my case, I did consider the possibility that a narcotic may essentially cure my paranoia. However, after experimenting with an illicit drug, I still lacked insight with respect to the true nature of my condition.

This self-medicating behaviour may also provide some severely ill patients with a reason to feel normal. If the use of cannabis did mimic a state of psychosis, this could then enable the patient to establish a connection with other mentally healthy persons. Thus, some schizophrenia patients will feel less isolated if other persons experience mental states that are similar to their own, through the abuse of a substance. This type of connection essentially addresses many social problems related to alienation and withdrawal. From my experience, I knew that some of my paranoid thoughts were not common among the average healthy human being. For this reason, I believe that some schizophrenia patients may abuse illicit substances because they would rather be labelled as a drug addict, over a mentally disabled individual.

Indeed, many individuals will fear the possibility that they are mentally disabled over the possibility that they are guilty of substance abuse. The main difference between these two stereotypes remains the fact that drug addicts choose to enter into their irregular mental states, while mentally ill persons have no such choice. Thus, the act of self-medicating could provide a severely ill patient with a false perception of control over his state of mind.

There are similarities between schizophrenia and alcoholism. In fact, abnormal DA release within the striatum has been observed in both schizophrenia and alcoholism patients. Accordingly, some patients may choose to self-medicate themselves through alcohol, to regain a sense of reward that may be lost due to their illness.

In summation, the DA hypothesis is based on the confirmed findings that prefrontal and subcortical function improves following treatments through antipsychotic medicines, by way of enhanced DA activity. All of these findings seem to indicate that dopamine has some type of role in the psychotic symptoms that are characteristic of schizophrenia.

Recent scientific discoveries suggest that the glutamatergic system may also be involved in the cause of schizophrenia. In the glutamate theorem, researchers believe that a decrease in glutamatergic neurotransmission contributes towards the cause of schizophrenia. In fact, decreased quantities of glutamate receptors, within the brain, have been consistently discovered in the schizophrenia patient. Reduced levels of glutamate are also believed to be a contributing factor in Alzheimer's disease and other forms of memory disturbances (Weiten, 1995). Similar to dopamine, there also exists pharmacological evidence that associates abnormal glutamate neurotransmission to the pathophysiology of schizophrenia. Other researchers theorize that abnormal NMDA-receptor-dependent synaptic signalling could also cause schizophrenia.

Glutamate is the major excitatory neurotransmitter within the human brain. When it activates a group of NMDA receptors (NMDAR), these receptors need to be precisely localized to points of neuron-neuron contact, known as synapses. NMDA receptors bind glutamate and regulate the stability of these synapses by way of a physical interaction with other proteins. NMDA receptors also change the strength of the brain's synapses between neurons, and this shapes the individual's cognitive abilities.

The NMDA receptor is a glutamate receptor subtype labelled as the most important excitatory transmitter in the brain. Its primary function is to mediate communication between brain cells. The correct activation and expression of the NMDA receptor also plays a role in the normal development of the cortex. Other researchers have drawn a correlation between the glutamate receptor kainate and schizophrenia.

According to other research, the molecular composition of the NMDA receptor is altered in schizophrenia. Patients will also possess high levels of an NMDAR subunit, known as NR3A, within their prefrontal cortex.

The connection between behavioural symptoms and NMDA receptor deficits has also been studied. NMDA receptors are known to generate voltage-dependent postsynaptic potentials (EPSPs). EPSPs are believed to play a special role in the hippocampus and in memory abnormalities. Other studies seem to indicate that when NMDA channels are compromised in schizophrenia, very specific deficits in the recall of sequences will result. Therefore, a correlation may exist between memory and abnormal NMDA channels.

The NMDA receptor is scientifically classified as an ionotropic glutamate receptor. Various drugs that act upon the NMDA receptor are known to increase and worsen the symptoms of psychosis. Other medications, that affect glutamate function, may alleviate some of the psychotic symptoms observed in patients with abnormal glutamatergic systems. Similarly, several drugs that enhance NMDA receptor activity have also improved a state of psychosis. Accordingly, drugs that affect the NMDA receptor can both cause and treat a state of psychosis. This implies the possibility that a genetic defect in glutamate receptor function may act as a fundamental cause of schizophrenia.

It is known that several NMDA receptor antagonists, like ketamine, can induce transient schizophrenia-like-symptoms. These symptoms include paranoia, delusions, affect flattening, cognitive deficits and withdrawal. According to a further study, ketamine use may cause unpleasant dreams (Blagrove *et al*, 2009). The drug phencyclidine (PCP) can also block a class of glutamate receptors, which thereby produces schizophrenic-like states. When properly regulated, NMDA receptors are involved in developmental, physiological and pathological processes within the brain. When unregulated, however, NMDA receptor endocytosis could lead to the hypofunction of NMDA receptors (Huang, 2008). This type of hypofunction has been implicated in schizophrenia.

Other evidence demonstrates that PCP induced cognitive defects may be reversed by group 2/3 metabotropic glutamate receptors. Cystine-glutamate antiporters will then regulate these receptors. These antiporters will further regulate the synthesis of antioxidant, which is essential to the survival of brain cells. Consequently, other studies suggest the possibility that cystine-glutamate antiporters may also be altered in schizophrenia.

Recent discoveries further indicate a positive clinical efficacy for a drug that stimulates the metabotropic glutamate receptor LY2140023. Patients who were treated with this drug demonstrated improvements in their negative and cognitive symptoms (Sodhi *et al*, 2008).

Other researchers have found that low levels of the enzyme glutamate carboxypeptidase II (GCPII) will result in impaired folate absorption, and low serum folate levels have been linked to the negative symptoms of schizophrenia. This could provide a reason why there is low glutamate NMDA receptor activity in schizophrenia.

The peptide N-acetylaspartylglutamate (NAAG) has also been linked to the glutamatergic neurotransmitter system. NAAG actively binds two glutamate receptors in the brain, which are involved in psychosis and psychotic states. Abnormal levels of this peptide have also been observed in the schizophrenia patient.

Recent evidence reveals the possibility that the dopamine and glutamate systems may interact with each other. Dopamine turnover is known to increase when specific glutamate receptors are either stimulated or blocked. Other scientists have discovered that interactions between glutamate receptors and the dopaminergic system may affect mood and states of psychosis. Dopamine D1 and glutamate NMDA receptors have been further observed to take part in complex interactions, where the acute blockade of NMDA receptors may induce D1 receptor internalization.

Reduced levels of the brain chemical n-acetyl-aspartate (NAA) are also prevalent within the hippocampus of schizophrenia patients and their healthy siblings. NAA is a neuronal cell marker in schizophrenia, and it serves as a neurochemical measure that is responsible for the integrity of glutamate neurons. This discovery could connect the genetic and glutamatergic etiological theories of schizophrenia together.

Conversely, gamma-aminobutyric acid (GABA) is the major inhibitory neurotransmitter within the human brain. Actually, excitatory and inhibitory neurotransmission must be balanced for proper neural circuit function. GABA interneurons are also a major target of dopamine fibres.

Within the cerebral cortex, GABAergic interneurons are the main source of inhibition. Researchers have consistently observed losses of GABAergic cells within the schizophrenia patient. Other researchers have discovered that a subpopulation of inhibitory neurons down-regulates the expression of markers of the GABAergic neuronal phenotype, in schizophrenia. This dysfunction is limited to a subclass of GABA neurons that express parvalbumin, within the prefrontal cortex. Alterations in GABAergic synapses, including the parvalbumin-basket subtype, have been further linked to some of the memory impairments observed in schizophrenia.

According to other findings, enhanced GABA activity at alpha(2) subunit containing GABA(A) receptors has improved the behavioural and electrophysiological measures of prefrontal function, in the schizophrenia patient (Lewis *et al*, 2008). GABA may also contribute towards the regulation of anxiety related symptoms (Weiten, 1995).

Scientists have discovered that both typical and atypical antipsychotic medications seem to work on dynorphin GABAergic neurons located within the nucleus accumbens shell, the central amygdaloid nucleus, and the midline thalamic central medial nucleus. These neurons are known to have a substantial binding affinity for antipsychotic drugs. The down-regulation of an enzyme that produces GABA has also been commonly observed in the schizophrenia patient, during several postmortem studies.

Serotonin (5-HT) is another important neurotransmitter that has been linked to schizophrenia. Scientists have discovered that serotonin suppresses activity within the dopamine system. As a result, diminished function of the serotonin 5-HT2C receptor could lead to a hyperactive dopamine and norepinephrine system. Serotonin may have additional effects over the regulation of a specific class of GABA interneurons.

Serotonin reduces the function of certain sodium currents in dissociated cortical neurons. These sodium channels have a major role in nerve transmission and in the integration of nerve impulses. Decreases in density of the serotonin transporter (SERT) have been discovered within the frontal cortex of the schizophrenia patient. Reduced RNA editing and expression of 5HT2CR has also been observed in schizophrenia.

According to other studies, several 5-HT receptor subtypes have been linked to both depression and suicide. More specifically, serotonin may have some effects over the individual's mood levels. Nonetheless, the expression of these receptors differs across various brain regions, and is moderated by sex (Anisman *et al*, 2008). This neurotransmitter also seems to have an effect over the individual's sleep patterns. Researchers have discovered that the activity of serotonin-releasing neurons is highest when animals are awake. Similarly, this activity declines during deeper stages of sleep (Weiten, 1995). A reduction in serotonin neurotransmission has also been consistently observed within the forebrains of suicide victims.

Accordingly, boosting levels of 5-HT has been a successful mode of treatment for depression. In addition, serotonin systems may interact with dopamine systems within the striatum. In view of that, the 5-HT1A and 5-HT2A receptors could be correlated to the pathophysiology of schizophrenia. Other scientists theorize that schizophrenia may result due to alterations in 5-HT signalling during brain development.

5-HT6 serotonin receptors are G protein coupled receptors with a high affinity for several atypical antipsychotics. Some of these medicines include olanzapine and clozapine. In theory, these receptors may enhance cognitive functioning in the patient.

According to Clarke, the newer atypical antipsychotic medications emphasize blockade of serotonin 2 receptors (5-HT2A and 5-HT2C subtypes), with weaker antagonism at D2 receptors. Recent research also seems to indicate that many types of antipsychotics act as inverse agonists at 5-HT2A and 5-HT2C receptors. As a result, the role of ligand independent receptor activity may be correlated to the etiology and treatment for schizophrenia. Clarke also asserts that the capacity of some cells in the brain to edit the 5-HT2C mRNA may be reduced in schizophrenia patients and increased in patients who had committed suicide. All of these findings seem to correlate serotonin to the pathology and inner workings of schizophrenia.

The neurodevelopmental theory of schizophrenia also has many proponents. According to this theory, the cause of schizophrenia may be due to developmental abnormalities that occur within a foetus, during the prenatal phase. Abnormal development within the hippocampus has been linked to both schizophrenia and autism.

The hippocampus undergoes substantial maturational changes through infant and juvenile life. Therefore an early insult to these changing structures will result in abnormal brain development, and the altered function of distant neural systems. Some type of vulnerability could then develop soon after birth. According to some researchers, a foetus, during the prenatal phase, is most vulnerable to such impairments.

Other evidence suggests that schizophrenia may evolve during development due to a disruption among certain groups of neurons within the cerebral cortex. This disruption is presumed to be caused by alterations in the migration of terminal differentiation of interneurons, which are responsible for the proper synchronization of cortical activity.

It is also possible that an early brain insult could come about through a viral infection. Exposure to a viral infection during the prenatal phase may be one possible cause of schizophrenia. This theory is based on the increased incidence of craniofacial asymmetries and dermatoglyphic irregularities that reflect an abnormal development of the ectoderm and the neural crest. Researchers believe that this may result due to a viral infection incurred between the first and second trimester of pregnancy. An endemic virus could also initiate schizophrenia via a direct brain lesion or by triggering an autoimmune response, during the neurodevelopmental stage of a genetically susceptible brain (Fruntes and Limosin, 2008).

There may be a correlation between viral infections and the etiology of schizophrenia. First of all, it is known that patients who suffer from autoimmune diseases, like rheumatoid arthritis, are half as likely to develop schizophrenia when compared to the general public. Other findings suggest that there is an immune system dysfunction within the schizophrenia patient. Therefore, a viral infection during pregnancy could influence the abnormal brain development that is consistently observed in schizophrenia.

Other studies suggest that persons are at a higher risk to develop schizophrenia when their mother has had an infection during pregnancy. Some possible infections can include influenza, measles or pneumonia. This theory is based on the knowledge that the human body produces cytokine chemicals in order to counteract infections of these sorts. Cytokines can produce fever, increase sleep, and decrease activity and appetite in the individual. According to other evidence, cytokines can also affect brain development and function of brain dopamine systems.

Lower membrane levels of polyunsaturated fatty acids (PUFA) have also been discovered in both men and women with schizophrenia. PUFA are provided to foetuses maternally and are crucial for normal brain function and development.

Maternal glucocorticoids may be a common pathway linking a variety of insults to the risk for psychiatric disorders. This latter mechanism is believed to work by way of a neurogenesis disruption at critical periods, or by altering the brain's sensitivity to stress. The risk to develop schizophrenia may be linked to the second month, while other psychiatric diseases may be linked to peaks at twelve weeks, fifteen weeks, or later gestational ages. The sex of the foetus could have some influence over these risk factors as well.

In theory, interstitial white matter neurons (IWMNs) are human cells that are believed to be adult remnants of an embryonic structure. An altered density of these cells should be taken as evidence of the subplate, and, therefore, of a developmental anomaly. Thus, this evidence suggests that schizophrenia could have an embryonic origin.

Other research indicates that many risk factors for schizophrenia can occur either prenatally or perinatally. An insult to an immature brain could also alter the normal developmental progression of changes in the neural networks.

An disruption among neuronal connections within the hippocampus, after birth, could lead to the development of schizophrenia. In fact, the connections between glutamate and GABA neurons are primarily established during this period of development. Therefore, developmental abnormalities during a period after birth may also contribute towards the development of schizophrenia.

In theory, problems with the neurosteroid regulation of GABA receptors could cause schizophrenia. Neurosteroids are potent modulators of the receptors that regulate development. Brain levels of neurosteroids vary with stress, anoxia and infection, and all of these factors are future predictors for schizophrenic psychopathology. Neurosteroids may also be responsible for long-lasting structural, functional and behavioural changes within an individual's brain.

Another possibility is that N-methyl-D-aspartate receptor hypofunction (NRH) may occur early in life and give rise to the later development of schizophrenia. Disturbances in working memory (WM) could also indicate a possible neurodevelopmental origin of schizophrenia. Siblings at risk for schizophrenia who go on to develop the manifest illness demonstrate worse WM in childhood as compared to their siblings who do not go on to develop schizophrenia. This finding seems to suggest that persons with schizophrenia lack certain developmental features within the brain, correlated to working memory.

Central nervous system infections during childhood, like meningitis, may also be significant. Childhood meningitis can worsen an individual's cognition, and this is a known risk factor.

Furthermore, the offspring of women with schizophrenia are 10 times more likely to develop schizophrenia, in comparison to the average citizen. There is a great deal of evidence in which obstetric complications are associated with later schizophrenia. Other findings indicate that persons with schizophrenia, and the offspring of women with schizophrenia, consistently have lower birth weights than control subjects.

Nevertheless, the frequent occurrence of neurological soft signs in the patient, and in high-risk subjects during early life, implies the possibility that schizophrenia is a 'brain disease' reflecting pre- or perinatal insults during development (Krebs and Mouchet, 2007). Neurological soft signs, otherwise known as neurological examination abnormalities, may further characterize a subgroup of high-risk offspring who are at an elevated risk for psychopathology (Prasad *et al*, 2009).

Several proteins may also be linked to the development of schizophrenia. Scaffolding proteins are important regulators of 5-HT(2A) receptors (JA Allen, Yadav and Roth, 2008). Another protein of interest is the catechol-0-methyltransferase (COMT) enzyme, because it regulates dopamine within the prefrontal cortex.

It is believed that brain-derived neurotrophic factor (BDNF) may have some role in the birth of new neurons. Other researchers have found increased levels of BDNF protein within the frontal cortex of persons who were treated with antidepressants or antipsychotics. Furthermore, elevated C-reactive protein levels have been frequently observed in schizophrenia. Some researchers believe that this elevation may be associated with an evolution toward [sic] cognitive deficit and neuronal loss (Perron *et al*, 2008).

The Eph protein family influences neuron to neuron communication. These proteins control the structure of neurons known to be affected in schizophrenic patients. Eph proteins also control the ability of schizophrenia related neurons to efficiently respond to glutamate-induced signals. Some Eph family genes are also located in genomic regions that have been linked to schizophrenia.

Changes in the expression of postsynaptic density (PSD) proteins have also been discovered within the prefrontal cortex of the schizophrenia patient. Several alterations have been found in PSD protein expression, within the dorsolateral prefrontal cortex, that are lamina- and cell-specific in schizophrenia. PSD proteins mediate synaptic proteins and receptors at the cell membrane of the glutamatergic synapse. These proteins may alter receptor sensitivity to glutamate and modulate signaling cascades in glutamatergic synaptic transmission.

The G72 protein is also being studied because it activates D-serine oxidation through the D-amino acid oxidase (DAAO) enzyme, and excessive D-serine metabolism is known to disrupt glutamate signalling. According to other research, the protein dysbindin (DTNBP1), which plays a significant role in synaptic functioning, may also be connected to schizophrenia. A decrease of dysbindin protein expression in glutamatergic presynaptic terminal fields, within the hippocampus, has been discovered during studies conducted on the postmortem brain tissues of schizophrenia patients. Researchers are also interested in the dystrobrevin binding (DTNBD1) protein. This has been correlated into 'three high-risk haplotypes in DTNBD1' to schizophrenia.

Disturbances in the structure and function of the Homer proteins have also been linked to the pathophysiology of schizophrenia. Scientifically, they are a class of structural proteins that provide the selective segregation of proteins to the synapses.

Synapsin III is another protein that has been associated to schizophrenia. This protein coats vesicles containing neurotransmitters, and it has a role both in brain development and in the regulation of neurotransmission. The synapsin III gene is located on chromosome 22, and this area is theorized to be a schizophrenia susceptibility locus. Lower levels of synapsin I and II have also been consistently observed in the schizophrenia patient.

Proline dehydrogenase (PRODH) is another important protein in schizophrenia research. The gene for PRODH may increase the individual's risk to develop schizophrenia (Koike, 2008). Decreases of the RGS4 protein have also been discovered in the brains of schizophrenia patients.

The neuronal protein kinase Cdk5 could also be significant. This protein is involved in synapse formation and loss, and this is a mechanism that has been linked to adult brain function and neuropsychiatric disease. Stathmin is a substrate of Cdk5, and a tubulin-binding protein. There are abnormally high levels of stathmin and phosphor-stathmin within the schizophrenia patient's brain.

Likewise, lowered levels of reelin have been observed in patients with schizophrenia, depression and bipolar disorder. Reelin has a role in the normal migration of brain neurons, and in the positioning of nerve cells during development. Furthermore, this protein and the receptors that bind it are necessary for normal nerve cell function and cognitive processes. According to some studies, patients with schizophrenia have 50% less reelin in their bodies, when compared to persons with good mental health. Decreases of reelin have also been associated with decreases of the enzymes that metabolize glutamate.

Centrosomal proteins may also be important, because they have a role in cortical development. Some scientists theorize that the perturbation of centrosomal function could contribute towards the development of schizophrenia and other mental disorders. The 14-3-3 family of proteins have also been correlated to schizophrenia and bipolar disorder.

Furthermore, elevated levels of the amino acid glycine have been discovered within the cerebrospinal fluid and postmortem frontal lobe of schizophrenia patients. Glycine has been used as an adjuvant therapy for schizophrenia. Increases of glycine may improve symptoms because it activates the NMDA receptor. A schizophrenia susceptibility locus may also be located within or nearby the glycine transporter gene SLC6A5 (Deng et al, 2008).

The amino acid derivative homocysteine has also been linked to schizophrenia. Elevated levels of homocysteine will increase levels of the amino acid methionine, which in turn controls the expression level of many genes that have been linked to schizophrenia. Homocysteine may have some further influence over the NMDA receptor as well.

Schizophrenia researchers are also studying the neuropeptide Y (NPY). Neuropeptides are strings of amino acids. Researchers have discovered reduced levels of NPY within the schizophrenia patient's central nervous system. They have also uncovered evidence which suggests that antipsychotics may actively increase levels of NPY within the body.

The main NPY receptor, YI, may be associated to the hyperactivity of dopaminergic pathways in aggression and anxiety related domains. This receptor may also have effects on the human immune system.

Scientists have produced further evidence linking glial-cell dysfunction to schizophrenia. These cells provide structural support and insulation for neurons (Weiten, 1995). They may also mediate the function of glutamate, and this contributes towards the alterations in glutamatergic transmission that have been observed amid several major mental disorders. A significant reduction in glutamate neurotransmission is also known to involve the glia, which is regulated by several genetic markers of schizophrenia.

Likewise, the neurotransmitter acetylcholine (ACh) has been correlated with several symptoms in schizophrenia. ACh is the only transmitter between motor neurons and voluntary muscles. This transmitter is believed to affect attention, arousal and memory (Weiten, 1995). Inglis postulates that a deeper insight as to the inner workings of antipsychotic medicines may be attained through further studies of this neurotransmitter.

The stress-induced over-expression of acetylcholinesterase (AChE) impairs glutamatergic synaptic organization and function, which then impairs cognition. This theorized hyperfunction of AChE is based on the observation that anti-AChE therapies may improve cognition. The over-expression of AChE is also known to decrease the number of surface glutamate receptors in an individual's brain. Therefore, altered AChE expression may also have some role in the pathology of schizophrenia.

A significant reduction in histamine 1 and muscarinic 1 receptor expression has also been observed in schizophrenia. Accordingly, genetically mediated histamine and muscarinic mechanisms, which have a major role in the functions of memory, attention and learning, are also important elements in schizophrenia research.

Modern studies indicate that the individual's nitric oxide (NO) system is dampened in schizophrenia. This is due to the discovery that the plasma levels of NO metabolite (NOx) are significantly lower in schizophrenia patients, when compared to control subjects. After treatments through risperidone, the schizophrenia patient's plasma levels of NOx increased significantly.

The hypothalamic-pituitary-adrenal (HPA) axis is also a target of schizophrenia research. Both stress and the dysregulation of the HPA axis could contribute towards the development of schizophrenia and depression. Other evidence suggests that the transition to psychosis, and the initial phase of psychosis, may be linked to the hyperactivity of the HPA axis. The glucocorticoid receptor may also be important in schizophrenia research, because it regulates HPA axis activity.

The human olfactory system has also been correlated to schizophrenia. In particular, abnormalities in olfaction, olfactory bulb morphology, and olfactory-evoked response potentials have been observed in both patients with schizophrenia and their first-degree family members. This subgroup is also known to suffer from odour identification deficits. Since olfactory deficits have a high heritability, such deficits could serve as a biological marker in an individual's genetic liability to develop schizophrenia.

Scientists have also noted that changes in olfactory function occur in direct temporal relation to the onset of psychosis. A person who suffers from schizophrenia may also demonstrate poorer performance than controls on measures of olfactory function. Accordingly, persons with severe olfactory deficits may be at a higher risk to develop a schizophrenia spectrum disorder.

Schizophrenia can be conceived as a disorder that is characterized by deficits in early information processing, which then leads to difficulties in the inhibiting or filtering of irrelevant internal and external stimuli. These deficits may cause the individual to become overloaded with excessive stimuli which in turn could lead to a breakdown of cognitive functioning and in distinguishing of self from non-self.

P50 gating deficits have also been implicated in schizophrenia. In fact, auditory sensory gating deficits are widely considered as a leading endophenotype for schizophrenia (Hall *et al*, 2010). Other researchers have discovered deficits in prepulse inhibition (PPI) among patients that suffer from chronic schizophrenia. PPI is the ability to filter sensory inputs. Patients with PPI deficits will usually remain in a state of cognitive fragmentation and sensory inundation.

Increasing evidence suggests that cognitive dysfunction is a more reliable and sensitive predictor of long-term outcome than clinical symptoms. The patient's prognosis may also be determined through context processing, which is an executive control function related to the ability to maintain and use context information to guide appropriate responses. Many schizophrenia patients demonstrate context processing impairments over a range of tasks. There may be a link between context processing and the social outcomes of the schizophrenia patient.

An important aspect of cognitive control is the ability to detect and correct performance errors. This process is known as error-related negativity (ERN). The schizophrenia patient's ERN is abnormally reduced, even in cases when he is aware of his errors. Consequently, there may be further abnormalities located within the anterior cingulate cortex region of the brain.

From my own experience, I would have to conclude that the mental state of dreaming resembles a state of psychosis. Possibly either brain lesions, or a chemical disruption within two highly specific brain regions could selectively modify both psychotic and dream-like states.

The analysis of tens to hundreds of genes for hundreds of patients may be necessary in schizophrenia research. This seems to imply that current research, in the area of genetics, is truly at its infancy and that schizophrenia is an extremely complicated disorder.

8

Treating Schizophrenia

The main mode of treatment for schizophrenia is through antipsychotic medications. Although there is no cure at present, antipsychotic medicines have proven to be very effective in reducing the symptoms experienced by schizophrenia patients. Each individual possesses a unique biological makeup, with unique biological attributes. As a result, while a specific type of medication may be effective for one patient, it may not be equally effective for another patient. Therefore, psychiatric treatment is not a universal science.

Each schizophrenia patient will respond differently to the same antipsychotic medication. Therefore, there is no universal medicine for the schizophrenia patient, and likewise, there is no universal dosage. Every antipsychotic also differs with respect to potency. From my experience, 7.5 milligrams of olanzapine had more or less an equal effect on my body when compared to 300 milligrams of clozapine.

Antipsychotic medications have been divided into two main subgroups. Typical antipsychotics have been utilized since the middle of the twentieth century. Some typical antipsychotics include Haldol or its generic name haloperidol, Thorazine or chlorpromazine, Loxitane or loxapine, Trilafon or perphenazine, Mellaril or thioridazine, Navane or thiothixene, Stelazine or trifluoperazine, and Prolixin or fluphenazine. Typical antipsychotics are also labelled as first-generation medications, and in general, they have been known to cause more side effects. Some of these side effects include rigidity, persistent muscle spasms, tremors, and restlessness (National Institute of Mental Health, 2008). Impairments in sexual functioning, the experiencing of seizures, and possible liver or eye damage are other known side effects (Torrey, 1995). Side effects such as dry mouth and a fast heartbeat are some relatively tolerable side effects. Some researchers also hold the belief that typical medications are less effective, therapeutically, than atypical antipsychotics.

Atypical antipsychotics include Clozaril or its generic name clozapine, Risperdal or risperidone, Zyprexa or olanzapine, Seroquel or quetiapine, Serdolect or sertindole, Geodon or ziprasidone, and Aripiprazole or abilify. Introduced in the 1990's, atypical medicines were created to produce fewer side effects than typical antipsychotics. Torrey hypothesizes that while typical medicines target dopamine receptors, atypical medicines additionally target serotonin receptors. Accordingly, atypical antipsychotics have the capacity to affect multiple receptor types (Kim *et al*, 2009).

Nonetheless, it is still possible that atypical medicines will cause the same extrapyramidal side effects associated with typical antipsychotics. For example, risperidone caused me to experience muscle pains and rigidity. I also felt extremely restless at bedtime, because of this medication. Other atypical medicines have produced less painful side effects, like weight gain and a high degree of fatigue.

Next to denial, being subjected to an intolerable side effect is a main reason why many patients stop taking their medications. However, problems with memory can also pose a problem. When the side effects of an antipsychotic become too intolerable, the patient's psychiatrist will usually prescribe a different form of medication. Yet, every antipsychotic that I have ever taken caused some type of negative side effect in me.

When a patient experiences the side effect of sedation, he will usually be ordered to take his prescription at bedtime. In my case, both olanzapine and clozapine causes me to feel sedated, even throughout the entire day. The sedative effects of these medicines will force me into a state of deep sleep, within approximately one hour after I ingest them. Accordingly, it could be very dangerous for me to, for example, drive a car after I have taken these medicines. Every schizophrenia patient must also acknowledge any possible negative side effects on his daily life. In my case, the side effects of these medications will affect me to the point where I cannot remain awake for an extended period of time after I have taken them.

Weight gain is another predominant side effect of many antipsychotic medicines. According to a study conducted in Japan, there are genetic risk factors linked to olanzapine induced weight gain. Scientists have also associated weight gain with hyperlipidemia or type II diabetes (Carnahan *et al*, 2007). On a further note, a scientific correlation has been drawn between obesity and impaired cognitive functioning, even in mentally healthy persons. Other researchers have discovered a significant inverse association between body mass index (BMI) and metabolic activity, within the prefrontal cortex and cingulate gyrus (Volkow *et al*, 2009).

Moreover, scientists have discovered that newer atypical antipsychotics, like olanzapine and clozapine, may cause cardiovascular risks like ischemic heart disease, or diabetes (Tang, 2008). According to other research, an autonomic dysregulation within both the heart and pupil seems to be prevalent in schizophrenia (Bär *et al*, 2008). In view of that, every schizophrenia patient should also undertake a routine diabetes screening. It may also be necessary to monitor the patient's blood pressure, sugar glucose and weight.

Another study links antipsychotic medications to an increased risk for stroke. Researchers indicate that this risk may be higher in patients who are treated with atypical antipsychotics, as opposed to typical antipsychotics. Persons who suffer from dementia also seem to be at a higher risk for stroke, when compared to individuals without dementia. As a result, the use of antipsychotics for patients with dementia should be avoided when possible (Douglas and Smeeth, 2008).

Other studies suggest the potentiality that patients who suffer from type 2 diabetes and schizophrenia may exhibit more cognitive impairments, when compared to individuals that are affected by either schizophrenia or diabetes alone (Dickinson *et al*, 2008). Actually, schizophrenia patients with diabetes exhibit greater impairments in both physical and mental-health quality of life. They often report less satisfaction with their health, but not in other domains of life (Dickerson *et al*, 2008).

In my case, I experienced substantial weight gain while taking olanzapine and clozapine. These medicines effectively treated my symptoms, however, my body fat eventually increased and this caused me to become increasingly unhappy with my self-image. At one point, I gained approximately 55 pounds since the time when I was first diagnosed with schizophrenia. Mathematically, this works out to be approximately 44% of my previous body weight.

This increase in body mass also eventually caused me to hold the belief that I was physically unattractive. Nevertheless, this side effect was much more tolerable than any of my previous experiences with muscle stiffness and pain. Therefore, I decided to accept the side effects of my newly prescribed medicines, and I dealt with this problem by taking up some athletic hobbies. It all worked out in the end though, because I actually prefer the larger and more muscular physique that I have today.

Researchers theorize that obesity, due to olanzapine, may be associated with arcuate hypothalamic nucleus (Arc) H1 receptor expression and a downregulated ventromedial hypothalamic nucleus (VMH). Clozapine has an additional risk factor in that one of its side effects could produce agranulocytosis, which is a loss of white blood cells. During the preliminary stages of my clozapine treatments, I had to have my blood work checked every two weeks to monitor this potentially lethal side effect. Today, after being stable on that medicine for several years, I am only required to check my blood count on a monthly basis.

Clozapine effectively blocks the serotonin receptor 5HT-2A. The negative symptoms of schizophrenia are believed to be linked to the abnormal functioning of this serotonin receptor. Clozapine treatments have also been associated with the potentiation of GABA(B)-inhibitory neurotransmission and reduced GABA(A) inhibitory neurotransmission (Liu *et al*, 2009). In fact, clozapine has effectively treated patients who do not respond to other typical or atypical antipsychotics. According to another study, low discontinuation rates were observed with respect to the use of clozapine, and the continuation of clozapine treatments were correlated with real-world improvements in functional and clinical outcomes (Wheeler *et al*, 2009). Treatment by way of clozapine is also known to be superior in cases of treatment resistant or refractory schizophrenia. As a result, lowering serotonin expression may also have some beneficial effects.

On the other hand, the antipsychotic ziprasidone may prevent weight gain. However, patients who experience problems with weight gain should maintain a regular exercise program, if their current prescription is effective.

One of the worst possible side effects is muscle pain and stiffness. An acute dystonic reaction is the stiffening of muscles on one side of the neck and jaw (Torrey, 1995). I experienced sharp pains in my mouth and jaw while taking loxapine and risperidone. Patients who experience these side effects should immediately consult with their psychiatrist.

Bodily twitching and tremors are other possible side effects. On a positive note, all of the latter side effects can be reversed within several minutes, through the administration of an anticholinergic drug (Torrey, 1995). A lack of spontaneity, or akinesia, can be a further side effect of either an antipsychotic medicine or the disease itself.

When I was taking risperidone, Dr. Lupton wanted to test its efficacy. She also prescribed another medicine to counteract the side effect of muscle pains. After some time, and an increase in dosage, that antipsychotic caused feelings of akathisia within me, and I would begin to experience feelings of intense restlessness. In effect, I could not remain still during bedtime, and I needed to continually move my limbs to counteract these feelings. I lost feelings of inner peace due to that medicine. These side effects, alone, were powerful enough to make me dread the treatment of my illness.

I never became drowsy or fatigued during the day when taking either loxapine or risperidone, though conversely, I had problems with insomnia. Nevertheless, it is also possible that the disease itself could have caused my problems with sleeplessness. In any case, Dr. Lupton prescribed a small dosage of ativan to help me sleep at night. I did not notice any negative side effects from this medicine at that time.

The antipsychotic quetiapine was actually quite effective in the treatment of my symptoms. I felt a greater overall sense of awareness while taking this medicine. However, similar to risperidone, this medication caused extreme nasal congestion as a side effect, during bedtime. This time, my sleep patterns were mainly disrupted through this possible allergic reaction. Even though I felt substantial improvements with my attention and cognition, I would experience too many problems while trying to sleep. Disruptions in my sleep patterns would eventually become too difficult to endure.

Somnambulism is another possible side effect of quetiapine. This impairment emerges in normal mechanisms of arousal where motor behaviors are activated without full consciousness (Hafeez and Kalinowski, 2007). Patients may sit up, fumble with objects, or mumble, all while in a state of deep non-rapid eye movement.

On a general note, antipsychotics can also cause constipation. This side effect usually occurs when the individual is taking a new prescription. Over time, the severity of this side effect usually decreases to a tolerable level (Torrey, 1995).

Neuroleptic malignant syndrome is another possible side effect. This illness involves severe muscle stiffness and tremors that can lead to fever and other severe complications. Side effects impeding cognition are also possible. Typical antipsychotics are more likely to cause these problems, when compared to atypical medicines (McEvoy *et al*, 2010).

The worse possible side effect, though, is the eventual development of tardive dyskinesia. Patients with tardive dyskinesia experience random and involuntary movements within their tongue and mouth. Jerky and purposeless movements in other body parts may accompany these uncontrolled movements. Tardive dyskinesia can also become a potentially permanent side effect. Scientists theorize that dopamine-type 2 (D2) receptor up-regulation may be the primary root behind this disorder. Probably only a continuously high D2-receptor blockade will cause this type of receptor up-regulation. Parkinsonism is another possible side effect of antipsychotic medicines, which also affects the individual's motor skills.

Even so, both of these movement disorders have been observed in un-medicated patients. Tardive dyskinesia may be correlated to the negative symptoms of schizophrenia and executive or frontal lobe impairment. Thus, although tardive dyskinesia is a serious condition, it is not believed to be solely caused through antipsychotic treatments.

According to one case study, a 24-year-old woman of African descent developed tardive dyskinesia, after 9 months of treatment with fifteen milligrams of aripiprazole. When the patient discontinued this treatment and switched to quetiapine, her tardive dyskinesia related symptoms disappeared rapidly (Abbasian and Power, 2008).

Individuals who take antipsychotic agents are also at risk to develop hyperprolactinemia. As a hormonal abnormality, elevated prolactin levels can interfere with the reproductive, endocrine, and metabolic systems. Other consequences of this condition include menstrual disturbances, galactorrhea, gynecomastia, breast cancer, infertility, decreased bone mineral density, and possible sexual dysfunction (Bostwick *et al*, 2009). First generation antipsychotics are more likely to cause this side effect, though risperidone and paliperidone may also increase prolactin secretion. The risk of developing hyperprolactinemia can sometimes be minimized by using the lowest effective dose of a particular medicine.

Generally speaking, psychiatrists must utilize the method of trial and error to find the best combination of medicines for each individual patient. Moreover, antipsychotic medications can be ineffective in the treatment of negative symptoms. In these cases, the combined use of antipsychotic and selective serotonin reuptake inhibitor (SSRI) antidepressant medications may solve this problem (Kapur and Remington, 2001). Finding the most effective and tolerable set of medications is a process that many schizophrenia patients must endure, before they achieve a state of remission.

The patient's psychiatrist must also monitor possible psychological complications. Patients who experience problems with aggression may be ordered to take a high potency conventional or typical antipsychotic. Other patients that exhibit high levels of agitation or excitement may be treated through adjunctive medicines. Clozapine can address problems with psychogenic polydipsia, which is a problem where the individual drinks water in a compulsive fashion (McEvoy *et al*, 2010).

The majority of medical experts believe in the policy of prescribing newer atypical antipsychotics as the first line of treatment. Conventional antipsychotics are mainly prescribed in three situations. First, typical antipsychotics are prescribed to patients who have exhibited a good clinical response to these medicines, without experiencing any major side effects. Secondly, they are prescribed for patients who require intramuscular medications (IM). IM medications are administered by way of an injection into the muscle, and at present, there are no atypical antipsychotics available in this form. Lastly, typical antipsychotics are utilized in cases where the acute management of aggression or violence is needed, especially in patients who need depot medications (McEvoy *et al*, 2010).

Depot medications are released into the patient's body over several weeks, and are also administered through a medical syringe (Journals of the Royal College of Psychiatrists). This method is usually utilized for patients who do not comply with oral forms of treatment, or those who hold a persistent denial of their illness (McEvoy, 2006). Patients with high relapse rates, those who are open to drug treatment, and those with a high level of insight may also qualify for depot treatments (Heres *et al*, 2008). In other cases, an antipsychotic may be administered intravenously for the purpose of dose reduction. This method is also used to improve the efficacy of a medication, or it may be used to reduce the prevalence of any extrapyramidal side effects.

Anticholinergics are another category of medicines that are used in the treatment of schizophrenia. Their major side effect decreases the efficacy of an antipsychotic medication. Therefore, anticholinergics are usually withheld, and are mainly used to treat the ill side effects of an antipsychotic (Torrey, 1995).

Atypical medicines are recommended for patients who experience problems with dysphoria. Atypical medications can also address problems with suicidal behaviour or comorbid substance abuse (McEvoy *et al*, 2010). Nonetheless, in all of these cases, professional psychological counselling will also be necessary, in conjunction with antipsychotic treatments. This is necessary because the surfacing of some psychological problems may not be due to the illness itself. Hence, the patient's attitude or life experiences can also cause many psychological problems.

Another study, conducted in Germany, indicates that atypical antipsychotics are more effective for severe cases of schizophrenia. In this study, patients treated through atypical antipsychotics received significantly less prescriptions for anticholinergics. In contrast, typical antipsychotics were more effective in reducing re-hospitalization rates (Stargardt *et al,* 2008).

However, in Malaysia, researchers have observed a similar quality of life among patients who were treated with either conventional or atypical antipsychotics. Clinical and health outcomes, extrapyramidal side effects, and patient employment statuses were also similar after one year (Chee, 2009). Contrarily, a study conducted in Canada connects the greatest advantage of atypical medicines to a reduction in motor side effects (Agid *et al*, 2008).

It appears these newer atypical medicines are more effective for improving cognition and executive functioning, and in reducing negative symptoms. Furthermore, these medications are believed to increase prefrontal cortical dopamine. The atypical antipsychotic drug-induced augmentation of glutamatergic neurotransmission is sensitive to blockade by dopamine depletion and dopamine D1 receptor antagonist. This is a mechanism which makes atypical antipsychotics more effective than typical antipsychotics.

Another difference between typical and atypical medicines is based on the release of acetylcholine (ACh) within the brain. Atypical antipsychotics are known to preferentially increase ACh and dopamine release in the medial prefrontal cortex and hippocampus. An antagonist to the M1 muscarinic receptor may be a source of this release, and that the M1 antagonist telenzepine and a 5HT-1A antagonist may attenuate this release. It is theorized that this is a biological mechanism that could be correlated to the schizophrenia patient's ability to reverse cognitive dysfunction.

All scientists agree that both typical and atypical medicines effectively antagonize D2-dopaminergic receptors. However, most atypical medicines also alter noradrenergic transmission. This may be important, because mesocortical and mesolimbic dopaminergic neurons are differentially altered in schizophrenia and may participate in distinct aspects of the disorder. In effect, hyperactivity of mesolimbic dopaminergic transmission has been associated with positive symptoms, while hypoactivity of mesocortical dopaminergic transmission may be correlated to negative symptoms. These mechanisms may potentially explain the differences in efficacy between typical and atypical antipsychotics.

Even though it is widely known that antipsychotic medications target dopamine receptors, how the drugs actually produce their therapeutic effect is essentially unknown. Even though antipsychotics will block the effects of dopamine on the electrical activity of a neuron in seconds, a period of several weeks is needed to produce their remedial effects. Further improvements have also been noted following several months of treatment. Antipsychotics are theorized to work on dopamine pathways to override the abnormal circuitry in the brain that may have resulted during development. This hypothesis could explain why antipsychotic medicines take so long to become effective.

Additionally, antipsychotic drugs have not been formally approved for the treatment of children and adolescents. However, this subgroup is still prescribed antipsychotic medications for non-specific behavioral control. Consequently, the possible side effects of antipsychotic medications on non-adults still need to be further studied and examined.

Treatments for the elderly population, through clozapine, may also be problematic. Potentially fatal agranulocytosis, myocarditis, seizures, and adverse metabolic effects are some known side effects (Gareri *et al*, 2008).

According to many studies, 50% of patients that take antipsychotics will experience significant side effects. The individual's unique metabolism plays a major role in this respect. Persons who are ultrarapid metabolizers can fail to respond to a standard dose of antipsychotic medications. Similarly, persons who are poor metabolizers may be prone to adverse side effects at standard doses.

Antipsychotics can also interact with other drugs. For example, smoking cigarettes can increase the individual's rate of metabolism. To offset this effect, a higher dose may be required. Alcohol and illicit drugs can also have adverse effects, when combined with a prescribed medicine. Therefore, psychiatrists must know their patient's entire drug history, including other forms of prescriptions, to avoid any ill effects from multiple drug interactions.

Smoking cigarettes, in interaction with genetic risk factors, can also lead to the development of metabolic syndrome (Onat *et al*, 2006). Measuring the patient's body mass index may predict the development of this illness. An increase in abdominal obesity and a family history of diabetes may also be relevant factors (WD, 2008).

Changing a prescribed antipsychotic medicine is a viable choice for persons who experience intolerable side effects. The development of symptoms associated with tardive dyskinesia is another good reason to change one's prescription. Patients that continue to experience positive or negative symptoms, or those who have suffered from a relapse should also be treated with a newer antipsychotic. Likewise, individuals with cognitive problems, or those who want to improve their level of functioning may also need a change in their prescription. Patients who exhibit disorganized forms of behaviour, agitation, or mood related problems would also be strong candidates for a newer mode of treatment (McEvoy *et al*, 2010).

On the other hand, patients who are functioning well and those who experience few, yet tolerable side effects should continue to take their current prescription. Persons who could pose as a physical danger to either themselves or other persons, when extremely ill, should also temporarily remain on their current mode of treatment. Likewise, patients who have compliance problems and those who are taking depot medications should continue their existing treatments. Finally, patients who have recovered from a relapse within the last six months, and those who are enduring personal stress factors should also remain on their current prescription, until ordered to do otherwise by their psychiatrist (McEvoy *et al*, 2010).

There are three main methods that psychiatrists use when changing a prescription. Initially, the old medication may be stopped immediately, and a new one may be started in its place. The advantages in this method are a reduced risk of medication errors and intolerable side effects. Secondly, psychiatrists may gradually reduce the old medication, while systematically increasing the newer medication. This method reduces the possible surfacing of any withdrawal symptoms. Thirdly, a psychiatrist may discontinue the older treatment when a newer antipsychotic is prescribed at its full therapeutic dose (McEvoy *et al*, 2010). The advantage in this case is a reduced risk of relapse. Most medical professionals prefer the last two methods to protect their patient from a possible relapse.

From a technical standpoint, some high potency typical antipsychotics include haloperidol and fluphenazine. Psychiatrists usually prescribe a starting dose of these medicines at between 2 to 5 milligrams per day. The average target dose of these medicines ranges from 5 to 10 milligrams per day. For persons with recurrent episodes, doctors will usually prescribe between 8 to 12 milligrams of haloperidol per day, and between 10 to 15 milligrams of fluphenazine per day. The high potency atypical antipsychotic risperidone is usually started at around 1 to 2 milligrams per day. Its average target dose is 4 milligrams per day, and for recurrent episodes, the average target dose starts at approximately 6 milligrams per day (McEvoy *et al*, 2010).

Perphenazine, which is a medium potency typical antipsychotic, will be initially administered at a dose of 2 to 12 milligrams per day. Its target dose is 20 milligrams per day and a daily dose of 32 milligrams is recommended for patients with recurrent episodes. On the other hand, olanzapine is a medium potency atypical medicine. Its recommended starting dose ranges from between 5 and 10 milligrams per day, and its average target dose may vary at around 10 to 15 milligrams per day. In cases of recurrent episodes, psychiatrists will usually prescribe between 15 to 20 milligrams per day (McEvoy *et al*, 2010).

The low potency typical antipsychotic thioridazine has a starting dose of 50 to 125 milligrams per day. The average target dose for this medication ranges from between 250 to 300 milligrams per day, with a recurrent episode target dose of 400 milligrams per day (McEvoy *et al*, 2010). Quetiapine, ziprasidone, and clozapine are three low potency atypical antipsychotics. The average starting dose for quetiapine ranges at around 50 to 100 milligrams per day. Its average target dose is 300 milligrams per day, and its target dose for recurrent episodes is situated at between 300 to 600 milligrams per day. The medication ziprasidone has a recommended starting dose that ranges from between 40 to 80 milligrams per day. Its average target dose ranges from 80 to 120 milligrams per day, and its recurrent episode target dose is 160 milligrams per day. Lastly, the recommended starting dose for clozapine ranges from between 25 to 50 milligrams per day. The average target dose for clozapine is 300 milligrams per day, and its recurrent episode target dose ranges somewhere between 400 to 450 milligrams per day.

Most typical and atypical antipsychotics have a trial length that lasts for approximately six to seven weeks. Clozapine, on the other hand, has a trial length of 12 weeks. If the patient lacks a positive response to a proper dosage of medicines within an adequate trial length, his psychiatrist may prescribe a different medication. The next medicine of choice will be based on the patient's medical history, including both positive and negative symptoms, in addition to the type of response that the patient exhibited with respect to any previous medications.

It is possible that less frequent dosing could lower the patient's chance to develop any ill side effects. Many antipsychotics need not be administered on a daily basis. This theory is based on the findings that sustained D2 blockade is not required in the treatment for schizophrenia. Likewise, while the binding of D2 receptors is necessary, the optimal anti-psychotic may be responsible for D2 transience. Subsequently, daily treatments may be unnecessary. In contrast, other researchers have observed greater hostility in patients who have shorter lengths of exposure to antipsychotic medications (Betensky *et al*, 2008).

It is also possible that a particular antipsychotic will lose its efficacy. Even though current therapies are beneficial, they often lose their effectiveness. As a result, there is a chance that the patient may need a change in his prescription, even in cases where he has been healthy and stable for a long period of time. Thus, a relapse is always possible, under many different types of circumstances.

Accordingly, newer medicines are being constantly developed to address this potential problem. Some scientists categorize aripiprazole as a third generation antipsychotic. This class of medication functions as a dopamine-serotonin system stabilizer. Aripiprazole may be based on a new pharmacological profile, because it is differentiated by a partial agonist effect on the D2 and D3 dopaminergic receptors (Limosin *et al*, 2008). This medicine also effectively treats all of the dimensions in schizophrenia, including positive, negative, depressive, and anxious symptomatologies. Furthermore, it has significant advantages in tolerability when compared to typical antipsychotics (Bhattacharjee and El-Sayeh, 2008). Though currently used as a substitution for other antipsychotics, scientists are researching its use as an initial mode of treatment, based on its beneficial effects in the area of cognition.

Paliperidone is another promising antipsychotic. A recent study in Greece compared treatments with paliperidone extended release (ER) to treatments through risperidone, olanzapine, quetiapine, aripiprazole and ziprasidone, over a one year period. Patients treated with paliperidone ER had a higher number of stable days when compared to the other patients. Their treatment costs were also lower in comparison (Geitona *et al*, 2008).

Studies are also being conducted on glutamate antagonists. As an add-on treatment, patients who were treated with topiramate experienced a significant decline in negative symptoms, positive symptoms, and schizophrenic psychopathology. This medicine also had a further benefit in controlling the side effect of weight gain (Afshar *et al*, 2009).

A further study was conducted on the non-classical prescriptions of antipsychotic medicines. These prescriptions were usually inherited from another clinician, regardless of any efficacy factors. More than 60% of these prescriptions were clinically sound. Prescriptions that were not clinically sound appeared to reflect upon a problematic relationship between the doctor and his patient. Therefore, the relationship between a patient and his doctor is also essential to a good prognosis. In my mind, an unconditional form of trust must be established between the patient and his psychiatrist for a full recovery (Veronese *et al*, 2008).

As a psychological adjunctive mode of treatment, cognitive behavioural therapy (CBT) can also be an effective form of treatment for patients that exhibit problems with persisting symptoms. According to some studies, a strong correlation exists between patient insight and the severity of his symptoms (Granholm *et al*, 2007). Other studies further suggest that temperament is linked to cognition. Subsequently, CBT can address problems related to patient insight and quality of life.

CBT teaches patients how to assess their psychotic symptoms and psychologically cope with these symptoms. Patients will learn to test the reality of their thoughts and perceptions, how to 'not listen' to their voices, and how to shake off the apathy that often immobilizes them (National Institute of Mental Health, 2008). The techniques involved in CBT include reality testing, normalization, the enhancement of coping strategies, the development of trust, and work on behavioural reactions to symptoms of psychosis (Favrod *et al*, 2004).

Additional studies have proven that CBT is effective in treating negative and positive symptoms, and in ameliorating the severity of an individual's symptoms. Thus, patients who experience complications with standard forms of treatment may benefit from CBT. Other research indicates that CBT may be used to attenuate negative thoughts and emotions tied to the formation, expression, and maintenance of verbal auditory hallucinations (England, 2006). In fact, the best treatment known for persistent negative symptoms is centred on the combination of an optimal dose of a medicine and some form of psychosocial therapy (Carpenter, 1996).

In one particular case, a patient has improved his self-management skills, in relation to his delusions and hallucinations, through CBT. In other cases, patients have reported a decrease in the frequency of their auditory hallucinations, and they were also able to acknowledge the fact that these voices were formed internally. Psychological problem solving modules have further motivated patients to maintain their personal hygiene, and result in an increase in their overall self-esteem. Moreover, CBT has been proven to effectively treat suicidal thoughts, in patients that remain in a state of psychosis.

Other research demonstrates that CBT can improve the self-functioning of elderly patients who suffer from chronic schizophrenia. This mode of therapy has also effectively decreased depression, anxiety and hopelessness in some patients (Warman *et al*, 2005). Patients who suffer from acute psychotic episodes can also benefit through CBT. Equally, other evidence suggests that CBT may effectively reduce the risk of relapse, in patients who suffer from chronic states of psychosis. CBT has also increased medication compliance in both schizophrenia and bipolar patients (Marcinko and Read, 2004).

CBT is known to be an effective mode of treatment for unipolar depression, generalized anxiety disorder, panic disorder, posttraumatic stress disorder, obsessive-compulsive disorder, and some social phobias. Other studies indicate that CBT is superior to antidepressants in the treatment of some forms of adult depression (Butler *et al,* 2006).

Hence, CBT is a mode of education that improves the patient's personal insight into his illness. It improves the coping methods of schizophrenia patients through improved adherence and symptom management. Theoretically, CBT may also reduce hyperactivity within the amygdala.

Cognitive adaptation training (CAT) is another form of therapy. CAT has successfully improved the neuropsychological and functional abilities of adult patients. Psychoeducational programs, in general, may also reduce rehospitalization rates and the risk of relapse. Accordingly, inpatient-initiated psychoeducation may be a very cost-effective method of treatment (Vickar *et al,* 2009).

Treatments through clinical holistic medicine (CHM) have also been studied. CHM is a short-term psychodynamic psychotherapy that is complemented with bodywork and philosophical exercises. It differs from other forms of psychiatry in that it abides by the medical principle do no harm. In some psychiatric practices, the latter principle is not always followed. For example, the patient's freedom for autonomy may be overridden when involuntary modes of treatment are necessary.

Some researchers believe that with respect to risk, harmfulness, and side effects, CHM may be superior over standard forms of psychiatric treatment (Ventegodt *et al,* 2007). CHM was initially designed to treat patients with non-organic mental illnesses. Thus, patients who suffer from the residual side effects of a mental disorder may benefit from this mode of treatment.

CHM seems to heal the patient, as opposed to treating his symptoms. According to one study, CHM is neither dangerous, nor harmful, nor does it have any side effects which may put the patient at risk to commit suicide. There is also no danger that the patient may develop psychosis as a direct result from CHM. Consequently, some researchers conclude that CHM is an efficient, safe and affordable cure for a broad range of mental illnesses (Ventegodt *et al,* 2007).

Other effective modes of psychosocial therapy are based on governmental vocational programs. Programs like the Indianapolis Vocational Intervention Program (IVIP) will have a positive impact on many patients. In a group of 50 participants, with either schizophrenia or schizoaffective disorder, 25 patients were enrolled in IVIP and the other patients were offered standard support services. Participants in the IVIP group worked significantly more weeks and had better average work performance when compared to the other group. Likewise, their levels of hope and self-esteem also increased, and contrarily, these elements had decreased in those who were enrolled within the standard support group (Lysaker *et al*, 2005b). Consequently, specialized therapies have proven to be extremely effective.

Occupational therapy, for persons with psychosis, was also studied in the United Kingdom. After a 12 month period, patients who were enrolled within an occupational therapy group demonstrated clinically significant improvements in the areas of relationships, independence performance, independence competence and recreation. Other patients exhibited a decrease in their negative symptoms (Cook *et al*, 2009).

Persons with a disability may also seek help through religion or other spiritual resources. A study conducted in Cambodia reveals that most patients primarily seek traditional or religious forms of medical treatment, when suffering from psychosis. This may be due to a lack of knowledge regarding mental health care and mental health facilities. According to some researchers, the development of psychiatry, in Cambodia, will be easier to facilitate if the general public were educated in the areas of mental illness and mental health services (Coton *et al*, 2008).

Personally, my faith in God has strengthened through my experiences with schizophrenia. This increase in spiritual faith is probably centred on my ability to recover from my illness, in addition to my high level of functioning. Other patients may have other reasons to build a strong foundation through religion. Entering into a religious community can offer the individual comfort, support, and a sense of belonging. An increase in spiritual beliefs can also be a highly effective coping mechanism when one battles a lifelong illness.

The amino acid D-serine can also alleviate some of the symptoms observed in schizophrenia. As a naturally occurring compound in the brain, D-serine is theorized to increase NMDA receptor activity. When NMDA receptor function is increased, the brain's capacity to form new neuronal connections and strengthen existing connections will also increase. The addition of D-serine to antipsychotic treatments has also been correlated with significant improvements in the areas of negative symptoms and cognitive defects. Excessive amounts of D-serine in the brain may protect the subject from a decrease in NMDA receptor activity. Accordingly, persons with an abundant amount of D-serine may be less vulnerable to develop an illness like schizophrenia, when compared to individuals who have relatively low amounts of this amino acid.

Scientists have also linked D-cycloserine (DCS) to treatments for schizophrenia. DCS is a safe and partial activator of the excitatory glutamate receptor. Wright believes that DCS may be a useful therapeutic agent in anxiety, schizophrenia and depression. Treatments with DCS may also decrease amygdala activity, and produce a rapid extinction of fear responses.

Repetitive transcranial magnetic stimulation (rTMS) can also effectively treat schizophrenia and depression. Moghaddam theorizes that high frequency stimulation of the dorsolateral prefrontal cortex, which is known to alleviate the symptoms in depression, increases the release of serotonin and dopamine in the amygdala and limbic striatum. Similarly, low intensity stimulation of the parietal cortex, which is known to alleviate the hallucinatory symptoms of schizophrenia, may reduce dopamine and serotonin release within the amygdala and limbic striatum.

Nicotine is an ACh agonist that may also have therapeutic effects (Weiten, 1995). According to Anand, heavy smoking could essentially be an act of self-medication, which alleviates schizophrenic symptoms through the nicotinic receptors. Nicotinic agonists may also relieve neurocognitive deficits in the domain of behavioural attention. These deficits are known to be extremely disabling and difficult to treat. DMXB-A is both a pharmacological agent and a nicotinic agonist that is defective in many schizophrenia patients. During a clinical trial, Freedman has proven that DMXB-A may significantly improve attention and psychosocial dysfunction.

Lambe *et al* (2007) have has discovered that nicotine and the peptide hypocretin (orexin) directly excites the thalamocortical synapse. This synapse, located within the prefrontal cortex, is critical for executive aspects of attention. Patterns of activation within the prefrontal cortex are known to be disordered in schizophrenia. Accordingly, an interaction between nicotine and hypocretin could have profound effects over the individual's faculty of attention. Therefore, it is possible that the act of smoking may alleviate some symptoms, and have a therapeutic effect on the psychological elements of attention and cognition.

Almost 90% of persons that suffer from schizophrenia smoke cigarettes (Steinberg *et al*, 2005). Some patients smoke cigarettes to regulate their mood and reduce possible forms of stress. However, according to one study, schizophrenia patients who smoke cigarettes and take antipsychotic medications have a significantly higher risk of colon cancer and a lower risk of respiratory cancer compared with patients without schizophrenia (Hippisley-Cox *et al*, 2007). In contrast, bipolar patients who smoke have an equal risk of developing cancer, when compared to the average person. Hence, the risk of developing cancer due to smoking is still quite valid.

Electroconvulsive therapy (ECT) was invented in the late 1930's, and is still used as a mode of treatment today. In ECT, electrodes are attached over the temporal lobes to induce an electric shock. The purpose of this shock is to bring about a cortical seizure, which is then accompanied by convulsions (Weiten, 1995). The convulsive seizure usually lasts for approximately 30 seconds. During this seizure, the patient usually loses consciousness and then wakes in about one hour.

According to some patients, ECT is quite painful. On average, patients will receive between six to twenty treatments within a hospital setting. Although it is utilized for a variety of mental disorders, at current times, ECT is mainly used for patients that suffer from depression. The negative side effects associated with ECT include memory loss, impaired attention, and other cognitive deficits. According to Small, ECT produces both short and long-term intellectual impairments. However, such impairments are not universal, and are temporary in most cases (Weiten, 1995).

According to many medical professionals, patients that do not respond to any forms of antipsychotic medications should be considered for electroconvulsive therapy (Meltzer, 1992). In one case, a 20-year-old male patient was characterized as pharmacologically treatment-resistant. He failed to respond to all forms of psychopharmacological therapies, including clozapine, and his mental health had continued to decline. After receiving ECT as a monotherapy, he demonstrated a marked reduction of symptoms (Neuhaus *et al*, 2007). ECT was then continued for seven months and the patient was eventually discharged from a psychiatric hospital. After two years of tapered continuation ECT, and without any forms of prophylactic psychotropic medications, the patient remained in a state of remission.

In another case, a patient with an extreme case of schizophrenia, who did not respond well to any typical or atypical antipsychotics for seven years, responded well to acute ECT treatments (Shimizu *et al*, 2006). The patient continued treatment through ECT and eventually sustained a positive therapeutic response. Thus, ECT may be an effective mode of treatment for patients who are diagnosed with serious cases of refractory schizophrenia.

Additionally, ECT may be a preferable mode of treatment for pregnant females. Psychiatric medications, while effective for the mother, could be harmful to the fetus. In one case, a 34-year-old Caucasian female, who was thirteen weeks into her gestation period, received ECT treatments until three weeks after the birth of her child. Her symptoms of depression responded well to treatment, and she reported no complications other than pelvic pains and transient fetal arrhythmias. Under these circumstances, acute and maintenance ECT may be the primary choice of treatment for severely depressed or psychotic pregnant patients (Bozkurt *et al*, 2007).

Electroconvulsive therapy was also effective in treating a 92-year-old woman who could not tolerate her medications. In this case, because the woman refused treatment, her doctors had to obtain an informed consent from her family members. This was necessary because of the patient's increasing degree of dementia. In this case, no cognitive side-effects were observed during and after the two ECT sessions (Katagai *et al*, 2007).

ECT can also be used to prevent the possibility of relapse in relapse-prone patients. It is sometimes used for patients with persistent depression, bipolar disorder, schizoaffective disorder, and Parkinson's disease. Patients with unipolar affective disorders, long duration of admissions, and no history of previous admissions may also be strong candidates for treatment through ECT (Munk-Olsen *et al*, 2006). However, in some patients, there is a short electroencephalographic seizure or no seizure at the maximum stimulus intensity. In this case, the desired therapeutic effect may not be achieved (Suzuki *et al*, 2007a).

Some doctors regard ECT as an effective and safe treatment option that is remarkably stable (Munk-Olsen *et al*, 2006). The mechanisms linked to ECT include serotonin, norepinephrine, and dopamine receptor expression (Taylor, 2007).

On the subject of inpatient facilities, several factors are considered during the admittance phase. Schizophrenia patients who could pose as a physical harm to either themselves or other persons should be admitted into a medical hospital. Likewise, if the patient exhibits signs of severe disorganization or acute psychotic symptoms, admittance into a hospital setting should also be considered (McEvoy et al, 2010).

In other cases, inpatient facilities may be critical to the treatment process. In South Africa, patient discharges due to bed shortages have been correlated with higher rates of readmission (Niehaus *et al,* 2008). Therefore, an appropriate length of treatment within an inpatient facility may be necessary, for some patients.

On the other hand, it is possible that an individual, who is diagnosed with schizophrenia, will have no need to be admitted into an inpatient facility. In my particular case, I was given several opportunities to be treated in the comfort of my home. However, during those times, I was in a state of denial and I refused treatment. Eventually, I was admitted into a ward to enable the active monitoring of my antipsychotic treatments. In cases where the patient adheres to treatment, admittance into a hospital ward may be entirely avoidable.

For my final point, medical intervention prior to the full onset of an illness will usually result in the best possible outcome. The use of medical interventions prior to disease-onset in schizophrenia may reduce symptom severity and chronicity during the course of the illness. Prodromal diagnosing techniques are highly consistent and reliable. Prodromal patients are usually highly symptomatic, functionally impaired, cognitively impaired, and treatment seeking. Accordingly, these patients constitute a new clinical population in need of effective treatment and definition of a standard of care.

Individuals who are at a high risk to develop schizophrenia will exhibit an attenuated level of emotion-processing deficits. More specifically, at-risk groups will suffer from reduced emotion perception, self-reported anhedonia, and increased negative affect (Phillips and Seidman, 2008).

Olanzapine is most effective in the treatment of prodromal patients and probably the increases of the amino acid glycine may potentially relieve NMDA receptor hypofunction and promote neuronal plasticity. As a result, treating patients who are mildly symptomatic, and those who are at a high risk to develop schizophrenia, could be the most effective mode of treatment possible.

According to other researchers, treating patients during the prodrome stage, or during their first-episode of psychosis would be the best time to combat neurodegeneration. Neurodegeneration is theorized to result from neurochemical dysregulation during the onset of schizophrenia. A psychotic episode is known to cause a loss of cell processes and grey matter volume, and apoptosis. It also results in persistent symptomatology and functional impairments. Scientists have noted that treatments during the patient's first episode of psychosis often results in a robust response. Likewise, treatment during the prodrome stage may best delay the onset of an illness, mitigate its severity after onset, and prevent the onset of some symptoms entirely (Lieberman, 2007).

Psychological modes of treatment, like education and CBT, during the prodrome stage can also be beneficial. However, treating patients who display false positives for prodromal schizophrenia could be harmful, and this issue also needs to be addressed.

Undeniably, reducing the stigma associated with schizophrenia will have a positive effect on the treatment of all sick patients. An increasing stigmatization of persons with schizophrenia is currently widespread within the popular media of many societies. On some occasions, persons with schizophrenia are portrayed as hostile, violent, threatening, angry, and criminal. In my mind, this discrimination can create a potential barrier in the treatment of many patients. If we were to abrogate and repel all forms of societal stigma, most established forms of treatment should also be generally accepted. Likewise, patients who suffer from a mental illness will essentially face one less challenge during their recovery process.

If it were possible to predict the development of schizophrenia prior to its full onset, the individual would be better prepared to handle the mental states that come about due to psychosis and psychotic thoughts. The problem of denial could also be addressed, if we teach our children ideals that will negate the effects of societal stigma. Likewise, a relationship would be established between the patient and a certified doctor before any problematic symptoms surface. If this disease is effectively dealt with before its onset, the possibility of permanent brain damage can also be averted.

9

Psychological Counselling

Counselling from a mental health professional is also an essential element of the treatment process. To start with, all patients who suffer from a mental illness must be regularly monitored for the possibility of a relapse. This is the best reason to see a mental health counsellor on a regular basis. Secondly, being affected with schizophrenia can, indeed, be a highly traumatic experience for any human being. Even though psychiatric medications may treat the symptoms of schizophrenia, the individual may still suffer from other forms of psychological problems. According to one study, variations in emotion regulation and social cognition are predictive elements that have been associated with the coping of psychotic symptoms (Bak *et al*, 2008). Therefore, professional psychological counselling is significant to a full recovery from schizophrenia.

Under some circumstances, a schizophrenia patient may not have a social net to rely upon. Psychological counsellors can fulfill this role for the patient. Every individual that suffers from a personally traumatic event will need some type of social network. A social network can provide forms of moral support, including guidance counselling, problem solving assistance, and peer-to-peer relationships. Each individual will face differing social challenges. In my opinion, mental health professionals may be best suited to help the patient in this respect.

I am quite lucky to have family and friends that I can depend upon, to help me recover from my illness. The professional counselling that I rely on comes in the form of a mental health nurse. Actually, I have seen several nurses who have helped me with differing personal issues. My first nurse, Sharon, eventually stopped counselling me because she wanted to treat patients who were more severely ill in comparison. I have built a relationship with two other nurses, who have left the profession for differing reasons, including retirement and maternity leave. During the early stages of my illness, I saw Sharon on a weekly basis. Her first priority was to make certain that my symptoms were being properly treated. On every visit, we would chat and she would analyze my demeanour. Even when I had mistakenly believed that I was feeling well, Sharon was knowledgeable enough to observe that I was still suffering from other psychological problems, related to social withdrawal and poor self-esteem.

All of the nurses that I have seen had the ability to recognize if I was either healthy or sick, by the way I spoke. The job of my psychiatrist, on the other hand, is to find a combination of medicines that will effectively treat my symptoms. When the patient's symptoms are properly treated, the primary role of a counsellor will change. In essence, a counsellor must help the patient with any emotional issues that may arise due to his illness. It would be irresponsible for a medical system to treat an illness without providing any services to follow the patient's course and outcome.

As my health improved, my need to see a nurse diminished. The most important issues that I had discussed with Sharon usually related to Dr. Lupton's prognosis. In particular, I experienced problems with my self-perspective. After experiencing many extreme delusions, I would have problems differentiating my delusions from real world experiences. I shared my emotional responses to these delusions with Sharon. In reply, she taught me how to center my focus on the real, physical world.

During that period, I experienced significant problems while trying to distinguish real world events from my schizophrenic delusions. Therefore, I still had problems with delusions that I falsely believed were true. This is where problems with my self-confidence had evolved. Even after my symptoms were treated, I still possessed memories of many radical paranoid thoughts. After becoming relatively healthy, I still faced the problem of differentiating my psychotic thoughts, from my memories of the actual world.

Throughout my previous states of psychosis, the paranoid thoughts that I generated would often take full control over my identity, perspective of life, and overall attitude. I continued to occasionally experience problems with paranoia, even while my illness was in the process of being treated. The paranoid thoughts that I experienced at that time, though, did not have the same severity or control over my mind. My paranoid thoughts, during this period, were probably equal to purely random thoughts that any person could dismiss from his mind at will. By attending counselling sessions with

Sharon, I eventually learned how to analyze and differentiate these mild paranoid thoughts, from my normal thought processes.

Improvements in my self-confidence would eventually help me with this problem. As a primary step, I needed to acknowledge the fact that my prescribed medications were beneficial to my health. My problem with self-esteem originated from the period when I believed that I was healthy mentally, but was actually seriously ill. Being wrong about my previous states of mind caused me to lose confidence in my cognitive abilities, even after my symptoms were fully treated. Working with a counsellor helped to reinforce the belief that I was currently in a state of good mental health.

This was not an easy process though. At times, I would be able to recognize that I was healthy mentally, solely through Sharon's reactions. For example, when I was seriously ill, she would often take notes during our conversation. Dr. Lupton would then read these notes, to gain a better perspective over my present state of mind. On the other hand, when I was healthy, Sharon never seemed to be too concerned with my thoughts or statements. Instead, she taught me how to analyze these thought processes.

Whenever I wrongly believed that my normal thoughts were paranoid thoughts, Sharon would make me aware of the fact that I was not paranoid, and that my concerns were reasonable. Alternatively, when I wrongly believed that my illogical thoughts were rational, Sharon would correct me. Having a high level of confidence meant knowing when my thoughts were coherent, and when my thoughts were unintelligible.

Realizing the fact that some of my thoughts were rational boosted my overall self-esteem. It also alleviated some of the fears that I held with respect to experiencing a schizophrenic episode while in public. Deep in my mind, I held the fear that I may act strangely in public, in the same manner that I did during my college studies. I also feared that I might cause some kind of commotion while in public, due to my paranoid thoughts. In fact, I am a bit of a perfectionist. From what I had previously seen in the media, I believed that all persons with schizophrenia could potentially pose as a danger to other persons, even though I knew that I am, for the most part, not a violent person at heart. I feared the worst-case scenario, and this gave me enough reasons to withdraw from many social situations.

Having confidence in my state of mind also meant having confidence in my society's mental health care system. If my antipsychotic treatments were effective, this would necessarily entail the fact that I am also healthy mentally. Similarly, if these medicines were effective in alleviating my symptoms, perhaps psychological counselling could further help me with my illness. However, I still held the fear that I may experience a relapse, and this deeply affected my way of life.

After becoming stable on olanzapine, I realized that trial and error was a common element of the treatment process. I also subsequently realized that there could be many other treatment options for my illness. This gave me faith in the abilities of scientific researchers around the world. In time, I was able to establish hope in the possibility that they will produce a permanent cure for my disease, at some point in our future. This, in turn, gave me hope for a better future, and it enabled me to believe in the fact that I could still live a healthy and prosperous life.

My hope for a long and healthy life further reduced many of my anxieties, and this enabled me to live with a greater sense of comfort. I was then able to open up to Sharon about other troubles that I had in life. I eventually became fully confident in the abilities of both Dr. Lupton and Sharon. If Dr. Lupton's prescription became ineffectual, I knew that she could prescribe a newer and a more advanced form of medication. However, living a long and healthy life was not enough for me. I needed to live a life that would be similar to the life that I would have lived, had I not become ill with schizophrenia. In other words, I wanted to live the life that I had dreamed about during my youth, before I ever experienced any major problems with paranoid thoughts.

This meant that I would accomplish a university degree, at the very least, and work in a field according to my volitions. I always wanted to experience the life of a university student, and I knew that completing a degree would help me in almost all aspects of life. Likewise, I knew that a higher level of education will result in more career options. As a child, I first dreamed about becoming an astronaut. After many years, my desires changed and I wanted to study law. In order to achieve this, I would need to complete a four year Bachelor's degree, followed by a three year post-graduate degree in law.

I put this dream on hold when my cognitive abilities began to diminish, during my high school years. After grade ten, I knew that it was possible that

I would never attain a degree in law. My studies had become increasingly more difficult, and I was not achieving the grades necessary to study at the university level. At this point, I narrowed my goal, and decided to pursue a university degree in any specialty. After I accomplished this, I would then assess my possible career options. Yet, after I was diagnosed with schizophrenia, I did not know if I was still capable of completing any post-secondary studies at all.

I decided to test my intellectual abilities and return to college after my mental health became stable. Studying at the college level was more difficult this time around though. I still had troubles with attention, concentration, and memory. I also experienced problems while trying to complete many of my assigned readings. As a result, I began to doubt myself. At one point, I held the firm impression that I would never be granted entrance into any university level institution. This is where my counselling sessions fit in. Sharon did not necessarily improve my cognitive functions. However, she provided a social network that I could rely on.

At that time, I was extremely preoccupied with achieving the goals that I had set out for myself, prior to being diagnosed with schizophrenia. What I did not recognize, at first, was that my identity as a human being had essentially changed after this diagnosis. I was no longer the same person that I was during my adolescence. My identity had changed both spiritually and intellectually. Sharon taught me how to accept the human being that I had become, after achieving a state of remission. In effect, I was an older and more mature adult. Through Sharon's help, I also realized that it is fine to change one's goals in life. She helped me to understand that I had changed as a person because of my disease, whether I liked this or not. She then helped me to focus on the person that I could become, after I survive this devastating illness.

Probably the most significant reason why I had insisted on focusing on my past was due to the problem with accepting the fact that I had a chronic illness. During my youth, I was quite an overachiever. After some time, I then became a schizophrenic. It was difficult to accept the fact that I had become something that was never really within my control. I needed to stop identifying myself as the academic scholar who had so much potential, and realize that I had become an individual who must battle a lifelong illness. This was particularly difficult for me. In my mind, living with a mental illness meant living a less independent way of life. I also had to accept the possibility that some of my intellectual capacities may be lost indefinitely.

All of these thoughts gave me enough reasons to fear what my life would be like, in the long-term future.

After I talked to Sharon about these fears, her understanding and compassion enabled me to gain some insight and envision an entirely new perspective of life. Sharon always understood my feelings, whether they were morally confused or relevant reactions to my current condition. Actually, at that time, all I really needed was somebody who would listen to my feelings and frustrations. I needed someone who would understand the predicament that I was in, and I needed someone who would care about my well being unconditionally. Through something as simple as a compassionate heart, I began to accept my illness and all of the negative aspects that may be associated with it.

I could only accept the fact that I was ill, after Sharon's counsel. Of course, my extended family members and close friends would accept me as I am, with or without good mental health. However, having the support, from an individual who had no prior relationship with me, helped me to recognize that I was not alone in the world. At that time, I did not know anyone else who was diagnosed with schizophrenia. Yet, I did accept the fact that there may be millions of other persons in the world, like me, who must also overcome a demoralizing and chronic illness.

I eventually needed more than this though. I needed to know that there are other persons in the world, who live a prosperous life, despite the fact that they are schizophrenia patients. Being alone and secluded is a very frightening concept. A sense of belonging will usually come about when the individual realizes that he has peers who face similar challenges. When Sharon told me that there are doctors and lawyers who also suffer from schizophrenia, this began to alleviate my feelings of alienation. This knowledge enabled me to address my feelings of denial, which is also essential to a good prognosis.

Schizophrenia is an illness that is widely misunderstood within the general public. It is hardly talked about within the media, and when it is a topic of conversation, the media usually focuses on criminals who are affected with this disease. Hearing imaginary voices or having the delusion that one is a famous rock star can frighten a mentally healthy individual. Losing the use of one's legs could be equivalently frightful.

In the case of depression, every human being has felt sadness at some point in his life. However, with respect to schizophrenia, very few have ever experienced a schizophrenic delusion. This results in a poor understanding of schizophrenia in general. The average person may have reason to associate schizophrenia with negative connotations, because he lacks certain life experiences and does not understand what every schizophrenia patient must endure. This lack of understanding can also fuel a lack of acceptance towards schizophrenia, as an illness altogether.

After I accepted my illness, I needed to understand what it exactly means to be a patient with schizophrenia. Sharon provided me with the answers to this question. Professional counsellors are mainly educated at the university level. They understand the scientific facts on mental illness, and they understand the ramifications that may be associated with a mental disease. When Sharon taught me that schizophrenia is caused by a chemical imbalance, I understood that there was a physical problem within my brain. Through this knowledge, I was able to negate some of the stigmatized beliefs that I, myself, had previously held towards schizophrenia patients and the illness in general.

During my youth, I held the belief that persons acquire schizophrenia mainly through the abuse of illicit substances. I was wrong. In fact, the individual does not develop an illness like schizophrenia because of his life choices. Schizophrenia is a brain disease. The symptoms of schizophrenia are mainly the product of faulty or defective mechanisms within the brain. Shortly after I was diagnosed, I continued to believe that I had acquired schizophrenia, due to my life choices. Sharon helped me to understand that persons become affected with schizophrenia through no fault of their own. This enabled me to establish a newer sense of inner peace within myself.

Coming to terms with an illness is not easy to achieve. When people think about devastating illnesses, we automatically fear the worst-case scenarios. Actually, this is a very natural reaction. Individuals who discover that they have cancer may immediately associate their condition with possible mortality. Similarly, persons that are affected with schizophrenia may believe that they will never live a normal life.

This line of thinking is usually true with all other forms of illness. Accepting the fact that one is ill is, indeed, difficult universally. Envisioning a good prognosis can be equally difficult. Before my diagnosis, my identity was based on factors such as the fact that I am male, I have a Chinese ethnic background, and that I am a Canadian citizen. After my diagnosis, my identity changed to a Chinese Canadian male, with schizophrenia. Accepting this new identity meant accepting the possibility that I may never attain a state of permanent remission. As the worst-case scenario, it is possible that I could live the rest of my life as a delusional human being. It was also difficult to accept the possibility that I may become extremely sick, without ever being truly aware of this fact.

Professional counselling, from a psychologist with an objective point of view, can be very helpful when one faces a chronic illness. In fact, Sharon never answered any questions concerning my near future. Her reaction told me one thing. In time, I was able to realize that my future was never certain, in any respects. Thus, it is possible that I could live either a poor or a well-lived life. I also eventually came to understand that this was still under my control. If I had maintained focus on the barriers that exist against mental illness, my life would be less fulfilling. However, if I focused on my health and rehabilitation, it may still be possible to achieve some of the things that I had dreamed about as a youth. The main question for me was to find out what abilities I had lost, and what abilities I still possessed after my experience with a mental disease.

Sharon always had an ethical response to all of my questions. She helped me realize that many schizophrenia patients do live a healthy life. I then concluded that I would also try my best to live a well life. Sharon taught me that my future still depended entirely upon myself, and that I still had the power to act. I held this belief before I was diagnosed with schizophrenia, and Sharon helped me to retain this belief after the fact. In time, I finally realized that it was entirely in my power to survive a major illness.

Afterwards, I decided that I would try to live the lifestyle that I would have lived, as if I was never diagnosed with schizophrenia. Before experiencing my worst psychotic episodes, I was studying in college and I intended to complete a university degree. After I was confident that my illness was in a state of remission, I consulted with Sharon for her professional opinion. She agreed with my assessment, and I then decided to return to college during the next semester. Sharon told me to be cautious though. I listened to her advice and enrolled as a part-time student.

At that time, I had no awareness with respect to the true level of my intellectual functioning. Furthermore, I did not know if I would be overwhelmed by any forms of stress. It was very possible that I had permanently lost many of my cognitive capabilities. A part-time course load would enable me to assess my cognition in the areas of attention, concentration, memory, and logic. I would also have more time to spend on my readings and assignments. At that time, I felt that my mind had essentially worked at a slower pace, when compared to my youth. Subsequently, I knew that my post-secondary studies would be more difficult this time around, and also that I would probably need to work harder to achieve a satisfactory level of academic understanding.

Completing my assigned readings was the most difficult challenge that I faced at that time. Whenever I read a page of my assigned texts, I would experience problems while trying to remember what I had just read. In class, I would experience further problems with attention, and I often daydreamed. I also frequently experienced problems with concentration. When I spoke to Sharon about these problems, she gave me every assurance that my current prescription was still effective. However, we discovered that the side effect of fatigue could be affecting my ability to study.

Probably the most important role that Sharon fulfilled was to serve as an intermediary between Dr. Lupton and myself. It took eight years to find the best possible combination of medicines that would effectively treat my unique ailments. Within that period, I needed a mental health specialist to assure me of the fact that my symptoms were still in a state of remission.

Relapse prevention is the most essential issue for any patient who achieves a state of mental stability. The best predictor for a relapse is the patient's nonadherence to a given medication. Reasons for nonadherence will vary among differing individuals, and over differing periods of time. Long-term treatments are recognized as an effective method of treatment, but little else is known due to a lack of long-term studies. A recovery from schizophrenia is contingent on the stabilization of symptoms, and on the acquisition of necessary life skills. Scientifically, psychosocial interventions like professional counselling, an educated family, and social skills training are effective in helping to prevent symptom relapse (Schooler, 2006). These components will also improve deficits in social cognition.

Regular contact with a professional counsellor is also necessary for patients that concurrently suffer from a substance abuse disorder. Substance abuse is currently the most frequent and clinically significant comorbidity among schizophrenia patients (Drake, 2007). Alcohol or illicit drug abuse can have adverse effects on the treatment of many mental disorders. In some cases, psychotic symptoms can reappear due to substance abuse. In other cases, complications like intolerable side effects may arise.

Patients who face problems with substance abuse should understand that this is also a disorder, which will have direct effects on their mental health. Group interventions during the appropriate stage of treatment are particularly effective in helping patients with their addictions (Daughters *et al*, 2008). However, if the patient fails to overcome his substance abuse disorder, a longer period of recovery may be required. In this case, the patient should be regularly monitored by a mental health professional who is knowledgeable in the complications related to a dual-diagnosis. A newer form of treatment, based on the integration of mental health and substance abuse treatments may also be necessary.

According to some studies, persons with psychiatric disorders are twice as likely to abuse alcohol or other illicit substances, when compared to the general population. Other studies indicate that between 35 to 65 percent of patients abuse substances during the early phases of their psychotic disorder.

Cannabis is the most frequently used substance, and the risks associated with its use include a relapse of positive symptoms, toxic psychosis, and an increased risk to develop schizophrenia when used during early adolescence (Bonsack *et al*, 2007). According to another study, cannabis abuse is a component risk factor for the onset and poor outcome, during the early course of schizophrenia (Dekker *et al*, 2008). Another study has linked cannabis use, in adolescents, with the prodromal symptoms of psychosis (Miettunen *et al*, 2008). Heavy cannabis users also have bilaterally reduced hippocampal and amygdala volumes (Yücel *et al*, 2008). Nevertheless, many of these findings are still a topic of controversy among the medical and scientific communities.

Interventions against the use of cannabis are most effective when they are adapted to the specific needs of each individual patient. However, there may be many complexities involved. Primarily, some patients will fail to recognize any hazards related to cannabis use. Youths may also exhibit feelings of distrust or cognitive disturbances linked to psychosis. In addition, the stigmatization of psychiatry and the use of dangerous substances for socialization purposes can also create barriers against the treatment of a dual diagnosis (Butler and Sheridan, 2007).

Effective interventions are based on the principle of empathy, and are conducted through a non-judgmental approach. Moreover, these interventions are mainly aimed at developing insight, regarding the potential consequences of cannabis abuse. This is accomplished through the exploration of all positive and negative factors. The intervention should also be adapted during the patient's stage of motivation for change (Bonsack *et al*, 2007).

Successful interventions can also establish a trustful relationship between the patient and his therapist. After this trust is achieved, patients can explore the ambivalences related to cannabis abuse. It may also be necessary to explore any motivational elements, while acquiring an awareness of any possible links between cannabis use and psychosis.

A study conducted in the Netherlands demonstrates that most patients who abuse cannabis ceased using it after they became psychotic and after their first contact with psychiatric services. Researchers further found no differences in patient characteristics between patients who continued to use cannabis and those who did not. As a result, this study seems to suggest that, in the mind of the patient, the start of psychiatric treatment could be related to the cessation of cannabis abuse (Dekker *et al*, 2008).

Some psychiatric patients may also abuse cocaine for the reason of self-medication. According to a study conducted in France, psychostimulants activate extracellular signal-regulated kinases (ERKs) in the striatum through the combined stimulation of dopamine D(1) receptors (D1Rs) and glutamate NMDA receptors. Antipsychotic medications activate similar signalling proteins, by blocking dopamine D(2) receptors (Bertran-Gonzalez *et al*, 2008). Subsequently, cocaine abuse could produce effects that may be similar to the effects produced by antipsychotics.

According to a further study, there may be a causal relationship between psychosis and substance abuse. A shared psychotic-like experience may best describe this relationship. In the case of psychosis, the individual may experience a sense of alienation from his society. However, when in a hallucinogenic state, the individual may experience a sense of mystical union and revelation (Nelson and Sass, 2008). In view of that, the abuse of an illicit substance could provide the patient with an ad hoc cure, when he experiences extreme states of psychosis or paranoia.

As a matter of fact, I did experiment with cannabis during my high school years. In my case, I used marijuana mainly for recreation and social purposes. However, I was experiencing problems with cognition, delusions, and paranoia at that time as well. My poor academic performance may have also given me a substantial reason to smoke marijuana. In any case, I quit using cannabis after my grade 12 year, when I was free from the pressures and demands related to high school life.

After I was diagnosed with schizophrenia, I only abused substances in the form of coffee and nicotine. While first stable on olanzapine, I would experience copious problems with fatigue, and this interfered with my daily functioning. During the entire day, I would suffer from problems with attention and concentration, because of my low energy levels. Most afternoons I felt exhausted, and this forced me to take a nap on a daily basis. These feelings were immensely overpowering, and accordingly, I could no longer function during the day without taking a lengthy nap.

My daily naps at that time usually lasted for approximately four hours long, and in my mind, this was unacceptable. Feelings of fatigue had essentially taken too much control over my daily routines. From my perspective, I lost many years of my life while in a delusional state, and I felt the same way about my constant need to take a nap. I was also motivated to live a more fulfilling life, because of my good health. Personally, I felt that I could not live a better life if I spent the majority of my day in a state of deep slumber.

To address this problem, I began to drink between three to five cups of coffee per day. Most mornings, I would go out for a coffee and end up spending another hour having a second cup. After I ate lunch, I would drink an additional cup of coffee to feel alert. During the afternoon, I would sometimes drink two more cups of coffee to counteract feelings of drowsiness.

In actuality, coffee is barely a harmful substance. Therefore, a caffeine addiction will have far less repercussions when compared to either a cocaine, or heroin addiction. However, my caffeine dependence may be similar in another respect. If I did not have at least five cups of coffee per day, I would have lost some ability to function. Having to depend on caffeine forced me to focus on my disability, despite the fact that most of my symptoms were in a state of remission.

My high caffeine dependency lasted for several years. What bothered me the most was probably based on the fact that I needed to depend on another substance, other than my prescribed medicines, for daily life. When I spoke to my doctors about this problem, they did not seem to be too concerned. They made me aware of the fact that many other persons drink coffee on a regular basis. Sharon further made me realize that drinking coffee is not necessarily a bad habit. Nevertheless, I still felt that I was abnormal in some way, because of the large amount of coffee that I needed to consume. I eventually decided to reduce my coffee consumption, to build some self-esteem. After a change in my prescription, through the addition of other medications utilized to boost my energy levels, I was able to reduce my caffeine intake. Today, I am no longer dependent on coffee to the same degree that I was at that time. My fatigue is less of a problem today, and I usually drink no more than two to three cups per day.

Nicotine is another substance that is commonly used by many schizophrenia patients. I started to smoke cigarettes during my teenage years, after my academic efforts started to degrade. At worst, I smoked one pack of cigarettes per day during my youth. My nicotine consumption then fluctuated from between 10 to 20 cigarettes per day, until I was diagnosed with schizophrenia.

During that period, I was not working, nor studying. Existing in a delusional state could be comparable to existing in a constant dreamlike state. When smoking a cigarette, I would be better able to focus my mind on things other than my delusions or hallucinations. As a result, while in a state of extreme psychosis, I increased my daily consumption of nicotine.

At one point during my stay at the inpatient unit, I started to give out my cigarettes to other patients. In time, I ended up giving out entire packages of cigarettes every day. My mother eventually realized what I was doing, and consequently, the inpatient nurses then started to ration out my cigarettes on a daily basis. I only became conscious of the fact that I was supporting the smoking habit of other patients within the unit, after my mental health had improved

Currently, I smoke approximately 10 cigarettes per day. My reduced nicotine consumption is mainly due to the medication wellbutrin. Also known as bupropion, wellbutrin is an antidepressant that further acts as a nicotinic antagonist. As an antagonist, wellbutrin inhibits the nicotinic receptors. Dr. Freedman did not prescribe this medicine for reasons related to mood or depression. He believed that the medicine's insomnia-like side effects could potentially address my problems with fatigue. However, this medicine also has positive effects on my addiction to nicotine.

During a pilot trial, researchers discovered that bupropion caused a significantly greater reduction in smoking. Patients have also reported improvements with their negative symptoms, an increased stability of their psychotic and depressive symptoms, and a significant loss in weight (Evins *et al*, 2001). Although I have not quit smoking altogether, I should have a better chance of quitting while taking a medicine like wellbutrin.

Today I continue to smoke cigarettes for three main reasons. Above all, I still enjoy the act of smoking. Secondly, I use cigarettes to address feelings of fatigue. In truth, I feel more refreshed and alert after smoking a cigarette. Lastly, I smoke cigarettes as a means of reducing stress. When smoking, I am better able to gather my thoughts and focus on subjects other than daily life stressors.

If I were to quit smoking today, this would affect my bodily metabolism. Accordingly, Dr. Freedman may have to lower the dosage of my antipsychotic treatments, when I eventually quit. This is another reason why patients should keep in constant contact with a counsellor. If I increase my consumption of nicotine, it may also be necessary to increase the dosage of my prescribed medications. Other daily habits could also affect my metabolism. Therefore, a medical professional is needed to monitor problems related to the potency of their patient's prescribed medications. In some cases, it may be unpredictable how a patient's bodily metabolism will react, in conjunction with other substances.

A final reason to maintain contact with a professional counsellor is to help one address any possible suicidal thoughts. On a worldwide scale, there are approximately one million suicide victims each year (Dracheva *et al*, 2008). It is evident that patients with mood disorders, such as depression or bipolar disorder, may often have thoughts related to suicide. However, suicidal ideations can be common among patients with thought disorders, like schizophrenia, as well. A schizophrenic individual who suffers from hallucinations, for example, could hear voices that are telling him to harm himself in some manner.

Persons who are healthy mentally will most often be able to comprehend the full ramifications associated with the act of suicide. Conversely, persons with a mental illness may suffer from deficits in their cognition. Accordingly, mentally sick patients could mistakenly rationalize an act of suicide, because they cannot analyze their thoughts through a sound and coherent frame of mind.

According to other studies, there is a high prevalence of suicidal behaviour among schizophrenia patients. The greatest risk for suicide occurs during the early courses of the individual's illness, though the risk factor still lasts throughout his entire lifetime. The most evident risk factors include depression, psychosis, and substance abuse. Previous deliberate self-harm, compulsory admissions into an inpatient unit, work stresses, living alone, and being out of contact are other risk factors. These risk factors have been correlated to an act of suicide immediately after the patient is discharged from a psychiatric unit. Guilty thoughts, depressive mood, suicidal ideations, and a suicide attempt one month before admission have also been identified as risk factors.

Researchers furthermore assert that the overall number of risk factors have a greater screening efficacy for suicide, over any single factor. Thorough treatments which address the circumstances that lead to these risk factors, and the systematic assessment of suicide risk are recommended measures to take. Professional counsellors can identify other significant, yet less apparent factors related to suicide risk as well.

Scientifically, the serotonin 2C receptor (5HT(2C)R) has been implicated in suicidal behaviour (De Luca *et al*, 2007). The abnormal functioning of extracellular signal-regulated kinase 5 (ERK5) in the hippocampus, which has been observed in suicide subjects, is also believed to be a pathogenic mechanism linked to suicide (Dwivedi *et al*, 2007). Reduced functioning of tropomyosin receptor kinases (Trks), and increased expression ratios of pan75 neurotrophin receptors (p75(NTR) to Trks have also been consistently observed within the hippocampus of suicide subjects (Dwivedi *et al*, 2009).

Researchers have discovered other evidence linking genetic factors to suicide. One study demonstrates that suicide runs in the biological families of suicided (as well as schizophrenic or affectively ill) adoptees, but not in those of demographically matched healthy control adoptees (Voracek, 2007). Therefore, an individual`s risk for suicide resembles his biological relatives over his adoptive relatives. Other studies demonstrate that socio-cultural factors like ethnicity, and other environmental influences like family or social characteristics may also play a significant role in suicidal thoughts and behaviour.

Statistically, 10% of schizophrenia patients will commit suicide. In comparison, only 1% of persons in the general population will commit suicide (Caldwell and Gottesman, 1992). Therefore, a substantial gap in mortality rates exists between persons with schizophrenia and the general public. Researchers have also found that the associated risks for suicide are significantly higher in younger persons, though marked risk persists until the age of 70.

Patients at most risk tend to be young single males with post-psychotic depression who have a history of substance abuse and previous suicide attempts (Pompili *et al*, 2007). Elements like feelings of defeat, a lack of rescue, social isolation, an awareness of illness, and experiences with hospitalizations are some reasons that could motivate a patient to commit suicide. Schizophrenia patients have also reported that a decrease in mental functioning, a recent loss or rejection, limited external support, neuroleptic-induced akathisia, and severe psychosis are further motivational elements (De Leo and Spathonis, 2003). High dosages of antipsychotic medications and positive symptoms have also been associated with an increased risk of mortality by way of suicide.

There is also a high prevalence of suicidal ideations and attempts among women with post-partum onset psychosis. A study conducted in India indicates that women with an insidious onset of this illness, or those who suffer from depressive symptoms are at most risk to commit suicide. In this study, suicidal ideations were significantly associated with other ideas based on some harm to their infant as well (Babu *et al*, 2008). In addition, the offspring of mothers with psychotic disorders are also at an increased risk for suicide.

Evidence of prior familial suicidal behaviour seems to be vital for suicide risk assessment in young psychiatric inpatients (Mittendorfer-Rutz *et al*, 2008). In general, suicidal ideations can often indicate a recent suicide attempt, while a remote suicide attempt can sometimes be indicated by aggressive traits and depression (Mann *et al*, 2008). Elevated levels of impulsive, aggressive behaviours have been further linked to suicide across all major psychopathological categories (McGirr and Turecki, 2008). Short durations of an illness are also a significant predictor for suicide. At present, scientists believe that lower concentrations of serum cholesterol and platelet 5-HT may help estimate the individual's risk to commit suicide (Marcinko et al, 2007).

Early recognition and professional modes of treatment, like a psychosocial intervention, can prevent suicide attempts in younger individuals. Suicidal thinking is best addressed by effectively treating positive and depressive symptoms, eliminating substance abuse, negating feelings of akathisia, disavowing stigma and demoralization, and by instilling hope for a better future. Additionally, newer atypical antipsychotics have proven to effectively treat suicidal thoughts and behaviour. CBT has also reduced suicidal ideations in some patients (Vitiello, 2009). On a further note, restricted emotions have been correlated with a reduced risk to commit suicide.

According to a study conducted in Australia, patients with schizophrenia, and other mental disorders, communicate their suicide intent more frequently than those with no psychiatric diagnosis. Schizophrenia patients are also more likely to communicate this type of intent, in comparison to patients with other psychiatric diagnoses (De Leo and Klieve, 2007). The patient's willingness to communicate his suicidal thoughts seems to suggest that he may be contemplating many moral issues related to the act of suicide. Under these circumstances, there is a clear opportunity for a health advocate to intervene and work with the individual towards suicide prevention.

From my perspective, professional counselling is a necessary mode of treatment for any patient that exhibits suicidal thoughts. Psychiatric inpatient facilities are also in a position to establish suicide prevention programs. Active screening during the inpatient hospital stay and continuous monitoring following the period of discharge may be important precautions to take.

In general, patients who received help from counselling services have usually found them to be adequate. Concepts like resilience, recovery, and hope are best communicated via medical professionals who understand the patient's emotional states, and any problems that may be associated with the patient's disorder. On the other hand, some patients have voiced the fact that they do not receive the right type of help for issues like information, psychotic symptoms, intimate relationships, and sexual expression (Grinshpoon and Ponizovsky, 2008). As a result, advances in treatment techniques may be needed to address these additional concerns.

10

Re-socialization

The next step towards a full recovery from schizophrenia is to take a proactive approach to life, and re-enter oneself back into a community setting. Most disabilities force the individual to leave his social network, for an indefinite period of time. During this phase, the individual focuses mainly on therapy and rehabilitation. After his symptoms are fully treated, it is up to the individual to re-take his life and focus on a full recovery. This can be accomplished in several ways. The easiest method to reintegrate oneself back into a community setting is to take up a hobby. It is probably best to start an activity that will provide the individual with a different perspective of life.

Starting an enjoyable hobby should be the first aim of any recovering patient. A hobby will turn out to be a success simply if the individual benefits positively from his chosen activity. Volunteer work is another method that can aid the individual with his rehabilitation. The main objective in volunteer work is to dedicate one's time and energy towards some type of constructive cause. Persons who volunteer will help some type of foundation achieve certain goals within either his community or another society around the world.

An additional method of resocialization can be something as simple as enjoying leisure time with other persons. Maintaining contact with one's established social network is also an essential element of the recovery process. Many patients do not realize that the individuals within their social network feel an equivalent need for social connections and friendship.

If the patient wants to be challenged, completing an academic degree can also be a valid mode of resocialization. In many cases, the onset of a mental disorder occurs at an age that disrupts the individual's education, either at the high school level or during post-secondary studies. Under these circumstances, it may be difficult to resume an educational goal, after one is diagnosed with a mental illness. I recommend that all patients should seek to be educated within a field of interest, as opposed to a field that may be chosen because of any other extrinsic factors. An educated society has much to offer to the individual, and likewise, an education will enable the individual to take a greater role within his society. Knowledge is probably the most essential element of a prosperous life.

Another challenging method of resocialization is to acquire some type of formal employment. A loss of employment due to a mental illness can be extremely discouraging. In the western world, disability in the workplace due to a mental illness or addiction is more common in comparison to other forms of illnesses, like cancer or heart disease. On a worldwide scale, schizophrenia, unipolar depression, bipolar affective disorder, obsessive-compulsive disorder, and alcohol use disorder are among the 10 leading causes of a disability (Kirby and Keon, 2004).

Although it may be difficult, gaining meaningful part or full-time employment can be extremely rewarding for any persons who are diagnosed with a mental illness. Through employment, the individual will be able to contribute towards something that is important within his community. The patient will regain a structured lifestyle, and he will also benefit through an increase in social interactions. The compensation gained through employment can also provide the individual with a greater sense of independence. This level of independence will, in turn, bolster his self-esteem and demonstrate a sign of personal strength during times of extreme adversity. However, functions like memory and executive processes are significant in both instrumental and social dimensions of community functioning (Proteau and Doron, 2007).

Patients with a mental illness can face three other major problems related to paid employment. First, the individual may be subject to direct discrimination from a potential employer. Under the Canadian Charter of Rights and Freedoms, it is illegal to discriminate against persons with any type of disability (Canadian Heritage, 2008). Therefore, persons with a disability should be free from discrimination, at least within the public sector.

Secondly, the patient may require special needs, such as a leave from work due to an illness, which may not be granted by his employer. The Canadian Human Rights Act ensures that federally regulated employers accommodate persons with disabilities only to the point of the employers' undue hardship (Canadian Heritage, 2009). This type of regulation was created to provide an equal footing for persons with disabilities, and not as a form of preferential treatment. Yet, problems with health, safety, and economic concerns may make such accommodations too difficult to provide. Thus, although providing accommodations for persons with disabilities is encouraged, some businesses within the private sector will fail to provide such accommodations.

Thirdly, patients who have been severely ill, for a long period of time, may lack the credentials and work experience required for highly competitive forms of work. Under the Employment Equity Act, no person should be denied employment opportunities or benefits for reasons unrelated to ability. The purpose of this act is to correct the conditions of disadvantage in employment experienced by women, Aboriginal peoples, persons with disabilities and members of visible minorities (Department of Justice Canada, 2008). Although the objective of this act is to promote an equal opportunity for all persons, there currently exists no system of checks and balances which ensures that a potential employer will abide by this law.

According to some studies, the international unemployment rate for individuals who are affected by a severe and chronic mental illness is situated at around 90%. In contrast, approximately 50% of persons with a physical or sensory disability are unemployed (Kirby and Keon, 2004). As a result, although it is extremely rewarding, gaining some form of paid employment may be exceedingly difficult for most patients that suffer from a mental disorder.

In my opinion, the individual should acquire an enjoyable hobby as the first step towards his personal rehabilitation from a mental illness. Almost everyone in the world enjoys some type of hobby. The best type of hobby will provide the individual with some form of relief from everyday stressors. A hobby can be something as simple as going for a walk, to something more complex like writing poetry.

The first major hobby that I took up was based in the field of personal computing. I started this hobby after I was well enough to permanently leave the inpatient unit and live at home. During that period, my mental health could have still improved, and I was still experimenting with different combinations of medications. From my memory, I no longer had problems with positive symptoms, but I still suffered from negative symptoms. Dr. Lupton felt that I was healthy enough to leave the hospital ward, though personally, I did not feel well enough to socialize with other persons. Perhaps this feeling may have been due to a lack of self-esteem, and not any factors that may be directly related to my illness. At that time, I lost confidence in myself because I still doubted many of my perceptions. I did not trust my frame of mind. Working on a computer enabled me to work in a private environment, should it be the case that I experience any further problems with psychosis.

From this time to my first semesters back at college, I probably spent more time on the computer than I had watching television. After learning the intricacies of the internet, I started to spend time in several online chat rooms. There were many persons socializing there, from all around the world, with varying backgrounds. The conversations that I engaged in were based on a variety of topics. However, I did not spend time in these rooms mainly to socialize with other persons. One of my other objectives was to learn keyboarding skills. Participating in an online chat room helped me to both achieve this task, and rebuild my social skills.

In time, I knew that I would eventually give my best effort to achieve a degree at a post-secondary institution. However, I did not know if I still possessed the skills and raw ability to complete a degree. I also knew that I would need to use a computer upon my return to college. What started out as a hobby for me, turned into a self-learning activity with both practical uses and implications.

I also spent time playing video games on the computer. I had a few friends who also played computer games, so I decided to spend some leisure time with them. Soon enough, we played on a nightly basis. In my mind, the aspects of friendly competition are quite enjoyable, whether it is in the area of athletics or academics. My friends and I would play competitive games from about ten o'clock at night, until six o'clock in the morning. It felt good to know that I could still enjoy recreational activities again. When my friends won a game, I would be motivated to beat them in the next game. This concept of friendly competition had fuelled my love for video games. I also developed a unique social bond with these friends, as a direct result.

Still, there were other video games that I had enjoyed while playing alone. My circle of friends played only one game at that time. They had other commitments, including post-secondary studies. Thus, I spent time playing computer games with other persons around the world. Through the internet, I could find players during all times of the day. The global network that I joined further enabled me to re-build my social skills.

Playing computer games eventually became a full-time hobby of mine. After spending several hours per day on the computer, I discovered that I still had the ability to learn new things. My newly learned skills with computers gave me a new reason to hold a sense of trust in my intellectual capacities. I then decided to increase the range of my personal hobbies.

After some time, I chose to learn the sport of golf. I chose an athletic hobby for many reasons. Initially, I wanted to start a hobby that would help me to become more physically fit. I gained much weight due to my prescribed medications and I wanted to improve my physique. My experience with weight gain also had a negative effect on my self-perspective. Accordingly, I chose an activity that would potentially address this problem of mine.

Learning the sport of golf also helped me mentally. Every hour that I spent at the driving range would be recreational time that I spent away from my personal troubles. Focusing my mind on things other than my illness enabled me to envision a greater perspective on life as a whole. Returning home from a good workout also revitalized my energy levels during the day.

After some time, my golf technique eventually improved from a beginner's level to an intermediate level. I never took any formal lessons because they were too expensive. Instead, I studied lessons on the internet, and I read golf books and magazines. The time I spent practicing my golf swing gave me another opportunity to assess my mental capabilities. I picked up the sport of golf in a relatively short amount of time. I took this to be a good sign with respect to my overall mental health.

During my youth, I always understood academia in a quick and coherent fashion. Most of my schoolteachers helped me to become aware of this. After spending time at the driving range, I discovered that I could still learn at a fast pace. In time, I refined my golf swing into a longer and straighter shot. This, in turn, boosted my confidence and it enabled me to hold a greater sense of trust in my cognitive abilities.

Achieving a level of expertise in the game of golf went far beyond any of my expectations. Golf is not an easy sport to learn. It took me approximately a period of over one year, on a daily basis, to learn the proper technique on my own. When the game started to become less of a challenge for me, I knew that I could still achieve success in other areas of life, through hard work and determination. Golf is not merely a physical sport. The best golfers in the world are talented athletes, but there is more to the game than pure physical strength. Perfect hand eye coordination is possibly the most essential element of a good golf swing. This requires the golfer to focus, and remain in a total and absolute state of concentration. Becoming a good golfer implicated the fact that I still possessed the ability to concentrate and focus my attention on a subject matter that was new to me.

The final reason why I chose to play golf was based on my love for friendly competition. However, I probably would have enjoyed this hobby, even if I never learned the proper technique. The driving range became an environment which provided me with an escape from my personal troubles. I would be free from any external stressors at the driving range, and I was free to focus on something that was enjoyable. Once I became a fairly competitive player, the success that I had achieved was purely an unexpected bonus. As a person with a mental illness, I knew that I had developed a level of skill in a sport that the average person will never achieve.

In fact, many persons are not athletically inclined. Under these circumstances, a weight control program can have many similar benefits with learning a new sport. In Korea, a program based on diet therapy, exercise, education, and behaviour modification therapy effectively decreased the rate of weight gain in female inpatients, who were taking atypical antipsychotics. This program also ended up decreasing obesity, while increasing the patient's sense of control over her dietary behaviours (Hong *et al*, 2008b). Therefore, undertaking similar programs can also effectively address the problem of weight gain.

The final hobby I chose was to watch films. When I was first released from the inpatient unit, I wanted to test my cognitive abilities. I believed that I could test my attention span through watching a full-length movie. I usually rented one movie per day. On some occasions, I would watch more than one film in a day. This usually happened when I rented movies with sequels. Often, I would be too anxious to wait another day for the second instalment. The best movies that I have watched always taught me something different about life and the world in general. While extremely ill, I basically lost contact with the outside world. For this reason, I believed that I could regain much of what I had lost, by being knowledgeable in the recent cinematic arts.

The primary purpose of a hobby is not to learn a new skill, nor is it to improve one's self-confidence. These elements are merely further benefits that come along with developing a new hobby. From my point of view, the most important reason to develop a hobby is to regain a sense of happiness in life. When the individual is recovering from a disability, he may enter into a state of depression, due to his poor health. Once a medical professional has treated his illness, the onus is on the patient to retake control over his life. Finding happiness through a hobby will enable the individual to live a lifestyle according to his own choosing and volitions.

Spending leisure time with my friends also helped in my recovery from schizophrenia. On occasion, I would enjoy a cup of coffee with a friend on a nice day. Going to see my friends would also cure my occasional feelings of loneliness. Some of our conversations were meaningful. At other times, we met purely to enjoy each other's company. Most of my friends range in an age that is approximate to mine. Issues like employment would be a common topic of our conversations. We would also chat about future endeavours. The most important part of these outings, though, was based on the fact that my friends have benefited from my company, as much as I have benefited from theirs.

I also have other friends who enjoy athletic hobbies. Although I mostly went to the driving range alone, I would sometimes go there with another friend who also enjoys the sport. When I was with company, I usually concentrated more on socializing over anything else. However, I also spent much time at the driving range alone, so that I could learn the sport and play at a competitive level.

I also enjoy rollerblading around my city during a nice summer day. There are many specialized routes for bicyclists and persons who rollerblade, in the city that I reside in. When I rollerblade, my main aim is to enjoy the natural beauty that my city has to offer. Along with a wide variety of parkland and lush vegetation, there are also many beaches and waterways to view. For the most part, I never went rollerblading alone. I feel that this experience is best enjoyed when in the company of a friend.

I also started to play basketball again, with another friend of mine from high school. In fact, I have been playing basketball since I was five years old. Although I love the sport of hockey the most, I had more opportunities to play basketball during my youth. At the elementary and high school levels, there are school teams available for the sport of basketball, but not for hockey. In addition, most of my friends preferred to play basketball over any other sport. As a result, I was able to develop skills in the sport of basketball, throughout much of my teenage years.

After I graduated from high school, a couple of friends of mine would continue to meet and play basketball on a regular basis. I would join them when I had the time and energy to play. The members of our group also included several acquaintances that we met on the basketball court. In the beginning, my friends and I would meet at an indoor basketball court as a team of three or four persons, to play against a similar group of individuals. After seeing these other individuals on a regular basis, we eventually organized a weekly get together.

After Dr. Lupton diagnosed me with schizophrenia, I would not return to the basketball court until a period of approximately three years. I never told my basketball contacts why I had left the sport for such a long time. Perhaps they believed that I got lazy or had other commitments to fulfill. This was not uncommon, and I was not the only player in our group who left the sport for a period of time. As adults, persons must undertake more responsibilities. Accordingly, commitments to work and school will usually be prioritized over leisure activities.

Even though the majority of persons in our group love playing basketball, I mainly played the game to maintain some old relationships, and for exercise. At present, I no longer play basketball. However, I did make some new friends while playing this sport, at that point in my life.

During my youth, I also learned to play the sport of badminton. As a game, I enjoy playing badminton more than basketball. Badminton is based more on individual skill. Basketball, on the other hand, is more of a team sport. At the recreational centres in my neighbourhood, I have seen many elderly persons who play badminton on a regular basis. Consequently, I knew that I could play this sport throughout my senior years. The same is true with the sport of golf. In contrast, I have not witnessed many elderly persons who continue to play basketball.

Basketball is a game for youths and young adults in their prime. Very few seniors play the game because it is easy to get injured during the course of a game. I joined my college's badminton team to improve my skills, because I knew that there would be a time when I would no longer be playing basketball. The sport of badminton also provided me with a newer social network. One friend that I met playing basketball also enjoys playing badminton. However, most of the people that I have met on the badminton court play this sport exclusively.

When I first became sick and left my college studies, I also left the school's badminton team. At that time, nobody on the team had any inkling of what happened to me. My old coach believed that I had contracted mononucleosis. In contrast, the athletic director believed that I had just quit the team. I told both my new coach and the athletic director that I suffer from schizophrenia. From my point of view, the athletic director looked quite surprised to see that someone who looked as healthy as me could suffer from a disease like schizophrenia. I was eventually welcomed back onto the team and I retained a slight leadership role there as well.

In my eyes, I felt that improving my skill in badminton would provide me with a lifetime hobby and a greater social network. Building a familiarity with persons who are not close friends is also an important aspect of human socialization. When the individual establishes a remote familiarity with strangers, a sign of mutual respect is usually established. This leads to a wider range of social contacts. Persons who are purely acquaintances will usually have very few things in common with the individual. In this case, a type of affection based on a slighter degree of connectedness is established, and this is also an important element of life within a community setting.

Indeed, I enjoy athletic hobbies. The majority of persons will usually concentrate on a single sport within their lifetime. In my case, I have learned to play three sports at a fairly competitive level. I have also recently learned the sport of snowboarding, and including rollerblading, I have developed five hobbies based on physical activities. My philosophy after leaving the inpatient unit was quite simple. At that time, because my mental health had improved, I knew that I could still live a fulfilling life. I did not know if I would be successful in this undertaking. However, I did know that I would try my best to accomplish this.

As a Canadian, I also watch hockey games as a personal hobby. On occasion, I will watch a hockey game in the company of a friend. We will also drink alcohol together during the course of a game. At other times, when my friends are busy, I will watch the game alone. I rarely miss a hockey game when my home team is televised. I believe that many other Canadians are similar in this respect. As it turns out, choosing a hobby with an established social network may be an extremely effective mode of resocialization.

An extended education can also help integrate the patient back into his society. Some patients drop out of high school because they are suffering from the preliminary symptoms of a mental illness. I know this because, although I did not fully drop out of high school, I did need to take another year of part-time schooling to complete my high school credits. I also had to drop out of my college studies, after I entered into a constant state of psychosis. Most patients will also discontinue their studies when they enter into a prolonged sickened state. Subsequently, poor academic performance in the years prior to the onset of a mental illness will usually be due to the disease itself.

In my opinion, once the individual has graduated from high school, a post-secondary education will be a further highly effective mode of resocialization. In Canada, some colleges and institutions require only a high school diploma for entrance. This is one reason why high school graduation is essential for all individuals. However, the main reason for completing a high school diploma is based on the acquisition of fundamental life skills. Individuals who finish their high school education will acquire basic life skills that are intrinsic to living in a cooperative fashion, within a community-based environment. Persons with a high school diploma will have the basic language skills, mathematical skills, and general knowledge crucial for interpersonal interactions within most social environments. Individuals who lack these skills may experience difficulties while trying to thrive within their community.

Once the individual has completed a high school education, he will have enough knowledge to flourish within most societies. However, I believe that persons who complete a post-secondary education will have an increased chance for success, within a complex society. When the individual completes a college degree, he will be knowledgeable in some of the intricacies that are characteristic of a developed nation. Determining an area of focus at the college level depends mainly on the individual. In high school, I was probably most successful in the field of mathematics. However, my main interests at the college level were based on the humanities and human civilization.

In terms of my specific preferences during college, I loved to study philosophy. I was particularly interested in the study of ethics, and moral values. However, I also had to take elements like my future career options into consideration. If I achieved high grades, I would then enter into law school. However, if I did not perform well academically, my studies in philosophy could be irrelevant to my future career. To solve this problem, I took formal courses in computer science, so that I would have a second career option.

After a few semesters, I began to realize that I enjoyed my philosophy classes over any other subject matter. I strongly believe that the individual should love his career, to be successful in it. Similarly, I believe that an individual will not prosper in a career that he detests. These latter thoughts, and my desire for ethical knowledge gave me enough reasons to continue my studies in philosophy. Along with ethical principles, studies in philosophy emphasize a strong understanding in the areas of reason and logic. In fact, my former success in the field of mathematics was mainly due to my aptitude in reason and logic. After I completed a college degree, I decided to pursue another goal. I wanted to transfer into university studies and complete a second degree. At that time, I believed that my academic background would be diverse enough to specialize in either fields of computing science or philosophy.

Studying in a field of interest is critical to the completion of a post-secondary degree. Choosing an area of specialization should be an easier choice to make, when the individual has specific career goals. My goal, after being formally diagnosed with schizophrenia, was to complete a university degree in any field. However, studying at a technical school may be more appropriate for some individuals. Most certificates and diplomas at a technical school, on average, take between one and two years to complete. The associate's degree that I attained at the college level also took approximately two years to complete. On the other hand, a university degree will take at least four years of studies to complete. In my particular case, I was able to transfer two years of my college credits towards a Bachelor's degree at the university level.

Even so, four years of schooling may be too much of a commitment for some individuals, especially if they are not motivated to complete a higher form of education. Technical schools mainly focus on the understanding of applicable skills, within the individual's community. Universities, on the other hand, stress an understanding in the areas of complex concepts and general principles. It is up to the individual to choose a form of education that is most relevant to his personal goals.

A two-year degree at the college level could be equivalent to a shortened version of a Bachelor's degree at the university level. Both accreditations emphasize a high level of knowledge and understanding within some area of human civilization. On the other hand, a certificate or diploma from a technical school will generally teach competence within a specific field of employment. Areas of specialization within a technical school can vary from learning how to cook, learning the field of computing, or learning skills within the theatrical arts. An education within a technical school will essentially provide the individual with a new ability. Therefore, studying at a technical school can be the most efficient mode of instruction for persons who are pursuing employment within a specific craft or trade. Individuals who wish to succeed in industries such as mechanics, electronics, or carpentry will benefit more from studies at a technical school over a university.

A university level education is available for persons who desire knowledge within the complex intricacies of a specific area in human civilization. In comparison to college and most technical schools, students must endure more demands while studying at the university level. College, from my perspective, had a relaxed and easy-going atmosphere. At the college level, students may freely study subjects according to their own choosing and pace. In university, course selection is more structured, and students are encouraged to specialize in a field quite early during their studies. Technical schools are even more structured than a university, because students will usually choose a specialized program of studies, mainly before any instruction is ever carried out.

Although the overall environment within a technical school is probably more stressful than the college environment, the overall environment within a university is probably more stressful than most technical schools. In university, students will have a larger workload of assignments and readings to complete. They will also face higher standards, in terms of grading. I would recommend a university education for highly focused students who desire knowledge and understanding over any other benefits from their post-secondary studies.

I eventually chose to study at a university for two reasons. Primarily, I wanted to invest my time in studies that would enable me to build a personally rewarding career. Secondly, I wanted to be educated in an academic field, according to my personal volitions.

I have learned more about our society and civilization as a direct result of my university studies. However, during the first semesters of my studies,

I discovered how difficult it truly is to achieve satisfactory grades at the university level. I also shortly realized that I would not be able to complete a degree in computing science, because of these difficulties. In fact, I chose the field of computer science mainly to acquire a well-paying job within that field. In the end, I eventually had to give up this dream and focus on completing a degree in philosophy, which was an area that I chose strictly through personal interests.

A Master's degree is the next level of education within the university setting, after one completes a Bachelor's degree. Upon completion of a Master's degree, the next level is a Doctorate of Philosophy (PhD). Both of these degrees are known as post-graduate degrees. The average student will usually have no need to complete a post-graduate degree, unless he is aiming to teach or conduct research within his field of interest. I wanted to attain a post-graduate degree because I was interested in conducting research within the field of philosophy. However, my grades were not high enough to enter into studies at the master's level. Despite my inability to enter into a post-graduate program, I eventually realized that the achievement of a Bachelor's degree was still a great accomplishment. My academic success has taught me that every person can still achieve his personal goals, even when facing extreme hardships. It also reinforced my belief in the principle of equality for all human beings.

A higher education will bequeath the individual with a broader understanding of life, and it will enable him to become a more active member within his community. A greater depth of knowledge should empower any human being. Realizing one's academic potential will lead to a kind of growth that cannot be achieved in any other manner. Therefore, in my opinion, seeking a higher form of education may be the best method of resocialization for persons with a mental illness.

Volunteer work is a more easily acquired mode of resocialization. When an individual volunteers his time and works for a worthy organization, both parties will benefit. Although there is no monetary compensation, volunteer work enables the individual to work towards something that is still constructive. Many different organizations need volunteer workers. As a result, the individual will usually have more options when considering volunteer work over paid employment.

Positions for volunteer work can range from helping animals at the SPCA, to helping persons at the Cancer Society. Some patients may want to work at the Schizophrenia Society to help their peers with common problems. Other organizations may require help with administrative duties. The most important aspect of volunteer work is to provide a service that will result in some type of personal benefit. Compassion may be an essential component of volunteer work. Many opportunities are centred on helping persons who are in less fortunate situations. As a result, volunteer work can often lead to rewards that cannot be gained through any other forms of socialization.

Personally, I have experience with volunteer work through my studies at university. I volunteered to act as the treasurer of my school's badminton club. My main duties were to help with club events, and record the club's financial transactions. In fact, I gained valuable leadership skills through this volunteer work. However, I soon discovered that I needed to spend more time on my studies, because this work was interfering with my overall academic success. I then resigned from my position as a club executive after one year.

The main difference between formal employment and volunteer work is the monetary compensation. According to most statistics, finding meaningful employment is more difficult for persons with disabilities, when compared to the average citizen. Therefore, volunteer work may be the right choice for persons who are finding it difficult to acquire paid employment. Organizations that accept volunteer workers will usually be more flexible in terms of scheduling. In some positions, the individual may set his own work schedule. As a result, having flexible hours may be one significant advantage that volunteer work has over paid employment.

Finding paid employment, when possible, may be most desirable though. Acquiring a rewarding full-time job may be as difficult, for some persons, as completing a post-secondary degree. Likewise, persons, with any form of disability, will almost always face a challenge when trying to find paid employment. In the acquisition of paid employment, the individual must satisfy several requirements. Initially, persons must have the educational background to be effective within their field of employment. Being well educated is a characteristic that all employers look for when hiring a potential employee. Secondly, the individual must have relevant work experience. Although prior work experience may not be required for an entry-level position, previous work and volunteer experience can make the individual more employable. Education and work experience are the two most important factors that employers look for when they hire a specific candidate.

According to some researchers, both employment and education are significantly related to a higher quality of life. However, persons with a mental illness have exceedingly high unemployment rates and, in many occasions, will face poverty. The two concepts of social underachievement and social decline also become relevant issues. Social underachievement occurs when the educational attainment of people with mental illness is low and entry to the labor market fails. Social decline is a loss of competitive employment opportunities after the onset of an illness. Individuals who face these predicaments will experience prolonged periods of unemployment and other difficulties upon their re-entry into the labour market (Nordt *et al*, 2007).

On the other hand, low numbers of psychiatric hospitalizations, higher levels of education, and years of work experience have been associated with an increase in vocational status. Higher rates of income have also been correlated with a higher age in the onset of an illness, competitive forms of employment, and no recent hospitalizations. Patients who hold forms of employment also report a higher subjective quality of life, when compared to those who are unemployed (Nordt *et al*, 2007).

When the schizophrenia patient considers his true employment options, he will be making his first step towards a more independent way of life. When steadily employed, a marked improvement in the patient's normal daily functioning and social interaction skills is usually evident. Securing one's material needs can also improve elements like subjective safety (Schomerus *et al*, 2008). From a community's perspective, improving employment rates may substantially reduce both the economic and personal impact of chronic mental diseases (Fitzgerald *et al*, 2007).

Employment resource programs, like cognitive training programs, have had an extremely positive impact on the lives of persons with disabilities. Over three years, patients enrolled in these programs were more likely to hold jobs, work more hours, and earn higher wages than patients who were offered supported employment services alone.

More specifically, the neurocognitive enhancement therapy (NET) program has had a positive influence on individuals with schizophrenia. Individuals who participated in this program, along with six months of paid work therapy (WT), worked more hours than persons who were enrolled in WT alone. During the follow-up period, these patients worked the most, and they were employed in positions with a competitive-wage (Bell et al, 2005). All of these results suggest that cognitive therapies have an immense impact on the employability of persons with schizophrenia. According to another study, though, social factors like the compelling need to be employed, a supportive work environment, and the number of years of formal education are more important elements relevant to higher levels of work functioning among schizophrenia patients (Srinivasan and Tirupati, 2005).

In China, a program called the Community Re-Entry Module (CRM) had a greater effect on social functioning, insight and psychiatric symptoms, when compared to standard psycho-education groups. The CRM program focuses on social skills training, and patients enrolled within this program have reported significantly higher re-employment rates, along with significantly lower relapse and re-hospitalization rates (Xiang *et al*, 2007). Furthermore, in another study, the participant's annual inpatient days had deceased precipitously, and the average relative cost of his mental health services had dropped by over 70%, following enrolment into a community based vocational rehabilitation program (Jaeger *et al*, 2006).

According to another study, schizophrenia patients living in France, Germany and the UK held jobs in all sections of the job market. These persons were more likely to be working if they experienced only a single episode of their illness, possessed a degree, or lived with their families (Marwaha *et al*, 2007).

However, researchers have discovered a substantial difference between patients with or without cognitive deficits in competitive employment status and vocational functioning. They have linked cognition to work performance and have characterized a cognitive deficit as a rate-limiting factor (Holthausen *et al*, 2007).

Moreover, the impact that employment services have on patients with mental illness is known to increase over time. This provides further evidence that improvements in cognitive functioning may be directly linked with optimal employment outcomes.

Another study based on data from the United States, during the year 2007, recorded a 17.2% employment rate for patients with schizophrenia. Only

57.1% of these individuals reported more than 40 hours of work during their past month of employment. Of these individuals, their mean wage was $7.05 per hour, while their mean earnings were $494.20 per month (Salkever *et al*, 2007).

In essence, psychiatric diagnoses are the main reason for disability income in women, while ranking as the third most prevalent reason for men. The average retirement age for males in this group is 39 years, while the average retirement age for females is 42 years. Moreover, schizophrenia is the most significant single reason for early retirement before the age of 40 (Clouth, 2004). In other cases, patients who are employed will face workplace discrimination, forms of abuse, and difficulties when changing professions. They may also exhibit a need for social support, and face a reduction in both career choices and working hours. Researchers have further discovered a negative association between patients that suffer from comorbid physical health conditions and their employment status (Waghorn *et al*, 2008).

The individual who finds paid employment will benefit not only financially, but also through a psychological standpoint. In truth, re-entry into a community setting, by way of a career, may be difficult for the majority of persons that are affected with a disability. Employment programs have removed barriers to job seeking, but success is mainly achieved through a positive focus and painstaking determination.

Acquiring a full-time career in one's field of choice is not an easy task to achieve, even for persons with good mental health. In my personal case, I have utilized online job boards for over a year, after I graduated from university, without acquiring any forms of employment. I also failed to impress any potential employers during the few job interviews that were offered to me. Considering all things, I believe that it was easier to find employment before I was diagnosed with schizophrenia, in comparison to present times, even though I have completed a degree at the university level.

Yet, resocialization by way of employment can enable the individual to achieve major life goals related to independent living. Choosing a form of paid work will reinforce important human values, like hope and empowerment (Corrigan, 2006). Scientifically, employment has been associated with less severe symptoms, improved neurocognitive functioning, and higher scores on psychological tests that measure motivation and empathy. Greater access to rehabilitation services was also associated with greater participation in both competitive and noncompetitive employment (Rosenheck *et al*, 2006).

Therefore, gaining employment may be the final step in the patient's journey towards a full recovery.

These are the many benefits linked to the employment of persons with mental illness. Vocational development is an important and natural condition of human growth for all persons, yet many clinically relevant improvements are also realized through this mode of re-socialization (Gioia, 2005). Achieving economic self-sufficiency is another element. Nonetheless, a higher education may be necessary for many forms of social independence.

Premorbid school functioning has been positively correlated with employment status. Alternatively, premorbid social functioning has been linked to a higher quality of life and higher global functioning (Hofer *et al,* 2006). Vocational functioning has been further linked to the elements of cognition, attention, learning, memory, and executive functioning (Ikebuchi, 2006). Accordingly, patients who do achieve vocational success will assess their mental health, they will maintain an active effort to improve their mental health, and they will also maintain an active effort to connect with other persons at the work place. However, symptoms, medications, and a potential deterioration of health are problems that can affect vocational functioning. As a result, although most patients want to acquire some form of work, the many complications that they face can affect their choice to seek employment.

In summation, researchers have linked social isolation to a poor prognosis in the schizophrenia patient (Schomerus *et al*, 2007a). Therefore, the act of resocialization is imperative for a higher global quality of life.

11
Stability

The most important advice that I could give to another schizophrenia patient is to always follow the counsel of a trained and certified psychiatrist. All accredited doctors have studied for many years, at the highest levels of our education system. Accordingly, only these individuals can be truly recognized as experts on mental illness. Psychiatrists are trained to know when it is appropriate to prescribe medicines, and also when not to take any forms of medical intervention at all. A psychiatrist's responsibilities will be mainly fulfilled when he finds a tolerable combination of medicines for his patient. At this point, it is up to the individual to become fully responsible for his mental health, by continuing his prescribed mode of treatment.

In Germany, only factors such as the patient's insight and trust in antipsychotic medications were correlated to treatment compliance. Therefore, neither the side effects of a medication, nor poor neuropsychological functioning was linked to medication compliance in outpatients (Klingberg *et al*, 2008). I believe that a lack of insight and trust in one's mental health care system is caused solely through societal stigmas.

The biggest regret that I hold today, with respect to my illness, is based on the fact that I did not listen to Dr. Lupton when she first diagnosed me with schizophrenia. The feelings of denial that I held were fuelled mainly by one fundamental element; I did not want to be labelled as a schizophrenic. Accordingly, I chose to believe in the delusion that I was not suffering from any illness, and I tried to rationalize the belief that Dr. Lupton was diagnosing a false positive. I now realize that these thoughts were misguided and highly irrational. In retrospect, if I had cooperated with Dr. Lupton from the very beginning, it is possible that I could have avoided my entire stay at the inpatient unit. I personally believe that I would have fully complied with Dr. Lupton's treatment plan, had I not been affected by any forms of societal stigmas.

To remain in a state of remission, the patient must always follow his doctor's advice and remain on a specific mode of treatment. If I were to forget my antipsychotic treatments for one day, I may not be able to sleep that night. However, missing a single dose of my medications could also have a minor impact on my cognition. Since I became stable on olanzapine, I have never purposely discontinued any of my daily antipsychotic treatments. I have also developed a system, using a pillbox, which makes it extremely unlikely that I will forget to take my prescription, at some time in the future. I speculate that I would enter into a state of extreme psychosis, should I stop taking my medicines for a period of less than a single week.

Once I experience the preliminary stages of a relapse, it may take over one month's time for my body to adjust and re-metabolize my antipsychotic treatments. Therefore, a permanent state of remission depends wholly on maintaining one's prescribed mode of treatment. Everyone, either healthy or sick, should concentrate on maintaining a state of good health. However, good health is also dependent on sound judgment and a rational frame of mind. As a consequence, the patient may require a form of support from an external party, known as a health advocate. A health advocate must be someone that is both reliable and trustworthy. The role of an advocate is to monitor the overall well being of a patient, and ensure that the patient remains in a permanent state of good mental health.

The primary duty of a health advocate is to monitor the patient's condition and watch for any possible signs of relapse. If the advocate should observe any problematic symptoms, then it is possible that a relapse may be occurring. This is why the relationship between the patient and his advocate is important. The schizophrenia patient must respect his health advocate, and thus, rely on his advocate to put his own medical needs above anything else.

Initially, the patient must trust a psychiatrist, who is previously unknown to him, for a preliminary diagnosis. The doctor's efforts will be fruitless if there is no sense of trust established between the patient and himself. On the other hand, if a sense of trust is established between a patient and his doctor, the doctor's opinion should be regarded as certain and unequivocal.

The same sense of trust established between a patient and his doctor must also exist between the patient and his health advocate. Under both circumstances, the patient must trust someone, other than himself, to make the most critical decisions regarding his overall health. The primary role of a health advocate is to monitor the individual's progress, during a state of remission. The health advocate should also make crucial decisions for the patient, in case of a relapse. However, if the patient is well and does not exhibit any problematic symptoms, his health advocate must also have an ability to recognize this. In other cases, the patient may realize that his symptoms have returned. When this occurs, the role of a health advocate changes to provide a form of social support, that is essential to the overall well being of the patient.

If a relapse is imminent, the patient may lose an ability to be self-sufficient. Similarly, because the patient may be delusional, he may also enter into a state of denial. Under these circumstances, the role of a health advocate increases to make decisions that are relevant to the patient's living conditions. Most importantly, though, a health advocate must make certain that his patient will follow the guidance of a trained psychiatrist.

A study, in Australia, was conducted on patients who were case-closed by community mental-health teams. These patients demonstrated significant impairments after a period of three years (Callaly *et al*, 2008). Hence, it is entirely possible that a patient's health may decline, even after he has achieved a state of remission.

Ideally, a family member or a close friend may be the best choice for a potential health advocate. However, if the individual has been socially isolated for a long period of time, these options may not be available to him. In this case, the individual may seek help from a governmental or community based service. In fact, Sharon served as my primary health advocate, until I was healthy and stable. Community services, including the Schizophrenia Society or peer-to-peer support groups, can also potentially fill a role as a health advocate.

The second, and equally important responsibility of a health advocate, is to ensure that resources such as food, shelter, and other finances related to everyday living are satisfied, especially during times when the patient is severely ill. From my personal view, the mental health care system in my society may be quite fragmented. It is essentially a complex array of services delivered through federal, provincial and municipal jurisdictions and private providers (Kirby and Keon, 2004). Moreover, it is institutionally driven as opposed to patient centred. As a result, in some cases, an acutely ill patient may experience troubles while trying to access health services that are readily available.

A fundamental right, for all schizophrenia patients, is the right to apply for social support mechanisms that are made available through a governing body. Once an individual has been formally diagnosed with schizophrenia, he has the right to apply for financial aid and other forms of social assistance. Disability income is a mode of support offered by many governments around the world, due to the difficulties that patients face when trying to find employment. In Canada, there are two levels of disability assistance. The amount of support offered depends on the individual's specific condition. The first level of support is available for persons with a temporary disability. A second, and higher level of support, is available for persons with a permanent disability. Accordingly, the amount of financial support available will vary on a case-by-case basis.

In my nation, individuals with a chronic mental disability currently qualify for an allowance of approximately $900 per month. Three hundred fifty dollars is allocated towards shelter, and the remaining five hundred fifty dollars covers all other living expenses. Personally, I feel that this allowance is insufficient for many reasons. Firstly, the average rental price for a one-bedroom apartment in my city is currently situated at anywhere between 550 to 1200 dollars per month. As a consequence, this allowance may not be adequate, if the patient has no further modes of support.

The current minimum wage in my province is eight dollars an hour. If the individual works forty hours per week, he will earn approximately 1400 dollars per month. Patients with a chronic disability are given roughly 65% of this total. Thus, persons with chronic disabilities must live well below the established poverty line, within both rural communities and major cities alike.

In some jurisdictions, there are low-income shelters available that specifically address this problem. From my understanding, there is also a lengthy wait list associated with these assisted living shelters, within my community. Some shelters are reserved specifically for persons with mental illness. Other shelters have been created for the general population, including low-income families. In cases where an emergency shelter is needed, temporary housing may also be available. From my perspective, I believe that the schizophrenia patient should remain in a state of remission, for a period of at least one year, before choosing a more independent way of life.

Individuals with disabilities may also require aid for their transportation needs. This need is quite evident for persons with a physical disability. However, persons with a mental disability will also require transportation aid, because of their low income levels. The income assistance that I currently receive barely covers finances related to food, shelter and clothing. Subsequently, a government subsidized bus pass is also available for persons with mental disabilities.

Quitting substance abuse, in the form of alcohol or a narcotic, is also essential to the patient's mental health. It is estimated that more than half of all schizophrenia patients will have a lifetime diagnosis, with respect to a substance abuse disorder (Tsuang and Fong, 2004). Both illegal drugs and alcohol will have clear effects on the patient's metabolism, which could negatively affect his prescribed mode of treatment.

Substance abuse is a major cause of relapse. Further, many illicit drugs can worsen the symptoms of a mental disorder. According to a study conducted in Oslo, there is a direct correlation between quantities of drug abuse and more severe symptoms (Ringen *et al*, 2008). Quitting all forms of illicit substance or alcohol abuse is, thus, vital to a state of remission. In Canada, the mental health and addiction treatment systems are not integrated together. This creates difficulties in the treatment of patients with concurrent disorders (Kirby and Keon, 2004).

Homelessness is another real issue for patients with mental illness. Persons with schizophrenia face homelessness mainly because they are addicted to illegal substances. Likewise, those patients who do become homeless will usually remain in a constant state of relapse. In the majority of cases, patients who are both ill and homeless will not receive the emergency social services that they urgently need.

The first step in combating homelessness is to ensure that the patient remains in a state of remission. If drug abuse leads to a relapse, then professional forms of intervention may be needed. On the other hand, if a patient is prone to relapse for reasons other than substance abuse, this can indicate a permanent need for third party support.

Two types of interventions can solve homelessness among persons with mental illness. In principle, the patient's health advocate may undertake a primary responsibility to become his caretaker. If the patient has no such advocate, then this responsibility should be passed on to a governing body. In fact, a significant flaw exists within any social welfare system where there is homelessness among the mentally sick. A society's governing body must take more responsibility in situations where a mentally sick patient lacks the social resources necessary for his everyday living and survival.

According to several studies, schizophrenia patients are over-represented within the homeless population. Between 80 to 95 percent of homeless persons in Canada, The United States, Australia, Norway, and Germany suffer from some type of mental disorder. Conversely, in Ireland and Spain, only 25 to 33 percent of homeless persons suffer from a mental illness (Martens, 2001). Homeless persons that remain in a state of psychosis are more likely to be male, single, and have some type of drug use disorder (Cougnard *et al*, 2006).

In France, researchers have conducted a study on the rate of homeless subjects who used emergency psychiatric services. Most homeless persons with psychosis had already been identified as individuals with a severe mental illness. This suggests the possibility that homelessness is a consequence of a break in contact with mental health services (Cougnard *et al*, 2006). This study also indicates that many patients will need third party support, with respect to the management of their psychotic symptoms. In a further study, homeless persons use more inpatient and emergency services, and fewer outpatient services (Folsom *et al*, 2005). In contrast, residents of board-and-care facilities had a greater use of outpatient mental health services. Therefore, a clear division exists between the mental health of patients who are homeless and other patients who utilize governmental support mechanisms.

Other studies have shown that homelessness may be a predictive element for nonadherence (Nyamathi *et al*, 2008). Many homeless patients have problems with both a history of medicine non-compliance, and substance abuse. They also have problems when trying to recognize their symptoms. Such individuals were less likely to have formed a good therapeutic alliance during hospitalization, and more likely to have family members that refused to become involved in their treatment (Olfson *et al*, 2000). All of these facts seem to suggest that a social bond has been broken between homeless patients and their community.

A study of 82 homeless men, in Stockholm, reveals a more in depth truth regarding this social problem. After five years, the mortality rate of persons with a drug addiction was recorded at 46%. However, there were no deaths recorded among any men who were diagnosed with a single psychiatric disorder exclusively, like schizophrenia. A 17% increase in substance abuse problems was recorded among those who still faced homelessness. Furthermore, at the end of this study, 75% of the survivors were still homeless (Beijer *et al*, 2007). According to this study, the majority of homeless schizophrenia patients will never improve their situation, and some may begin to abuse illicit substances as a direct result.

In Germany, a study was conducted on homeless women with psychiatric disorders. In this study, women mainly lost their home when leaving a violent situation. The main elements that differentiated male and female homelessness were precipitant situations, the need for help, and help seeking patterns (Torchalla *et al*, 2004). Another study suggests that symptom severity, among homeless persons with schizophrenia, appears as an interaction of symptom profiles and risk behaviors that are gender specific. Consequently, gender specific routes to homelessness have also been observed among mentally sick adults (Opler *et al*, 2001).

An increased exposure to adverse childhood events has also been linked to social problems and homelessness (Lu *et al*, 2008). Other significant predictors of homelessness include living in an unstable shelter, having a family history of mental disorders, having no sources of income, and having an unmarried, divorced or separated social status. Further, the risk factor for homelessness increases with an increased exposure to multiple risk factors (Ran *et al*, 2006).

The most effective precautionary measures used to combat homelessness are based on early intervention (EI) techniques. Many studies demonstrate that early intervention measures are positively correlated with a better prognosis. Early intervention patients are also more likely to remain living with their families. In a further study, more patients within an EI group stopped using illicit drugs, in comparison to those who were treated through a standard community mental health team (Agius *et al*, 2007).

Dual disorder modes of treatment have also shown some promise in addressing these issues. In principle, integrated treatment services combine both mental health and substance abuse treatments concurrently. The strategy behind an integrated service includes pharmacological treatment, intensive case management, motivational interviewing, individual and group psychotherapies, and family participation (Tsuang and Fong, 2004).

Patients with co-occurring schizophrenic and substance use disorders have indicated a high level of recovery through positive coping behaviours, based on their level of education. Improvements in schizophrenic symptoms, active remissions from substance abuse, increases in social contacts, an increased competitive employment rate, and a reduction in hospitalizations and homelessness has also been reported by these patients. Although they have reported improvements in their overall life satisfaction, there was no change reported regarding independent living conditions (Drake *et al*, 2006).

Integrated housing services may also be more effective than parallel housing services. In an integrated housing program, case management and housing services are provided to patients by a team within a single agency. In a parallel housing program, case management and housing services are provided by two independent agencies. One study indicates that an integrated housing service led to more days of stable housing and greater life satisfaction. Patients also reported greater reductions of their psychiatric symptoms, while enrolled within an integrated service (McHugo *et al*, 2004).

Integrated housing services have also been linked with greater gains in several outcome domains (McHugo *et al*, 2004). I theorize that this is due to the fact that schizophrenia patients require simplicity over complexity. Some social programs may be unknown to the patient, and thus difficult to access. This difficulty increases exponentially for patients who are presently struggling with the symptoms of an illness. The best solution may be the introduction of an assisted living facility that provides outpatient health services hand in hand. The creation of targeted services that are easy to access could address the problem of homelessness, among this sub-population.

Although homelessness is an international problem, some elements may be culturally based. Researchers have found significant cross-cultural differences in the prevalence of mental disorders diagnosed in homeless patients around the world. For example, homeless rates among patients with schizophrenia are exceedingly lower in high-income welfare societies.

Nevertheless, in these states, there were insufficient efforts directed towards social rehabilitative programs and vocational services (Melle *et al*, 2007).

Other studies indicate that homelessness is a state of flection. In this case, even if a mentally sick patient does own a home, there exists a high probability that he will lose it and become homeless. Moreover, according to some researchers, lacking a permanent home may be inherent to a mental illness (Melamed *et al*, 2004). If this is true, then another serious problem, in the form of civic discrimination, may be prevalent within our society as well.

A further study links homelessness and psychological symptom severity to non-violent crimes. Scientists have discovered that the severity of a patient's psychotic symptoms may partially mediate the relationship between a psychotic disorder and criminal activity (Fischer *et al*, 2008). Consequently, addressing the problem of homelessness for persons with mental illness, and providing efficient modes of treatment could further benefit a community through a reduction in crime rates.

Redlich observes the fact that individuals with mental illness are overrepresented within the criminal justice system. She theorizes that this may be due to the phenomenon of false confessions. There are three possible kinds of confessions. Voluntary confessions are motivated by a will to protect the true perpetrator. Coerced-compliant confessions are attained through stress, from intense police pressure. Coerced-internalized confessions occur when the suspect is led to remember that he committed the crime, and thus he falsely believes that he is the genuine perpetrator (Redlich, 2004).

From my perspective, many persons that suffer from a mental disorder are quite susceptible to coercion. This is due to the fact that their mental faculties are highly compromised because of their illness. Most schizophrenia patients cannot cope with intense degrees of stress in the same manner that a mentally healthy person could. Redlich's research could provide a greater insight into this social problem, which may then prevent failures like these within our justice system.

Migration has also been associated with mental illness and schizophrenia. This association appears to be mediated by psychosocial factors, including difficulties with establishing social capital in smaller migrant groups

(Kelly, 2005). The reasons for migration, the nature of entry, and the social position of immigrants within the host country are other relevant factors (Corcoran *et al*. 2009).

As a final point, patients with schizophrenia must strive towards reducing all forms of extrinsic stressors. Periods of intense stress will affect the mental health of any schizophrenia patient. Medically termed as sensitization, environmental stressors in interaction with epigenetic factors can induce psychological, or physiological alterations that facilitate the onset and persistence of psychotic symptoms (Collip *et al*, 2008). Other studies suggest that stress-related disorders may sometimes precede more severe psychological disorders (Hageman *et al*, 2008). Therefore, environmental stressors can also cause psychotic symptoms in some patients.

In a study comparing schizophrenia outpatients to non-psychiatric control subjects, the outpatients scored higher levels of trait emotional reactivity, arousability, and trait anxiety. The occurrence of potentially stressful life events also predicted an increase of psychotic symptoms in these patients, and likewise there was a significant interaction between the level of initial trait reactivity and the occurrence of life events in the prediction of these increases (Docherty *et al*, 2009). In other words, patients with schizophrenia have higher levels of trait reactivity when compared to the average person, and high levels of trait reactivity have been linked to an increased risk for a psychotic relapse due to stress.

A further study correlates stressful conditions to increases of paranoia, depression, and negative emotions in patients with psychosis. An increase of paranoia under stress is believed to be moderated by a level of vulnerability and mediated through anxiety. The participants of this study also demonstrated increases of anxiety under stress, and anxiety was linked to paranoia in participants with higher forms of baseline symptomatologies (Lincoln *et al*, 2009).

In fact, most dissociative reactions among schizophrenia patients result from traumatic experiences that lead to a loss of inhibitory control (Bob *et al*, 2007 b,c). Researchers have observed that a third of these patients may also suffer from posttraumatic stress symptoms. Therefore, an increase in the severity of one's symptoms has been consistently observed in schizophrenia patients who suffer from a comorbid posttraumatic stress disorder (Spitzer *et al*, 2007).

According to another study, the most significant increases of stress affecting schizophrenia patients are in areas such as their domestic environment, their driven behaviours, and a state of depression. Areas excluded from this subgroup include the patient's health, attitude posture, relaxation potential, role definition, and other elements related to time pressure, hostility, and anxiety (Betensky *et al*, 2008). Cases of depression were also correlated with greater negative symptom severity.

Scientists have also drawn a correlation between the patient's family history and his emotional distress. This study reveals that patients with a positive family history of schizophrenia are likely to suffer from long-term elevated levels of emotional distress. Thus, a relation has been drawn between an individual's persistently elevated emotional distress and his genetic liability to develop schizophrenia (Ritsner *et al*, 2007).

A genetically mediated abnormal sensitivity to stress may also play a large role in the onset, exacerbation, and relapse of schizophrenia. According to one study, siblings of schizophrenia patients demonstrated significantly greater responses to stress, when compared to a control group. The control group also demonstrated a significantly less pronounced response to stress. As a result, genetic risks for schizophrenia may also cause an enhanced sensitivity to stress (Brunelin *et al*, 2008).

Scientifically, the human brain responds to stress when it determines what is potentially threatening to the individual. Psychological stress is also known to increase dopamine release within the brain (McEwen, 2007). The brain then communicates with bodily systems, like the cardiovascular or immune systems, to produce a natural physiological and behavioural response. In turn, these responses can either be adaptive or damaging to the human body.

Some stressors will also produce a form of chronic stress that harms the human body over a period of time. The hippocampus, amygdala, and prefrontal cortex all undergo stress-induced structural remodeling as a response to this chronic stress. Thus, stress hormones can also produce both adaptive and maladaptive effects on the human brain, throughout the course of an individual's lifetime (McEwen, 2007).

Abnormalities in the expression of neurotrophins, which respond to stressful stimuli, have been consistently observed in the schizophrenia patient (Bernstein *et al*, 2002). Likewise, certain severe mental illnesses have been associated with genetic changes in molecules that regulate the intracellular signaling pathways that are activated through stress (Arnsten, 2007). Some forms of stress may further exacerbate a breakdown in cortical processing, with respect to certain kinds of incoming information (Lambe *et al*, 2007).

The glycoprotein M6A gene is also important in schizophrenia research. This gene modulates the influence of stress on the hippocampus in some animals. Scientists further believe that this gene may play a role in some stress-induced hippocampal alterations, which have been discovered in the brains of patients with schizophrenia and other psychiatric disorders (Boks *et al*, 2008).

Most individuals who are exposed to some form of adversity will maintain relatively normal levels of psychological functioning. However, persons with a mental illness will face an unduly more difficult challenge when exposed to forms of adversity. In a study conducted on schizophrenia patients with European and Arabian backgrounds, nearly every patient reported that psychosocial stress is an important factor underlying their illness (Conrad *et al*, 2007).

Non-compliance to treatment is also a relevant issue. According to one study, up to 50% of patients will discontinue their treatments because of social barriers, experiences with adverse events, and ineffective medications (Altamura and Goikolea, 2008). Of these elements, the individual only has the power to potentially avoid stressful life events.

Another study, conducted in the United States, indicates that treatment costs are greater for schizophrenia patients who have experienced a recent crisis. Patients who have problems with suicide attempts, prior criminal arrests, violent behaviour, and recent psychiatric hospitalizations have been linked with higher treatment costs.

Researchers have also correlated rehospitalization rates to demographic and social factors. A lack of outpatient services is a main reason why many schizophrenia patients re-enter a hospitalized setting. The patient's family status, social relationships, and level of insight are other factors that have been linked to the risk of rehospitalization (Postrado and Lehman, 1995).

Relapses in schizophrenia have been correlated to the side effects of a medication, the number of psychotic episodes, unemployment, and problematic life events (Chabungbam *et al*, 2007). In contrast, a full recovery from schizophrenia has been associated with a shorter duration of untreated psychosis, better premorbid adjustment, fewer negative symptoms at baseline, no issues with substance abuse, and the patient's adherence to his medications (Petersen *et al*, 2008).

Improvements in subjective well-being may fundamentally act as the major predictor for the chance of remission (Naber, 2008). Achieving good health should be the first objective of all schizophrenia patients. Maintaining a state of remission should be the second objective. A trustworthy health advocate will serve to safeguard the patient's well-being. Nonetheless, a society's governing body may also be needed to combat further problems related to poverty and homelessness among the mentally sick.

12

Living with Schizophrenia

Achieving a state of remission should be the most important goal for all individuals that suffer from a mental illness. After the patient mentally recuperates from schizophrenia, what comes next? In my opinion, the patient must then strive towards the principle of acceptance. Nobody welcomes illness into his or her life. A disability, on the other hand, may be viewed as a chronic illness. The state of being ill, according to the uninformed individual, may imply a biological weakness. In the same fashion, a mental disability may implicate a functional weakness. As a matter of fact, the concept of strange behaviour due to a personal weakness may be the most significant root behind many societal stigmas (Jorm and Griffiths, 2008). Accordingly, problems with accepting the fact that one is sick may be a difficulty that is created through the ignorance of an imperfect society.

After I accept the fact that I have schizophrenia, I will essentially empower myself to psychologically address and counteract any barriers that have been associated with my illness. It is true that my memory has degraded, since the time when I was first diagnosed with schizophrenia. The same may be true about my attention span and concentration. However, if I am able to accept the current situation that I am in, whether it is favourable or not, I will free myself from the effects of social discrimination. What I am, biologically, is something that I can never change. If I cannot accept the physical being that I am, then I will never have any idea of what I can possibly become in the future. If I accept the fact that I have schizophrenia, I will also be accepting my personal identity as an imperfect human being.

In defining the concept of acceptance, holding an awareness of my symptoms is not enough. Acknowledging any forms of societal stigmas that exist against mental illness also contradicts the principle of acceptance. Accepting schizophrenia involves having a positive outlook on life, despite the fact that one suffers from a devastating mental disease.

At present, schizophrenia is a highly treatable disorder. The principle of acceptance also requires the patient to realize this fact. This can then lead to hope for a cure at some point in our future. The patient must also acknowledge the fact that there are forms of social support created specifically to help persons with mental illness. Scientifically speaking, this method of coping is correlated with a greater awareness of illness, but not distress (Cooke *et al*, 2007). Acceptance requires the individual to have factual knowledge of his illness, a positive demeanour, and the desire to live a healthy and satisfying life.

Accepting who you are is essential to understanding what you have to offer to the world. It is true that gaining employment in a highly stressful work environment may not be the best situation for me. Nevertheless, I still believe that I can contribute something positive towards my community. No human beings are without faults. Accepting one's faults is a natural part of being human. Therefore, the schizophrenia patient should understand any implications that may be associated with his illness, and plan a life with both the best and worst case scenarios in mind.

Illness, unfortunately, is a part of human existence in our natural world. So is mental illness. However, ignorant persons may hold the mistaken belief that mental illnesses are a rare and isolated phenomenon. They may believe that the individual holds an absolute responsibility over his mental health, and that mental illnesses are acquired solely through the patient's own fault. Nevertheless, according to a myriad of scientific evidence, schizophrenia is caused by biological factors. Therefore, the stigma produced towards mental illnesses may be fundamentally based on a negative attitude towards persons with poor health, a lack of understanding, and social intolerance.

The negative aspects associated with psychiatry as a medical specialty, within the last 20 years, has also created a source for societal stigmas. Uncertain diagnoses and the deinstitutionalizing of services for patients may be underlying elements. Hence, negative attitudes towards psychiatry, and a lack of faith in psychiatric institutions could provide a further source for cultural stigmas.

A lack of social acceptance, within one's society, will generally cause feelings of denial in the mentally sick individual. Under these circumstances, persons who are fighting an illness must also overcome barriers that are created ad hoc within their own community. In many cases, individuals who experience the preliminary symptoms of a mental illness may avoid professional help, because of these stigmas. Therefore, social stigmas have a definite and direct impact on a patient's mental health. In fact, many problems that mentally sick patients face would not exist, if there were no forms of discrimination present within our society.

One common stigmatized belief labels all schizophrenics as persons who are prone to criminal behaviour. When a schizophrenia patient commits murder, this can sometimes lead to the belief that all persons with schizophrenia may also be capable of this act. However, according to a study conducted in Australia, personality factors, rather than symptoms or neuropsychological functioning are most significant with respect to the violent acts committed by schizophrenia patients (Fullam and Dollan, 2008).

Nonetheless, according to another study, there is some consistency on a small but significant relation between schizophrenia patients and violent acts. Yet, the researcher of this study also stressed the fact that many public fears targeted towards persons with psychotic illnesses are largely unfounded (Taylor, 2008). Furthermore, there exists a large amount of evidence which suggests that schizophrenia patients, themselves, may be the victims of violence. Consequently, there may be a pressing need to develop newer modes of therapy that will address this specific problem.

Other stigmatized beliefs are spawned when violent interactions occur between patients with mental illness and police authorities. According to a study conducted in Germany, the solution to this problem may come about through the special training of police officers on the subject of mental illness (Wundsam *et al*, 2007). It is theorized that this specialized training could reduce the occurrence of violent interactions, which will thereby reduce a significant source behind many societal stigmas.

A study conducted in the United States seems to confirm this theory. Officers in a crisis intervention team took part in a 40-hour training program, designed to help them better interact with mentally sick individuals. Upon completion, the officers reported improved attitudes regarding aggressiveness among individuals with schizophrenia. These officers also reported feelings of less social distance towards persons with mental illness. Therefore, educational programs may also effectively reduce some of the societal stigmas that are generated towards schizophrenia patients (Compton *et al*, 2006).

Patients with mental illness can also be stereotyped as unpredictable or dangerous. This label has further led to the social distancing of patients from their society (Lai *et al*, 2000). According to another study, individuals with schizophrenia are substantially over-represented amongst prison populations. This latter element may also give rise to some forms of stigma (Kelly, 2005).

Indeed, there are individuals with mental disorders who do commit crimes. Psychiatric patients that are diagnosed with antisocial personality disorder (ASPD) have been positively associated with criminal behaviour. These patients have also been associated with severe drug abuse and extensive homelessness (Mueser *et al*, 2006). On the other hand, criminal behaviour has not been linked to patients that suffer from both schizophrenia and a substance use disorder. This seems to suggest that psychiatric patients with substance abuse problems, who do not go on to develop ASPD, will pose no criminal harm to their society (Mueser *et al*, 2006). Dispelling the myths associated with schizophrenia can essentially diminish the prejudices and biases that are currently widespread within our society.

According to the World Health Organization, one of the greatest obstacles hindering the treatment of all mental illnesses is social stigma (Oral, 2007). Some researchers further believe that societal stigmas can affect elements like change and reform within the mental health care system. Likewise, social stigmas can affect both the patient and his family members alike. This often results in a varied range of beliefs towards the cause and treatments for schizophrenia.

In general, the patient's internalized stigma usually emerges through many faulty models and concepts that have been wrongly associated with mental illness. These false beliefs will cause considerable misconceptions towards his illness and psychiatry as a whole. Consequently, many false beliefs associated with schizophrenia can either mitigate or aggravate the effects of societal stigmas on the patient (Charles *et al*, 2007).

Levels of internalized stigma have also been correlated to the severity of the individual's illness. Social stigma is most problematic when the patient accepts and believes in the negative connotations that have been created through a misinformed public. For example, an extremely low rate of paranoid thoughts has been correlated to valid social persecution, during the early stages of psychosis. As a result, some scientists theorize that paranoid thoughts, relevant to justified persecution, may be primarily caused through societal stigmas and personal depression (Fornells-Ambrojo and Garety, 2005).

The patient's internalization of stigmatized beliefs is largely due to the pervasive incidences of social discrimination. Prejudices can affect elements like self-esteem and adaptive social functioning in the patient (Oral, 2007). Patients who experience high degrees of social anxieties can also attach a greater shame to their illness. They often feel that they are socially marginalized and that they have a low social status. The patient's limited access to important roles within his community may then propagate other forms of societal stigmas (Birchwood et al, 2007). Without a doubt, internalized stigma can have a direct influence on the social interactions of patients within their community.

In another study, aspects of self-esteem related to lovability were correlated with feelings of being alienated from others due to mental illness. Hence, social stigmas can also have a direct effect on the psychological well being of the schizophrenia patient (Lysaker et al, 2008 a,b).

Trait paranoia has also been associated with lower levels and higher instability of self-esteem. Therefore, decreases in self-esteem have been correlated with an immediate increase in paranoia. These findings seem to suggest that individuals with paranoia are also characterized by a lower level of self-esteem, and that fluctuations in one's self-esteem predict the degree of subsequent paranoia. Some researchers hypothesize that dysfunctional strategies of self-esteem regulation may also be linked to paranoid thoughts (Thewissen et al, 2008).

Self-esteem, in relation to independence, has been connected to the rejection of mental illness stereotypes. Conversely, reduced personal empowerment has been tied to depression and a lower quality of life. Researchers have also correlated aspects of self-esteem and personal empowerment to both the absence of discrimination, and the individual's ability to ward off stigma (Lysaker et al, 2008a). Accordingly, social stigmas may also have immense effects on the patient's independence and way of life.

Internalized stigma can also affect the qualities of self-experience, which is believed to be important in the recovery process from a mental illness (Lysaker et al, 2008a). In Australia, researchers studied artworks that were created mainly by schizophrenia patients. At the outset, these works were used for diagnostic and interpretive purposes. However, when a group of art historians evaluated these works, their criticisms were patronising and vulnerable to perversion by totalitarian regimes. The patients' artworks were often portrayed as degenerate art, which, in my opinion, illustrates an extreme degree of discrimination and social intolerance within our society (Rosen, 2007).

Internalized stigma has been associated with both social functioning and positive symptoms. Some researchers theorize that positive symptoms may be the most influential factor related to ongoing stigmatized experiences (Lysaker *et al*, 2007a). However, high levels of internalized stigma have also been associated with increases in the patient's cognitive insight, along with the attribution of personal responsibility towards the cause and onset of his illness. In all of these cases, cognitive restructuring may be necessary to alleviate the problem of internalized stigma (Mak and Wu, 2006).

Forms of discrimination against schizophrenia have also increased because of the socially undesirable side effects of antipsychotic medications. Some persons actually believe in the notion that antipsychotic medications have no beneficial or therapeutic effects (Sajatovic and Jenkins, 2007). Therefore, this false belief merely takes the adverse effects of antipsychotic medications into consideration. The patient's lack of awareness, regarding his symptoms during treatment, can also fuel stigmas towards psychiatric medications. However, improvements in biomarker technology and translational biology, in addition to a better understanding of psychopathology in the future may shed the stigma of 'dirty drugs' (Wong *et al*, 2008). Accordingly, the stigma associated with psychiatric medications may be mainly based on insufficient scientific progress.

Research indicates that early intervention modes of treatment, during the first psychotic episode, will generally result in the best possible prognosis. Nonetheless, the existence of social and cultural stigmas may lead to the refusal for treatment at this stage. Stigmas based on the negative effects of antipsychotic medications can provide a second reason why some patients will refuse treatment. One possible solution comes from a study conducted in 2007. These researchers state:

"At the time of first-episode psychosis presentation, it is crucial that clinicians select the most effective treatment option as immediate intervention offers the best chance for containing the illness" (Buckley *et al*, 2007).

The stigma created against psychiatric medications is mainly based on the often serious and painful side effects associated with typical antipsychotic medications. However, if the patient is treated with newer antipsychotics during the preliminary stages of his illness, and if he no longer has to endure the most serious side effects of older medications, this could negate much of the stigma that exists against antipsychotic medications altogether.

A second reason why psychiatrists should initially prescribe the best available medicine may be due to the fact that functional impairment occurs most rapidly during this early period, which can alter the patient's future prognosis, level of necessary treatment, and affect morbidity (Buckley *et al,* 2007). A more efficacious mode of treatment may give prospective patients enough reason to comply with their doctors, during the early stages of their illness.

The quality of mental health services can also provide a source for social stigmas. Many sick persons may fear the possibility that they will be committed into an inpatient facility. A loss of personal freedoms within these facilities could be comparable, by some persons, to formal incarceration. Poor representations of inpatient units on television and in the movies can fuel some forms of stigma linked to psychiatric hospitals.

Stigmatized attitudes towards mental illness are, in fact, a global problem. Many misconceptions are based on the media reports of criminal actions committed by individuals who are extremely sick. However, criminal behaviour does not typify all persons with mental illness. Individuals with a mental illness are, in most respects, much like any other persons within their society. We wish for the necessities in life like good mental and physical health, caring relationships, meaningful forms of employment, and a positive sense of identity. All of these factors have been associated with a more satisfactory quality of life. Yet, in order to acquire these life basics, individuals with a mental illness must be viewed as equals within a non-discriminating society.

National anti-stigma interventions have been effective within many regions of the world. However, these educational campaigns must be culturally targeted to be effective. These campaigns can often negate many false or contradictory beliefs that the average citizen may hold towards mental illness. For instance, in some parts of the developing world, non-biomedical beliefs are held with respect to the treatment of psychosis. In India, participants in a study viewed indigenous healing methods as complementary to allopathic treatments (Saravanan *et al*, 2008).

In Nigeria, supernatural factors and the misuse of psychoactive substances are believed to be the most common causes of mental illness. This belief was especially held by persons who were elder, those who were living within rural dwellings, and those who were less familiar with mental illnesses. On the other hand, persons who were familiar with mental illnesses, and those who lived in urban dwellings believed in a biological or psychosocial cause of mental illness (Adewuya and Makanjuola, 2008). This variation in etiological beliefs demonstrates the vast differences between stigmatized beliefs and scientific knowledge.

A study conducted in Pakistan also reveals the fact that some educated citizens hold superstitious beliefs towards mental illness. These participants mainly held the belief that psychosis is caused by the will of God, loneliness, and unemployment. Some individuals also held the belief that schizophrenia patients are generally dangerous. With respect to treatment, 40% of those surveyed viewed psychiatric consultation as the single most important management step. Other respondents believed in spiritual healing, social changes, and inaction. Therefore, because much of the population held non-biomedical beliefs towards the cause of schizophrenia, patients often did not seek appropriate modes of treatment, and this directly impacts the health and well being of schizophrenia patients in that nation (Zafar *et al*, 2008).

In a cross-cultural study, Japanese persons were more likely to hold stigmatized attitudes and be socially distant from individuals with depression, depression with suicidal ideations, early schizophrenia, and chronic schizophrenia. Conversely, Australians were more likely to perceive discriminatory forms of behaviour in other persons within their society. In both countries, personal stigma was significantly greater than perceived stigma. Likewise, in both countries, the average person held more stigmatized beliefs against persons with schizophrenia, in comparison to those with depression. There was also very little difference in the stigma generated towards persons with depression, and persons with depression who experience suicidal ideations. In Australia, a greater social distance was also observed towards patients with chronic schizophrenia, in comparison to those with early schizophrenia (Griffiths *et al*, 2006).

In a study comparing German and Russian cultures, 32% of individuals living in Germany associated split-personality disorder with schizophrenia. In comparison, only 2% of individuals in Russia held this belief. This study also reveals the fact that the association of schizophrenia with split-personality disorder has increased significantly in individuals with a higher education (Schomerus *et al*, 2007b).

However, according to a study conducted in Chicago, persons with a higher education were less likely to stigmatize than less educated participants. In addition, women were less likely to endorse stigmatized beliefs, while non-white individuals were more likely to endorse stigmatized beliefs (Corrigan and Watson, 2007).

In China, pervasive negative attitudes and discriminatory treatment towards persons with mental illness may be common. Stigmatized attitudes in this nation often resulted in direct individual discrimination, structural discrimination, and the internalization of stereotypes. Confucianism, the centrality of outward appearance, and pejorative aetiological beliefs linked to mental illness provides the main basis for societal stigmas in this nation (Yang, 2007).

According to another study conducted in China, stigmatized attitudes actively block the development of community-based services for schizophrenia patients. Moreover, many patients in China face a constant series of rejections and exclusions when applying for established services (Liu, 2007). Impaired access to social services through the negative effects of social, economic, and stigmatic factors is largely known as structural violence (Kelly, 2008). Consequently, cultural stigmas can also have a significant effect over the creation of support programs for patients with mental illness.

In fact, focus group patients in Hong Kong have reported stigmatized experiences in relation to both their clinical visits, and the side effects of their antipsychotic medications. These patients reported that they were the victims of structural discrimination, by way of the adverse treatment and experiences incurred during hospitalization. Patients had to deal with negative attitudes from staff members, excessive measures of restraint, inadequate information services, and limited personal rights. Hence, individual and structural based stigmas may be quite extensive within this part of the world.

According to this study, schizophrenia patients were also more likely to anticipate stigma, conceal illness, and default on clinic visits, when compared to patients with diabetes. Medication-induced stigma also resulted in an unwelcome disclosure of illness, workplace difficulties, family rejection, and treatment non-adherence. It is theorized that some societal stigmas may also be based on a difference of power between mentally sick persons and the community itself. This theory is based on the inequities observed in health policies, resource allocation, and the privileged control that is granted to service providers over users (Lee *et al*, 2006).

In Singapore, schizophrenia patients treated in a state mental hospital were less likely to be the victims of stigma, when compared to patients who were treated in a general hospital. In contrast, the converse was true regarding all other forms of mental illness. Stigma in that country was also more likely to be sustained by persons who were employed and those who were of a younger age (Chee *et al*, 2005). This study suggests that some forms of societal stigmas may be based on institutional and illness specific factors.

A study conducted in South Africa reveals that most patients with schizophrenia perceive a high overall degree of stigmatization within their community. Twenty-nine percent of those surveyed felt that many sources in the media actively delineate a negative attitude towards schizophrenia patients. Furthermore, 39% of those surveyed indicated that they had been the victims of physical abuse due to their illness (Botha *et al*, 2006). Patients who were male, those who spoke Xhosa, those who had more inpatient facility admissions, and those who had a longer duration of illness also reported excessive physical abuse.

In Israel, older patients have reported comparatively lower levels of self-stigma than younger patients (Werner *et al*, 2008). In this case, differences in age also suggest that the materialization of societal stigma is culturally dependent.

The odd behaviour of persons with mental illness could provide another source for cultural stigmas, in China. However, in the United States, the strange emotional states of patients with mental illness may provide a basis for stigma. Accordingly, social stigmas are mainly produced through differing factors among different cultures. If this is true and the problem of societal stigma is culturally based, then it is also true that there exists no universal reason why some persons will discriminate against the mentally sick. The only common element among stigmatized beliefs around the world is that these beliefs are based on prejudice and falsehoods, and not scientific fact. Under these circumstances, a possible solution to the problem of social stigmas may come about through a well-educated society.

A study conducted in the United States attributes mental disorders as the primary cause of a disability, over any other class of illness, in citizens who are between 15 and 44 years of age. Suicidal rates among persons with mental illness also peak at a higher annual mortality rate when compared to homicide rates, patients with AIDS, and patients with most forms of cancer. Moreover, according to this study, morbidity and mortality rates for persons with mental disorders have not changed within the past several decades. In effect, these researchers conclude that societal stigmas may be a key reason behind the lack of progress with mental illnesses relative to other medical illnesses (Insel and Scolnick, 2006).

Indeed, scientists have made progress in the form of cures, treatments, and modes of prevention for many illnesses. Nonetheless, in the treatment of mental disorders, researchers have only discovered drugs with fewer adverse effects. According to one study, the expectations and goals of the scientific community have contributed to this relative lack of progress (Insel and Scolnick, 2006). Personally, I would have to disagree with this assessment. I believe that a lack of progress in schizophrenia research may be due more to the complexity of the disease, and the absence of scientific knowledge with respect to the inner workings of the human brain.

According to other research, schizophrenia patients will also characteristically have a shorter lifespan, when compared to the general population. Higher rates of HIV, cardiovascular disease, diabetes, hepatitis, osteoporosis, obesity, altered pain sensitivity, polydipsia, dental problems, and sexual dysfunction have been consistently observed in schizophrenia (Leucht *et al*, 2007). Factors related to the disease, its treatment, the unsatisfactory organization of health services, the attitudes of medical doctors, and the social stigma ascribed to patients could be the quintessential roots behind this problem.

The relatives of patients with psychosis also want support in combating societal stigmas. According to one study, family members of patients with schizophrenia have reported more intense negative feelings, elevated levels of objective and subjective burden, less closeness and more shame in comparison to a control group. It is often the case that the stigma ascribed to all mental illnesses will create secondary victims (Barak and

Solomon, 2005). Therefore, the relatives of the schizophrenia patient may also suffer from anxiety or guilt, due to societal stigmas. These individuals can experience further problems with psychological suffering, sleep disturbances, poor social relationships, and a lower quality of life (Kadri *et al*, 2004).

In contrast, according to another study, societal stigmas directed towards the family members of patients with schizophrenia are uncommon. Moreover, discrimination against the family members of individuals with drug dependence problems may be worse, in comparison to other health conditions. In the latter cases, family members can often be blamed for the onset and offset of a relative's disorder, and they may be shunned within their community (Corrigan *et al*, 2006). In my opinion, this stigmatized belief may be similar to the impression that schizophrenia patients are personally responsible for their poor health. In both cases, responsibility and blame may be erroneously assigned to a guiltless party.

Societal stigmas mainly stem through false beliefs regarding the causes of mental illness. Elements like drug or alcohol abuse, evil spirits, radiation, the avoidance of life problems, and a form of punishment from God are baseless causal beliefs held by some individuals around the world. Other forms of stigma assume the notion that persons with mental illness are incapable of living an independent way of life. In fact, schizophrenia patients with high insight and a minimal amount of internalized stigma demonstrate significantly greater social functioning than any other subgroup. However, patients with high insight and moderate levels of internalized stigma have significantly lower levels of hope, according to the Beck Hopelessness Scale (Lysaker *et al*, 2005b). The existence of societal stigmas also forces the patient to conceal his illness from much of the general public. As a result, many patients may not be completely honest when engaged in a variety of social situations. This, in turn, creates a considerable barrier against the patient's recovery and rehabilitation.

In a comparison of six case studies, some schizophrenia patients believe that they are diminished relative to their former selves (Lysaker and Lysaker, 2010). My self-assessment may be similar. In fact, I know that my cognitive abilities were much greater during my youth, before I became seriously ill. However, I also have to acknowledge the fact that I can still live a satisfying life. Even though cognition is essential to gaining forms of competitive employment and achieving higher levels of education, these are but two elements in a large sphere of other qualities in human life. There is no universal key to living a prosperous life. Consequently, it is up to the individual to find meaning in his life, despite the fact that he is chronically ill.

Acceptance is a key principle that must be embraced by both the schizophrenia patient and his community. Primarily, the patient must adapt his lifestyle to a chronic, yet treatable disease. On the other hand, societies around the world must recognize the fact that mental illnesses are not an isolated phenomenon. Stigma and discrimination are unfortunate elements in our civilization. Education and resilience can neutralize these forms of injustice. Therefore, understanding the truths on mental illness should repudiate elements like prejudice and inequality. Alternatively, when the schizophrenia patient demonstrates resilience, social attitudes based on stigma and ignorance will ultimately be rendered as barren and powerless.

13

Responsibility

Living with schizophrenia necessarily entails living by way of self-determination. It also means reclaiming the power to act, and take responsibility over one's life. The schizophrenia patient must also accept further responsibilities, with respect to any future offspring. According to family, twin, and adoption studies, the heritability risk factor for schizophrenia is situated at approximately 80% (Carroll and Owen, 2009). Therefore, since the pathology of schizophrenia will include genetic causes, the patient should begin a record of illness within his family. A record of illness will help later generations better prepare for any adverse effects from a potential illness.

It is recommended that the individual should also keep a record of his emotional states, after he is diagnosed with a mental illness. Since problems with memory are a general symptom among many mental disorders, a personal mood diary can provide the patient's medical team with a more complete understanding of his mental state. This, in turn, can result in a more efficient mode of treatment.

A mood diary can also be used to record the individual's progress, from the time when he was first diagnosed, until the present day. If the patient's health has not improved, then his current mode of treatment may be ineffective. However, if the patient demonstrates some degree of progress, a personal diary will enable his doctor to refine his current mode of treatment, and prescribe a more tolerable and effective set of medicines.

One area of new research focuses on the early or childhood onset of a mental illness. From a personal perspective, I believe that early onset schizophrenia is an extremely significant problem within our society. This is due to my belief that all childhood and teenage suicides are due solely to a mental illness. At present, it may be impossible to prove that my theory is true. Perhaps in the future, as our scientific knowledge progresses, my theory can be tested and proved valid or invalid. However, if I am right, mental disorders should immediately become an exceedingly more substantial problem within our society.

I believe that all non-adult suicides are due to a mental illness because of my personal experiences with schizophrenia. One memory of a suicidal ideation of mine occurred due to my paranoid state of mind. While on a spring vacation during my teenage years, I traveled to the Caribbean on a cruise liner. I remember that, on one occasion, I was looking over the railing of the ship. In my mind, I was thinking about what would happen if I jumped into the ocean. After realizing that I may drown without anyone's knowledge, I eventually re-examined my thoughts. Being 14 years of age could have been a factor that influenced my poor thought processes. However, I strongly believe that there are other factors behind this suicidal ideation. I eventually perceived that suicidal thought as a strange and irrational thought. This experience gave me a further reason to consider the possibility that I may be suffering from some type of mental illness.

Actually, there is a considerable difference between suicidal conceptions and suicidal ideations. When an individual conceives suicidal thoughts, there are usually no motivational factors involved. However, when the individual conceives suicidal ideations, he will be motivated by some reason to commit this act. This additional element distinguishes random thought from planned action. In the case of an ideation, the individual may actually weigh the pros and cons relevant to committing the act of suicide. If the individual has more reasons to choose death over life, his next action may be drastic. Consequently, persons who do commit suicide usually act in a premeditated fashion.

I firmly believe that all non-adults, who actually do commit suicide, choose this action because they are suffering from some form of mental disorder. The reasons that motivate suicide, though they may be rational to the individual, will always be irrational from an observer's point of view. My theory is based on my belief that only a mentally sick individual will be able to rationalize an act of suicide. Although all healthy non-adults may lack the necessary life experiences which enables them to form sound judgments, I believe that this subgroup will still possess a high enough sense of insight to understand that the act of suicide can never be justified, under any circumstances.

Rationalizing the act of suicide, then, only comes about when defective reasoning, deficient thoughts, and an unstable frame of mind clouds the individual. In the act of rationalizing suicide, the individual values death over life in the physical world. Under these circumstances, the individual no longer has any reasons to live, and likewise, he may have many more reasons to die. I believe that this devaluing of one's life can only result through a form of precarious reasoning. I also believe that only a mental illness will cause an individual to believe that suicide is the only solution to his personal problems.

I exclude adults from my theory for one reason. Though I believe that many adults do commit suicide because they are suffering from some form of mental illness, other healthy adults may purposely commit the act of suicide. Under these circumstances, the adult understands the true ramifications associated with suicide, and likewise, he has access to a relatively healthy frame of mind. Hence, some adults commit suicide as a fully conscious and deliberate choice.

Some mentally healthy adults commit suicide because they believe that it is their social responsibility to take this action. When someone reaches the age of adulthood, he enters into his community as a citizen that is fully accountable for all of his actions. Adults freely choose their lifestyles, and are held fully responsible for all of their actions and behaviours. In contrast, non-adults are vulnerable to persuasion. Accordingly, under many circumstances, a non-adult should not be held fully responsible for his actions, including any acts related to suicide.

I argue that some adults may have an objective reason to commit suicide. In other parts of the world, some adults commit suicide as an act of warfare. These individuals, known as suicide bombers, understand the circumstances that they are in and they choose to commit the act of suicide, while possessing a full awareness over the implications of their actions. Thus, these individuals are able to rationalize an act of suicide, through a calculated and predetermined frame of mind. Suicide bombers will commit suicide in order to achieve some type of personal or collective gain. Under these circumstances, it is possible that the individual does not suffer from any form of mental illness.

The adult, then, has an objective reason to commit suicide, and this reason is based on an act of war. Personally, I theorize that only adults can be held fully responsible for an act of suicide, based on this particular reason. This is due to my belief that every youth will lack a clear and sufficient understanding concerning any ideals related to a social responsibility.

From a legal standpoint, youths are technically classified as minors, until they reach the age of majority. When a youth reaches this age, he is considered to have reached adulthood and is then considered to be legally responsible for all of his actions. This principle is based on the fact that all youths will lack necessary life experiences that will enable them to comprehend complex issues like dutiful action and responsible behaviour.

Accordingly, in most societies, youths are not granted the same rights and privileges that are granted to every adult. For example, in Canada, youths are not granted the right to vote in governmental elections, nor are they permitted the right to purchase tobacco or alcohol. In a similar fashion, adolescents are not granted the right to drive a vehicle, or get married, until they reach a certain age as a young adult. In truth, youths are not granted the right to vote because they will fail to achieve a certain degree of understanding, with respect to any political issues that may be involved. Other special rights are not granted to youths for a similar reason. Thus, non-adults are not granted some forms of liberties, because they lack a definite understanding in the areas of personal and social responsibility.

Therefore, I theorize that a youth suicide bomber will only commit suicide for reasons beyond any forms of a social responsibility. I hypothesize that every youth suicide bomber will be highly susceptible to coercion, and that this vulnerability is created exclusively through a mental illness.

Under this specific circumstance, I believe that a youth suicide bomber will fail to comprehend the concept of a social responsibility, which would subsequently enable him to objectively rationalize suicide as an act of war. In reality, no youth will be able to rationalize complex socio concepts, entirely through his own accord. If this is true, then all youths will necessarily lack a similar degree of accountability that we can attribute to a grown adult.

Hence, an authority figure has inevitably coerced a youth suicide bomber to become an enemy combatant. If this is true, then this youth should not be held fully responsible for his act of suicide. Nevertheless, I believe that there are further factors that must compel a youth to commit an act that is as far-reaching as suicide. From my perspective, I believe that it is impossible to coerce a mentally healthy youth into committing an action that is as radical as suicide. The act of suicide should always be an irrational solution to any given problem, even within the mind of an immature adolescent. Thus, the mentally healthy adolescent should have enough cognitive insight to foresee alternative modes of action to suicide, even while under a state of extreme duress. Therefore, I believe that my hypothesis still applies in the case of all youth suicide bombers.

In effect, I propose that a youth suicide bomber will only commit this act, when he is both coerced by a person of authority, and suffering from some form of mental instability. Steinberg (2008) argues that risk-taking behaviour increases during adolescence as a result of changes around the time of puberty in the brain's socio-emotional system. This then leads to an increased reward-seeking psychological state. He also theorizes that this latter condition is fueled mainly by a dramatic remodeling of the brain's dopaminergic system. His theory suggests that risk taking behaviours originate through physical mechanisms within the brain. Similarly, it is conceivable that an act of suicide may also be caused by similar structural or functional changes within the brain, due exclusively to a mental illness.

Adult suicide bombers, then, have a clear and objective reason to commit suicide. These individuals believe that it is their personal duty to engage in an act of war. As a morally debated topic, euthanasia may also provide an adult with an objective reason to commit suicide. By definition, euthanasia is the act of killing, or permitting the death of a hopelessly sick or terminally ill individual, in a relatively painless way for reasons of mercy (Merriam-Webster, 2008). Therefore, persons who contemplate about euthanasia suffer from perpetual and lasting pains, due to an incurable terminal illness.

Personally, I believe in the principles of freedom and personal autonomy. Thus, I believe that the act of euthanasia should be permitted under certain circumstances. Nonetheless, if the act of euthanasia were to be legalized in Canada, then it is highly probable that this right will be abused. For example, persons who are not terminally ill may believe that they should also have the right to commit euthanasia. Furthermore, the definition of terminal can be misinterpreted. According to Jack Kevorkian, a terminal illness is any disease that curtails life even for a day (Euthanasia.com, 2008). The concept of terminal may then encompass old age, or a condition from which death will imminently occur. As a result, exorbitant connotations associated with the concept of euthanasia would create many difficulties, if it were legalized on a worldwide basis.

In any case, these are two objective reasons why an adult may choose to commit suicide. I argue that any adult, who has no objective reason to commit suicide, will also choose this act because he is suffering from some form of mental illness. I further argue that no child will ever have an objective reason to commit suicide. All youths will lack an equivalent sense of social responsibility that we can attribute to a grown adult. Therefore, I hypothesize that all youths and most adults, who do commit suicide, may be suffering from some form of mental illness.

A schizophrenia patient can rationalize an act of suicide through two central reasons. One reason may be based on the concept of hopelessness. In this case, the individual believes that he has no more reasons to live. This reason is most common in the illness of depression, yet persons with other mental illnesses may contemplate similar thoughts. The second reason is based on an extreme reaction to a delusion or hallucination. In some instances, the patient may believe that he is a targeted member within his community. This can occur if the individual believes that he is someone famous. The individual can also hear voices, which are telling him to commit suicide. When the schizophrenia patient's mind enters into this condition, he will sometimes feel compelled to follow the commands of these imaginary voices. He may also believe that these voices represent the will of his entire community. Therefore, in this case, the individual will act upon falsehoods, which he believes are true, due to a state of psychosis.

On the other hand, persons who are diagnosed with any form of mental illness will sometimes experience the feeling of perpetual hopelessness. Feelings of hopelessness entail the belief that one's personal situation can never improve. The average mentally healthy person never really scrutinizes the concept of hopelessness, because his cognition is usually not impaired. Rational persons can feel depressed at times, though these feelings gradually weaken after some time. For patients with a mental illness, feelings of hopelessness may never fade away. Patients with a mental disorder will usually reflect upon the concept of hopelessness, at both the conscious and subconscious levels. Therefore, when the patient cannot conceive thoughts of happiness, he may be prone to rationalize an act of suicide, as the only solution to his problems.

The hypothesis that there is a weaker association between suicidal behaviour and stressful life events, in adolescent schizophrenia patients, was tested. In this study, control subjects reported fewer life events in general, and fewer negative events in comparison to the patients with schizophrenia. Similarly, suicidal schizophrenia patients reported fewer life events in general, when compared to non-suicidal patients (Fennig *et al*, 2005). Within the suicidal group, the proportion of negative life events to total life events was higher, and the perceived impact of these events was stronger. This seems to support the theory that suicidal behaviour is correlated less with the number of life events, and correlated more with the negative perception and personal impact of these events.

Another study comparing adolescents with schizophrenia, schizophrenia with post-psychotic depression (PPD), or major depression reveals some other serious implications. Adolescents with schizophrenia and PPD demonstrated fewer somatic and behavioural symptoms, but equally severe cognitive and affective depressive symptoms, when compared to those with major depression. Suicidal risk and behaviour was also prominent among this subgroup, and a positive correlation between suicide risk and an awareness of illness was drawn. Negative schizophrenia symptoms were also distinguishable from PPD symptoms, and a negative correlation between blunted affect and PPD was also observed (Schwartz-Stav *et al*, 2006).

A study conducted in Taiwan also confirms the theory that adolescents with depressive disorders commonly manifest suicide attempts. However, there are cultural differences with respect to the risk factors involved. In Taiwan, school related problems and prior suicide attempts play a significant role among adolescent suicides. Parent child conflicts, psychopathology, psychotic symptoms, and feelings of hopelessness are also common risk factors (Chiou *et al*, 2006). In addition, according to this study, considerably more females had attempted to commit an act of suicide, in comparison to males.

Alternatively, suicidal ideations due to a state of paranoia may be more difficult to comprehend. When a psychotic patient attempts to commit suicide, he usually believes that this action will better his society in some manner. The reasons behind this belief may vary on an individual basis. When I was in an extremely psychotic state, I never contemplated thoughts related to suicide, though I did, at times, hear voices that were telling me to hurt myself.

I was able to resist these voices for the most part. In addition, I never held the perception that these voices were authoritative in any manner. During that period, I did not believe that my society would benefit if I did hurt myself, but I did believe that these voices were endorsed by my society, and also that these voices would not stop unless I followed their orders. This latter thought may seem irrational to most persons, however, the average person will never experience an auditory hallucination. These voices caused feelings of anxiety within me. Patients with psychosis can easily rationalize seemingly irrational thoughts due to their superficial delusions and hallucinations.

A study conducted in the United States seems to corroborate my last point. Researchers have discovered that lower levels of emotional clarity were associated with more severe hallucination ratings, in schizophrenia spectrum patients and patients with mood or substance disorders (Serper and Berenbaum, 2008). Regarding severe delusions, mood or substance disorder patients had higher levels of attention over their emotions, though the converse was true of the schizophrenia spectrum patients. As a result, the delusions experienced by schizophrenia spectrum patients differ from the delusional states experienced by persons with other types of disorders. A lack of emotional awareness may explain some of the irrational behaviours committed by schizophrenia spectrum patients, including acts related to suicide.

In Israel, suicide attempts have been linked to the use of alcohol, inhalants, lysergic acid diethylamide (LSD), and methylenedioxymethamphetamine (MDMA) among adolescent schizophrenia patients. These patients were also observed to have more previous psychiatric admissions, greater levels of deliberate self-harm behaviour, and higher levels of suicidal ideations (Shoval *et al*, 2006). Yet, the severity of their psychotic symptoms decreased. Furthermore, no differences were observed among patients who used cannabis, amphetamines, cocaine, or opiates. Therefore, patients who abuse specific types of substances may be at a higher risk to commit suicide. In my opinion, the act of self-medicating oneself can sometimes be internally justified by the schizophrenia patient, given the fact that some substances may reduce psychosis. However, one of the adverse side effects of self-medicating behaviour includes an increased risk to commit suicide.

A case study was conducted on a young suicide victim whose antemortem course did not demonstrate apparent psychopathology to either his family or fellow students. A journal written by the deceased, however, revealed that he was suffering from extensive suicidal ideations, depressive symptoms, and possible delusions or hallucinations. The researchers of this study theorize that the individual was in the preliminary stages of psychosis, and that he committed suicide as a response to the awareness of his deteriorating mental status (Knittel *et al*, 2008). They also assert the possibility that prodromal psychosis could be the cause of many suicides that have no evident causal factors.

Unwanted pregnancies have also been linked to adult schizophrenia-spectrum and affective disorders, in offspring with a genetic risk for psychosis. The researchers of this study theorize that an unwanted pregnancy may be mediated by functional and discrete environmental psychosocial factors (McNeil *et al*, 2009). Perhaps an unwanted pregnancy may be comparable to a suicidal ideation, in that it may come about through structural and functional changes within the brain, which surface during the development of an illness.

Although at present, it may be impossible to prove that all youth and most adult suicides are due to a mental illness, my theory does have some serious implications. Today, as a mentally healthy adult, I could never rationalize an act of suicide, either for myself or for any other person within my society. Nevertheless, I have thought about suicide as an adolescent, and I strongly believe that these thoughts were due to my poor state of mind. I base this theory on my personal experiences with a mental illness. In retrospect, all of my radical thoughts, including thoughts related to suicide, occurred while I was in a state of paranoia or psychosis.

If my hypothesis is true, I believe that many societies around the world may possess the resources to solve a very serious social problem. Advancing techniques in the recognition of early risk factors for all mental disorders could be prioritized. Developing effective treatment options for at risk youths could also effectively address the problem of youth suicides. Medicines have enabled me to regain much of my personal health, and I believe that our current medical knowledge is also at a level to have a positive impact on many other forms of mental disorders.

Childhood onset schizophrenia (COS) is a rare disorder, and it is also a highly debated subject. Early onset schizophrenia (EOS) is defined as the onset of schizophrenia in individuals who are 17 years of age or younger. According to cognitive, phenomenological, genetic, and neuroimaging data, many scientists theorize that a continuity exists between early and adult onset patients (Kyriakopoulos and Frangou, 2007). However, diagnosing the symptoms of schizophrenia in children and adolescents can sometimes be problematic, and modes of treatment also have difficulties. This is due to the fact that there are a limited number of controlled studies conducted on the effects of psychotropic medications in children. This is one reason why some parents will hesitate to administer medications to children who are less than 18 years of age.

One diagnostic tool is an interview instrument known as the Kiddie Schedule for Affective Disorders and Schizophrenia (Kim *et al*, 2004). Research seems to indicate that infant and adolescent adjustment and global functioning is lower, when they are affected with a psychotic disorder. Severity of symptoms has also been correlated with general disability (Castro-Fornieles *et al*, 2007). As a result, poor childhood function is the most significant predictor of outcome in EOS (Vyas *et al*, 2007).

Premorbid developmental impairments in the areas of immediate verbal memory, motor deficits, and social deficits are also more frequent and pronounced in children and adolescents that suffer from early onset schizophrenia. These impairments, also known as pan-dysmaturation, are reported during the first months of life in more than half of the children who will develop childhood-onset schizophrenia (Masi *et al*, 2006). Researchers theorize that this may be due to a severe disruption during brain development. Negative symptoms are also largely predominant, while the most frequent positive symptoms are elementary auditory hallucinations. Equally, a marked deterioration in levels of functioning is universally present among all EOS cases, and an impaired outcome occurs in approximately 60% of all cases (Masi *et al*, 2006).

In childhood onset schizophrenia, patients have marked neuropsychological deficits in areas of attention, working memory and executive functions. When compared to adolescent and adult onset schizophrenia, COS patients have significantly greater deficits in the areas of IQ, memory and perceptuomotor skills. Researchers believe that these deficits may be present in the patient, even before the onset of his illness. Differences in age groups also imply the possibility that brain damage in children with schizophrenia is most severe, least severe in adolescents with schizophrenia, and that it ranges somewhere in between these two subgroups in adult schizophrenia (Biswas *et al*, 2006).

Adolescents with EOS are also impaired across several neurocognitive domains. Researchers have correlated problems in social, personal, communication, and community living skills with deficits in attention, working memory, vigilance, and verbal memory. Furthermore, all of these individual cognitive domains are more strongly related to functional outcome than a global measure of intelligence. These cognitive impairments usually remain relatively stable over time, which seems to indicate their pressing needs, with respect to the guidance and support from a proven health advocate (Cervellione *et al*, 2007).

Adolescents with schizophrenia are also known to have early visual deficits that contribute towards impaired working memory, and other deficits in future memory-related processes (Haenschel *et al*, 2007). Visuospatial memory, consistent with encoding impairments, is also significantly impaired in adolescents with schizophrenia (Vance *et al*, 2007).

Further, children with schizophrenia demonstrate impaired response inhibition and impaired spatial accuracy (Ross *et al*, 2005). Accordingly, they display saccadic abnormalities that are similar to those observed among adult patients. Sleep disturbances are also common among children with schizophrenia. A study was conducted on 61 medication free COS patients, within an inpatient facility. Patients who slept less than six hours per night experienced severe positive and negative symptoms both on admission and during the medication-free period (Mattai *et al*, 2006). Accordingly, difficulties with sleep were highly associated with symptom severity.

According to data collected from phenomenological, cognitive, neuroimaging, and genetic studies, patients with early onset schizophrenia have a similar profile of clinical and neurobiological abnormalities with adult onset patients. Early onset patients also have more severe premorbid neurodevelopmental abnormalities, more cytogenetic anomalies, worse long term outcome, and a greater family history of schizophrenia spectrum disorders, when compared to adult onset patients (Kumra and Schulz, 2008). As a result, some researchers hypothesize that EOS may reflect a more severe form of the disorder associated with a greater genetic disposition.

Patients that are diagnosed with COS and catatonia also appear to be more severely ill during the admission and discharge stages from an inpatient unit, in comparison to COS patients in nearly all clinical scores. In addition, their state of psychosis is usually longer in duration. A study conducted in Paris indicates that the average stay at an inpatient unit for patients with catatonic symptoms was 50 weeks, while the stay for patients without catatonic symptoms usually averaged at around 20 weeks. According to these findings, researchers theorize that catatonic COS differs from COS in ways that extend beyond motor symptoms (Bonnot *et al*, 2008). I would speculate that catatonia is more severe in children because their brains are in the preliminary stages of physical maturation and development.

In one case study, two teenage male identical twins exhibited severe catatonic symptoms. Upon admission into an inpatient unit, the brothers showed signs of stupor, catatonic posturing, rigidity, mutism, negativism, and they refrained from eating food and drinking liquids. Both were treated through electroconvulsive therapy to no effect. Improvements, however, were noted upon the initiation of olanzapine treatments. One twin demonstrated a marked improvement after two weeks, on a dosage of 10 milligrams per day. The other twin demonstrated improvements after four weeks while on a dosage of 15 milligrams per day. Both twins were discharged after eight and eleven weeks of antipsychotic treatments respectively (Dudova and Hrdlicka, 2008). This case study seems to demonstrate that individuals with similar biological attributes may have concordant resistances and responses, with respect to different modes of treatment.

A study was also conducted on 93 adolescents who were diagnosed with both a movement disorder and schizophrenia. All of the subjects showed pronounced global psychopathological signs, increased thought disturbances, predominant anergia symptoms, and an inclination towards higher anxiety and depressive related symptoms. Negative symptoms and anergia were further correlated with tardive dyskinesia and Parkinsonism symptoms. Likewise, symptoms of akathisia were associated with hostile and suspicious symptoms. The researchers conclude that the motor symptoms of schizophrenia could be triggered by antipsychotics, and that they co-occur with more residual symptoms within a long-term treatment (Gebhardt *et al*, 2008).

Another study compared youths with schizophrenia or schizoaffective disorder. One hundred nineteen youths ranging from 8 to 19 years of age were studied, and the mean age for the onset of illness was 11 years of age. Patients in both groups had similar ratings regarding their positive symptoms, negative symptoms, psychiatric ratings, and their clinical severity scale scores. High rates of symptoms and general psychopathology were also noted, along with equivalent levels of overall function (Frazier *et al*, 2007).

In essence, there are considerable differences among gender and age, with respect to schizotypy. Schizotypy is a multidimensional personality construct that appears to indicate psychosis proneness. Males differ from females in that they score higher in categories like physical anhedonia, social anhedonia, and impulsive non-conformity. Females, on the other hand, score higher in the categories of positive symptoms, negative evaluation, and social paranoia. On the subject of age groups, adolescents more frequently report social paranoia, negative evaluation, disordered thoughts, unusual experiences, and self-referent ideations (Fonsesca-Pedrero *et al*, 2008).

Childhood exposure to trauma may also be more common among patients with schizophrenia, in comparison to patients with a non-psychotic illness. This type of trauma has been correlated with poor communication skills and depressive symptoms. Researchers also believe that childhood trauma may be significant etiologically (Spence *et al*, 2006). However, the exact mechanism behind this theory remains unknown.

One biological marker of child or adolescent schizophrenia comes in the form of a more pronounced ventricular enlargement within the brain (Ferrari *et al*, 2006). The mitochondrial complex I is also theorized to be a potential peripheral marker in early onset schizophrenia (Mehler-Wex *et al*, 2006).

Another biological marker of EOS is the 22q11.2 genetic microdeletion. 22q11.2 microdeletion is a rare yet important risk factor in children and adolescents. Young patients with this deletion, in conjunction with evident psychiatric problems, will require a more specialized mode of care (Briegel, 2007).

Progressive losses of cortical grey matter volume have also been observed in COS. The adolescent's rate of cortical loss is theorized to plateau during early adulthood. Patients with first-episode adolescent schizophrenia also consistently show less marked progressive changes (Arango *et al*, 2008). In effect, researchers have discovered a greater loss of brain tissue in patients with COS, when compared to patients with either adolescent or adult onset schizophrenia. These changes have also been observed in non-schizophrenia early onset psychosis, though to a lesser degree. Other findings support the hypothesis that early onset schizophrenia is a progressive neurodevelopmental disorder with both early and late developmental abnormalities (Arango *et al*, 2008).

Other discoveries include widespread abnormalities characterized by a lower fractional anisotropy neuroanatomically associated with localized reduced grey matter. Researchers have further discovered a widespread reduction of anisotropy in the white matter, especially in the corpus callosum (Douaud et al, 2007).

Abnormalities in the primary sensorimotor and premotor cortices and in white matter tracts subserving motor control may also be prevalent. Scientists have further discovered significantly lower fractional anisotropy in the white matter of the parietal association cortex bilaterally and in the left middle cerebellar penduncle [sic] (Kyriakopoulos et al, 2007). These findings could serve as a potential marker of altered white matter maturation that is specific in adolescent-onset schizophrenia (Douaud et al, 2007).

Likewise, abnormalities in grey and white matter within the Heschl's gyrus, parietal operculum, left Broca's area, and left arcuate fasciculus also seem to be common in EOS. All of these discoveries seem to imply that there are more widespread changes consistent with a higher clinical severity in adolescent onset schizophrenia, when compared to the adult form (Douaud et al, 2007).

Adolescent patients were also discovered to have hemispheric symmetry in the anterior-posterior dimension, which is consistent with the data accumulated in adult psychosis. In contrast, a reversed pattern of hemispheric asymmetry has been observed in healthy adolescents and adults. Similarly, source locations, patterns of cerebral lateralization, and inter-hemispheric correlations were observed to be consistently different in individuals with psychosis and their healthy counterparts. Therefore, scientists have deduced that aberrant maturation may cause the reduction in cerebral laterality observed in patients with psychosis (Wilson et al, 2007).

The treatment process for childhood schizophrenia has also been carefully studied. Research seems to indicate that typical antipsychotic medications are more effective in the treatment of children and adolescents. Typical medicines also caused less weight gain. The average patient taking typical antipsychotics gained 1.4 Kg. In contrast, patients who took atypical medicines gained an average of 4.5 Kg (Hrdlicka and Dudova, 2007). Sedation was also more prevalent within the latter subgroup. Nevertheless, the rate of extrapyramidal side effects was equal among both groups.

In Canada, one survey indicates that the majority of child psychiatrists and developmental paediatricians prescribe atypical antipsychotics for their patients. Risperidone was the most commonly prescribed medicine. It was used to treat problems with mood, anxiety, the symptom of externalizing, and other psychotic or pervasive developmental disorders. Antipsychotics were also used to treat the symptoms of aggression, low frustration tolerance, and affect dysregulation. Twelve percent of these patients were less than 10 years old. However, no evidence-based guidelines nor a consensus on monitoring exists, concerning patients who are less than 18 years of age (Doey *et al,* 2007).

In comparison, the medication olanzapine may be equally as effective as risperidone, and more effective than haloperidol. However, weight gain was greater among patients who were treated with olanzapine. Sedation was also prominent. Other long-term complications include obesity and glucose dysregulation. Liver enzymes and blood sugar levels may also be slightly elevated within some patients. On the other hand, patients reported mild to moderate extrapyramidal side effects, in comparison to those who were treated with haloperidol (Frémaux *et al*, 2007).

When compared to clozapine, though, olanzapine was less effective. Yet, some potentially adverse metabolic effects have been linked to clozapine treatments. These effects include alterations in insulin sensitivity and hyperglycemia (Avram *et al*, 2001).

In a study conducted within the United States, 119 youths diagnosed with an early onset schizophrenia spectrum (EOSS) disorder were randomly treated with risperidone, olanzapine, or molindone. After eight weeks, these treatments resulted in a 20% reduction in baseline Positive and Negative Symptom Scale scores, along with significant improvements within the Clinical Global Impression scale. Secondary response criteria were based on assessments of psychopathology, functional impairments, quality of life, and medication safety. In some cases, treatments through olanzapine were cancelled due to excessive weight gain. Safety concerns that arose include higher rates of suicidality, and problems with the tapering of thymoleptic agents before randomization (McClellan *et al*, 2007).

Other antipsychotics have been studied in the treatment of COS, including aripiprazole. This medicine was more effective than a placebo in the acute treatment of adolescent onset schizophrenia. In terms of side effects, aripiprazole was also generally well tolerated (Findling *et al*, 2008). Quetiapine may also have beneficial effects in the treatment of COS. Equally, there were no unexpected tolerability findings observed during a trial of ziprasidone for children and adolescent patients (DelBello *et al*, 2008).

A further study compares differences in cortical thickness between COS patients who have reached remission, and COS patients who were newly admitted into an inpatient unit. Through MRI scans, recently discharged COS patients had a thicker regional cortex in left orbitofrontal, left superior, and middle temporal gyri and bilateral postcentral and angular gyri. This seems to indicate that a positive response to treatment could be mediated through these cortical regions within the brain (Greenstein *et al*, 2008).

Other studies reveal that EOSS disorders may be linked with significant cognitive impairments and a poor response to antipsychotic treatments. This theory is based on the fact that dopamine, and other neurotransmitter receptor systems, are in a stage of development during childhood. Therefore, the ongoing biological developments in adolescents could affect both the clinical response, and the rate of side effects associated with antipsychotic treatments (Kumra *et al*, 2008).

Some short-term studies also suggest that youths are more sensitive to the side effects of antipsychotic medications, in comparison to adults. In some cases, the use of second-generation antipsychotics has led to the development of diabetes (Kumra *et al*, 2008). However, an examination of clinical trials, conducted from 1980 to 2007, reveals that antipsychotic medications were consistently found to reduce the severity of psychotic symptoms (Kumra *et al*, 2008). Consequently, antipsychotic medications may have both positive and negative effects on youths who are diagnosed with a schizophrenia spectrum disorder.

Indeed, parental attitudes towards the prescribing of antipsychotics for children can conflict with the opinions of certified medical professionals. One study, comprised mostly of mothers between the ages of 25 and 45 years, indicates that some parents are afraid to administer psychotropic medications to their child (Lazaratou *et al*, 2007). This survey group also believed in the notion that psychotherapy is the most effective method of treatment for childhood mental disorders.

According to another study, many parents hold feelings of frequent ambivalence and lesser satisfaction towards their mentally ill child. Nonetheless, these parents also reported feelings that were equally strong related to their ill child as to his sibling (Burkhardt *et al*, 2007). This was especially true for the parents of adults with a substance abuse disorder. This latter fact seems to indicate that intergenerational ambivalences can add further complications in the treatment of children who are diagnosed with schizophrenia.

Another false belief is based on the notion that children who take psychotropic medications may develop an addiction to some form of narcotic. This belief has been correlated to the parent's level of education. Moreover, although 40% of those surveyed believe that there is a proper use for psychotropic medications, 20% think psychiatrists prescribe unnecessarily high doses of these medicines. In view of that, there is a strong need to educate parents, concerning the safe and proper use of antipsychotic medications for children. Most researchers and psychiatrists agree that responsible modes of treatment for children will sometimes involve the use of medications (Lazaratou *et al*, 2007).

Cognitive remediation therapy (CRT) may also improve cognitive deficits in adolescents with schizophrenia. Through CRT, the individual learns information processing strategies through mental exercises. According to a study conducted in the United Kingdom, CRT produces significant additional improvements in the realm of cognitive flexibility. Improvements within all domains of cognition are known to have a direct effect on social functioning, and result in overall symptom improvements (Wykes *et al*, 2007).

Electroconvulsive therapy is another possible mode of treatment. ECT may offer a fairly swift but a time-limited response. On a further note, the administration of ECT usually follows the same general principles among all age groups. ECT is also known to be most effective in cases of patient catatonia.

Other difficulties include a delay in the recognition of the syndrome. Reasons for this include an insidious onset in at least 75% of children, high rates of premorbid problems, and a hesitant attitude on the part of clinicians to diagnose a child with schizophrenia. Some diagnostic challenges further include differentiating COS from disorders like depression, bipolar disorder, and other developmental or personality disorders. In some cases, individuals with post-traumatic stress disorder, or obsessive-compulsive disorder are sometimes misdiagnosed with schizophrenia. In addition, 10% of children report nonpsychotic delusions or hallucinations (Masi *et al*, 2006). In other cases, some atypical psychotic features may not fit into a specific diagnostic criterion, and newer forms of categories may thus be required.

In a follow up study conducted between 1920 and 1961, seventy-six patients who had a suspected diagnosis of COS were admitted into the Department of Child and Adolescent Psychiatry at Philipps University, in Germany. The diagnosis of schizophrenia had only a 50% confirmation rate, while the other patients were diagnosed with other psychiatric disorders. The age of onset for these patients varied at between 5 and 14 years of age, while the average age at follow up ranged from between 42 to 62 years of age. Only 16% had a good outcome, and 24% had a moderate outcome according to the Global Assessment Scale. Furthermore, 10 out of 16 COS patients displayed moderate to severe depressive symptoms. The death rate among all of the patients surveyed was also significantly higher in the schizophrenia group. In this sample, 91% revealed a diagnostic stability retrospectively, while the other seven patients had a change in diagnosis. Of these seven patients, four were originally diagnosed with COS (Remschmidt *et al*, 2007).

Another follow up study was conducted during a two year period, on 24 patients who were diagnosed with early-onset psychosis. Their mean age was 15 years. In this study, schizophrenia had the highest prospective consistency at 100%. Conversely, the diagnostic stability for bipolar disorder was at 71%, while the diagnostic stability for schizoaffective disorder, schizophreniform disorder and brief psychosis was at a relatively low 50% (Fraguas *et al*, 2008). There was a 54% agreement rate between the original and one year follow up diagnoses, while there was a 95% agreement rate between the one and two year follow up diagnoses. Baseline negative symptoms were the single predictors for level of functioning, after the two year follow up period. Accordingly, a first-year follow up diagnosis is necessary for all cases of early-onset psychosis (Fraguas *et al*, 2008).

Age also plays a factor when problematic symptoms arise. In Australia, adolescents mainly seek help from family members, while young adults mainly rely upon their general practitioners. Parents also seek help from their general practitioners, when concerned about the mental health of their child. Embarrassment and social stigma were the main elements that stopped young persons from asking for help, and resistance from the child was the main barrier for parents (Jorm *et al*, 2007).

Treatment options are available for at-risk individuals as well. According to a study conducted in Germany, psychoeducation enabled some individuals to gain improvements in knowledge, global functioning, and other areas related to quality of life. Likewise, a significant reduction in psychopathology was observed among these patients (Hauser *et al*, 2009).

An interesting study conducted on high school students in China explores the effects of physical activity on substance abuse, suicidal behaviour, and psychopathological symptoms. Five thousand four hundred fifty three students participated through a self-administered anonymous survey. The results indicate that 22% of those surveyed are persons who enjoy high intensity physical activities. This was a known risk factor for binge drinking, hostile symptoms, suicidal ideations, and general psychological disorders. Thirty seven percent enjoyed low to moderate intensity physical activities. This trait proved to be a protective factor against depression and psychotic symptoms. Nothing conclusive was discovered among the remaining 41% of students who fit into the low intensity category (Tao *et al*, 2007).

Regardless of age, all persons that are diagnosed with schizophrenia will require aid from a third party. Children differ from adults in that they lack significant life experiences, which are necessary for making sound and reliable judgments. Therefore, the onus may be on either the parent, or our mental health care system in general, to make the right decisions with respect to a child's mental health. Parents with a family history of mental illness should especially monitor their children's behaviour, and identify any possible early warning signs. The early detection of symptoms will lead to the best possible prognosis. As such, when a patient cannot make any sound or rational decisions, this responsibility must be passed on to someone who can befit the role as an accountable and trustworthy caretaker.

14

Final Thoughts

Recovering from a disease like schizophrenia requires part focus and part determination. Persons who are diagnosed with schizophrenia will probably face the most difficult challenge that they will ever come across within their entire lifetime. Overcoming the problems associated with all mental disorders can be a difficult process. Some problems are exclusive to schizophrenia patients. In reality, the majority of persons around the world will never be diagnosed with schizophrenia. From their perspective, it may be impossible to truly understand the multitude of challenges that schizophrenia patients face on a daily basis.

The schizophrenia patient will experience psychological problems, both when in a state of psychosis and during the early stages of his rehabilitation process. The key paradigm under these circumstances is to readjust one's focus away from the concept of disability, on to the concept of ability. Having the ability to ignore extremely paranoid thoughts is small battle that must be won by every patient. Having rational insight with respect to the true condition of one's mental state is a further battle. Once this is accomplished, the patient will demonstrate a unique strength that can only be seen in individuals who are diagnosed with a mental illness.

One study indicates that schizophrenia patients base their recovery on low levels of symptoms, and the knowledge that taking medications will play a critical role in the management of their symptoms and in avoiding hospitalizations. The subjective sense that they will recover from their illness, and the belief that the quality of their lives will improve are other important factors (Jenkins *et al*, 2005). Many outpatients also report that the recovery process is slow, steady, and highly subjective. They hold the firm belief that a recovery from a mental illness requires some form of sacrifice. This is due to the fact that many outpatients will be labelled as either fat or crazy, or be subjected to other forms of societal stigmas (Jenkins and Carpenter-Song, 2005).

An analysis of 65 studies, conducted between 1980 and 2003, reveals that approximately half of the psychiatric patients surveyed did not know their diagnosis, and also that schizophrenia patients were the least informed. In fact, many patients have fairly limited knowledge regarding the cause and treatment for schizophrenia. Some patients also demonstrate problems while trying to understand the concept of a multifactorial cause. Other patients felt that their psychiatrists were mainly interested in the pharmacological aspects of the disease, and that they paid little attention to personal issues. As a result, this study concludes that a greater quality of communication between the doctor and patient will lead to a greater compliance with respect to treatment programs, and it may also serve to dispel some forms of internalized stigma (Paccaloni *et al*, 2004).

An awareness of illness necessarily implies an implicit understanding regarding the impact of a disorder on one's life. Researchers divided a group of 76 adults into three subgroups based on a full awareness, a limited awareness, and a superficial awareness of their illness. They found that persons within the superficial group had poorer executive functioning, poorer emotion recognition abilities, and a decreased capacity for social relationships. Yet, they also found that the superficial group had better verbal memory and more social contacts when compared to the limited awareness group (Lysaker *et al*, 2008b). As a result, differing degrees of awareness may be associated with distinct psychological symptoms.

Approximately 14% of persons affected by a disease worldwide are diagnosed with a neuropsychiatric disorder. In London, several researchers assert that the alienation of mental health from mainstream efforts to improve health and reduce poverty is due to a separation between mental and physical disorders . Some persons may connect mental illnesses to disability, and physical illnesses with possible mortality. However, the interaction between mental and physical illnesses may be protean (Prince *et al*, 2007). In other words, some mental disorders can increase the individual's risk to develop both a communicable or non-communicable disease, and contrariwise, some health conditions can increase the individual's risk to develop a mental disorder.

These researchers also recognize the fact that health services are not provided equitably to people with mental disorders. They assert the view that health care systems should be strengthened to improve the delivery of mental health services, through programs that focus on the treatment and prevention of other physical illnesses. Likewise, there is also a strong need to integrate mental health awareness into health-system planning, health and social policies, and the primary and secondary health care systems (Prince *et al*, 2007).

Kelly argues that although mental illness is widespread within the United States, mental health services remain poorly funded, mental illness remains misunderstood, and individuals with a recurring illness are constrained to live lives characterized by isolation, under-employment, stigma and denial of rights (Kelly, 2008). This may be, in part, due to the ways in which the freedom and power of the mentally ill are undermined. Kelly observes that there is a lack of political power, in the form of mental health interest groups, in proportion to the number of persons that are affected by a mental illness. Patients with mental illness are also subjected to structural violence, or they may be systematically excluded from civic, social or political life. Kelly notes the fact that many patients with a mental illness will experience difficulties when trying to recognize or articulate needs that may be absent within their mental health care system (Kelly, 2008). This leads to an absence of knowledge between mentally sick patients and the government services that have been primarily created for them.

The solution to this problem may be quite complex. According to Kelly, the enhancement of individual agency may be necessary to address this gap in political power. Thus, improvements in advocacy, empowerment and guardianship processes, and the implementation of rights-based approaches may be necessary. The creation of governance, accountability and quality procedures in mental health services may also be required. Further, Kelly stresses that there is a strong need to increase the element of accountability amongst all mental health services. Therefore, the creation of stronger advocacy programs could address this problem (Kelly, 2008).

The project titled Enhancing Quality of care In Psychosis (EQUIP) identifies some strategies that will increase the adoption and implementation of chronic illness care principles. An evaluation of EQUIP demonstrates that many problems related to schizophrenia are due to a lack of awareness, with respect to evidence based practices. Improving care for schizophrenia patients may require the creation of resources for physicians, which can help them implement practice changes. Intensive forms of education and the creation of product champions who will aid physicians with the utilization of these resources may also be needed. Furthermore, the addition of care managers and informatics systems can aid physicians in the identification of problems, in the monitoring of follow-up sessions, and with making referrals (Brown *et al*, 2008). As a result, the implementation of complex care models can potentially improve our current mental health care system.

Economically, atypical medications are more expensive than first generation antipsychotics. This could be one reason why I was never prescribed olanzapine or clozapine during the preliminary stages of my illness. In retrospect, I believe that this mental health policy could potentially create another source for societal stigmas. In fact, this policy creates many unneeded problems, related to intolerable side effects and medicine non-compliance. A recent study, conducted in the United States, indicates that the higher drug costs of atypicals for maintenance-phase treatments are at least partially offset by higher earnings among patients (Salkever *et al*, 2006). Thus, patients attributed with a faster recovery process will also have the potential to find work and become taxpayers within a shorter period of time. The researchers of this study also believe that these effects represent benefits to consumers as well as savings to taxpayer-supported income transfer programmes (Salkever *et al*, 2006). From my perspective, many problems associated with schizophrenia could be resolved if patients were prescribed the best medicine available, during the preliminary stages of their illness.

The recent downsizing of psychiatric hospitals is also a topic of major controversy. In Finland, researchers have discovered a reduction in post-discharge suicides, after the deinstitutionalization of psychiatric hospitals. They found that the risk for suicide was greater between the years 1985 to 1991, than the years 1995 to 2001 among patients who were discharged from a hospital after both one week and one year. A greater risk of suicide was further correlated to patients with schizophrenia or an affective disorder. Subsequently, at present times, hospitalized patients are less suicidal after discharge (Pirkola *et al*, 2007). This seems to indicate that the downsizing of psychiatric hospitals may essentially be an improved mode of health care.

In contrast, the costs associated with psychiatric hospitals are lower, when compared to psychiatric departments within a general hospital (Magnezi *et al*, 2007). Nonetheless, I believe that the use of a general hospital could offer a more regular or standard environment for mentally sick patients. The atmosphere of the inpatient unit that I stayed at could be comparable to a specialized halfway house. However, the older psychiatric hospital in my community may be comparable to a highly structured prison.

That inpatient unit was decommissioned a few years after I was permanently discharged. During that period, patients were treated in a dedicated psychiatric ward within a general hospital. It was made operational again after another several years. In my opinion, a general hospital environment may have other advantages over an inpatient unit. In essence, patients that suffer from a mental illness will not be segregated from the general public, and this could serve to diminish many forms of societal stigmas.

In fact, a two-tiered mental health care system was utilized before the deinstitutionalization of psychiatric hospitals in my nation. During the 1960's, general hospital psychiatric units tended to be voluntarily used by individuals with middle and upper income, while psychiatric hospitals were mainly used by poorer individuals on an involuntary basis (Kirby and Keon, 2004).

A two-tiered mental health care system is also being currently utilized in India. In that nation, patients are likely to abscond from treatment within an open psychiatric ward, because of the economic costs. Only persons who can afford to treat their illness will actually seek help for their poor mental health (Khisty *et al*, 2008). Consequently, inadequate government funding is a major problem within India's mental health care system.

Inadequate funding at the community level is a significant problem related to the deinstitutionalization of psychiatric hospitals. In actuality, patients receive fewer to no services while living within their community. This leads to a higher frequency of relapse, greater readmission rates, increased homelessness, and increased rates of criminal behaviour and incarceration (Kirby and Keon, 2004). Therefore, the creation of outpatient services is also vital to the deinstitutionalization of psychiatric hospitals.

According to a study conducted in Germany, differences among inpatient and outpatient prescribing behaviours result in a lack of continuity of care. Between the years 2000 to 2006, researchers discovered that the proportion of inpatient prescriptions for antidepressant and anti-dementia drugs had increased, while the proportion of neuroleptic and benzodiazepine prescriptions had decreased. They also found that the proportion of generic medicines prescribed to inpatients was significantly lower when compared to outpatients (Hausner *et al*, 2008).

Psychiatric units within a general hospital also have an increased potential to enable early identification, to facilitate preventative psychiatry, and to treat a wide range of less serious psychiatric disorders (Kirby and Keon, 2004). A study comparing an early intervention (EI) team to a standard community mental health team was conducted in the United Kingdom. The early intervention team was different, in that they were assertive in their approach. They also offered more relapse prevention services and psychosocial interventions. Likewise, the team had a universal policy of prescribing atypical antipsychotics, at the lowest effective dose (Agius *et al*, 2007).

Patients were randomly admitted into both treatment teams during their first psychotic episode. After three years, patients treated by the EI team were more likely to be taking their prescribed medications, they were more compliant with their medications, and more often than not, they were prescribed atypical medicines. EI patients were also more likely to have returned to work or their education, and live with their families. From a clinical standpoint, EI patients were less likely to suffer from depression to the extent of requiring anti-depressant medications, they were less likely to commit suicide, and they were also less likely to suffer from a relapse or be re-hospitalized (Agius *et al*, 2007).

EI patients were also less likely to be involuntarily admitted into a hospital, and they developed relapse prevention plans based on early warning signs. Furthermore, more patients in the EI group stopped using illicit drugs, in comparison to those who were treated by the community mental health group. From a social perspective, EI patients and their families also received more psycho-education. Consequently, after a three year period, EI patients were better able to independently manage their illness or vulnerability (Agius *et al*, 2007).

According to another study, the specialized Early Intervention in Psychosis program may effectively delay the transition to psychosis, reduce the duration of untreated psychosis, reduce suicide rates, reduce admission and treatment costs, and prevent relapses (Ricciardi *et al*, 2008). In Germany, early detection services supported through public awareness campaigns were well received by its users and private practitioners (Schultze-Lutter *et al*, 2009). Thus, newer modes of treatment through early intervention principles have proven to be more successful than traditional modes of treatment.

The hospitalization patterns of patients with all forms of psychiatric disorders were studied in Australia. According to these findings, discharge rates had decreased with age, while the length of stay had increased with age. They also found that hospital admission rates were higher, while the length of stay was lower for women in comparison to men. Hospitalization rates also decreased with age for conditions like schizophrenia, manic disorder, and some substance use disorders. In contrast, hospitalization rates had increased with age for organic disorders and they peaked at midlife for persons with alcohol abuse or mood disorders. A late-life increase in hospitalization rates for depressive and personality disorders, among men, was also observed. Accordingly, the creation of specialized psychiatric hospital services should take into account the mix of clinical needs by age, gender, and diagnosis (Low and Draper, 2009).

In Europe, a study was conducted to analyze the schizophrenia patient's quality of life. Patients who lived in France, Germany, and the United Kingdom were the main participants in this study. According to these researchers, individuals living in Germany had the highest subjective quality of life (QOL). The most important factors were country of residence, depression, accommodation status, and employment (Marwaha et al, 2008). Additionally, many correlates of subjective QOL in people with schizophrenia were similar to those in the general population. This study indicates the fact that differences in mental health and social services will directly affect the quality of life for schizophrenia patients around the world.

A further study, conducted in Chile, suggests that the quality of life for schizophrenia patients is greater in developing countries, when compared to developed countries. The sample studied related quality of life to perceptions of family functioning, over economic and community resources. Further, caregivers who participated in family psychoeducational programs obtained higher scores in family functioning (Caqueo and Lemos, 2008). As a consequence, schizophrenia patients will also necessarily depend on a reliable social network for a better quality of life.

A similar study was conducted in Japan. Depressive mood and uncooperativeness were correlated to self-esteem, and self-esteem was connected to quality of life. Therefore, self-esteem is also directly related to the patient's quality of life. Interventions that helped to alleviate psychiatric symptoms also often resulted in a greater quality of life (Kunikata et al,

2005). Likewise, the abolition of societal stigmas should positively affect the patient's coping skills and self-esteem.

Neurocognition is a strong predictor of social problem-solving. Researchers in Norway have associated emotional perceptions with the elements of neurocognition and social problem-solving. Accordingly, neurocognition and social problem solving is weaker in patients who try to control their emotional perceptions. This implies the possibility that emotional perceptions may act as a mediator between neurocognition and functional outcome (Vaskinn *et al*, 2008). In other words, emotional perceptions may play a key role in the functional outcome of many schizophrenia patients.

Subsequently, the widespread nature of societal stigmas only serves to complicate the lives of persons with mental illness. In Pakistan, just over half of the 294 medical students and doctors surveyed held negative attitudes towards patients with schizophrenia, depression, or a drug or alcohol disorder. Therefore, even citizens who dedicate their lives to helping sick persons may hold prejudices against mental disorders. However, most of those surveyed also held favourable views with respect to the treatability of mental disorders. These opinions are also generally similar to the opinions of medical students and doctors living within the United Kingdom (Naeem *et al*, 2006).

A survey completed by pharmacy students in Australia, Belgium, Finland, India, Estonia, and Latvia has similar results. Students in Australia, Estonia, and Latvia agreed with the statement that schizophrenia patients are difficult to talk to. In Belgium and Finland, pharmacy students held the belief that the individual is at fault when developing severe forms of depression (Bell, 2008a). Hence, stigmatized beliefs are also common among pharmacy students in some parts of the world.

In addition to misinformation, social stigmas may also be based on the individual's psychophysiological reactions. Fifteen male and twenty female participants exhibited higher brow muscle tension when exposed to the imagery of persons who were labelled as schizophrenia patients. This psychophysiological reactivity predicted global self-reported attitudes of stigma towards persons with schizophrenia. Researchers also believe that this form of arousal may be a negative experience. Accordingly, natural physiological responses may provide the common person with a further reason to avoid individuals with a mental illness (Graves *et al*, 2005).

Although childhood abuse is not considered to be a cause of a mental illness, schizophrenia spectrum patients who reported abuse have been associated with graver levels of symptoms and social dysfunction. A study of 12 patients with a history of sexual abuse, and 31 patients with no history of abuse, reveals that the abuse group had consistently higher levels of both symptom components and poorer participation in vocational rehabilitation. This group also worked increasingly fewer hours over a gradual amount of time, and they were more likely to perform poorly on tests related to their executive functioning. Similarly, the abuse group experienced higher levels of hallucinations and anxiety over an extended period of time (Lysaker *et al*, 2005a).

Other studies indicate that childhood adversity is directly related to poor overall health, within the general adult population. Five hundred sixty nine adults with schizophrenia were surveyed about their experiences with adverse childhood events. Elements such as physical abuse, sexual abuse, parental mental illness, parental separation, the loss of a parent, the witnessing of domestic violence, and experiences with foster care are some of the difficulties that these patients faced. An increased exposure to adversity was directly correlated with psychiatric problems like suicidal thinking, distress, frequent hospitalizations, and posttraumatic stress disorder. Problems with substance abuse, physical health problems, and poor social functioning were also noted (Rosenberg *et al*, 2007).

The individual's exposure to traumatic events has also been associated with a higher risk for re-victimization and re-traumatization. Patients within an inpatient unit can sometimes face seclusion or restraints, if they exhibit aggressive or hostile behaviours. In these cases, the patient may potentially experience further re-victimization within the hospital setting. A lifetime exposure to life-threatening traumatic events may then result (Steinert *et al*, 2007). From the average citizen's point of view, measures such as seclusion and restraint could also generate some forms of stigma towards psychiatric treatment or psychiatric patients in general. From the patient's point of view, though, these experiences can promote psychopathologic [sic] sequels, similar to the symptoms observed in posttraumatic stress disorder (Steinert *et al*, 2007).

The social and cognitive functioning of over 300 000 males with schizophrenia was examined in Israel. According to this study, the greatest risk of developing schizophrenia, within an urban environment, requires a pre-existing vulnerability. This study also suggests that there is an interaction between population density and poor premorbid social and cognitive functioning. Therefore, vulnerable individuals are at a higher risk when living in cities with greater populations. The need to cope with city life may thus be associated with a greater risk to develop schizophrenia (Weiser *et al*, 2007).

Consequently, stress also poses a significant problem for persons with mental illness. Reactions to acute stress can create survival responses within the neural, cardiovascular, autonomic, immune and metabolic systems. Chronic stress can also promote and exacerbate pathophysiology through the same systems. The brain regions affected by acute and chronic stress include the hippocampus, prefrontal cortex and amygdala (McEwen, 2008). These brain regions change in morphology and chemistry when the individual is subjected to chronic stress. It is believed that these latter changes are reversible in cases of short-term stress, though it is unknown if they are still reversible in cases of long-term stress.

Scientists have defined the burden of chronic stress, along with a change in one's personal behaviours or lifestyle, as an allostatic overload (McEwen, 2008). They observe the fact that reducing the effects of stress is just as important as pharmaceutical therapy. Thus, physical activities and social support mechanisms designed to reduce external stressors are also significant to a state of remission.

According to Seeman, some of the symptoms observed in schizophrenia may not be caused by any biological or brain irregularities. Therefore, some symptoms may be caused solely through psychological issues. For instance, a schizophrenia patient may struggle with interpersonal demands for subjective reasons. Due to his interpersonal inabilities, the patient may then protect himself from failure and avoid social conduct through isolation. From my experience, Seeman could be correct on this issue.

Seeman also hypothesizes that patients who suffer from cognitive deficits, are actually aware of their shortfalls and that they narrow their field of activities and compensate for deficiency by repetitive rituals and over-rehearsal. I would have to disagree with this point. While extremely ill, I did narrow the range of my daily activities, essentially because of my cognitive deficiencies. However, when I experienced repetitive thoughts, I believe that this was due entirely to my illness. Likewise, when I would find myself repeating a certain action, I believe that this was due entirely to a lack of consciousness or awareness, and my rapid and recurrent thought processes. Seeman also believes that eccentric behaviours such as unusual speech, unusual tone of speech, and the wearing of peculiar forms of clothing are mainly due to the patient's feeling that he is either side-lined or disregarded by his society. In fact, when I acted in a manner that could be viewed as socially odd, I did so mainly because of my fragmented thoughts and delusional frame of mind.

Furthermore, Seeman theorizes that the unsuccessful pursuit of happiness, in the areas of employment, material possessions and intimate relationships, causes patients to adopt habits and routines that are considered by others as impractical, illogical, and unfathomable (Seeman, 2007). Although he does not specify any examples, I would still have to attribute the cause of a patient's illogical and impractical actions to his hallucinations and delusional frame of mind. I understand Seeman's effort to reduce societal stigma and attribute a seemingly more normal or common reason behind irregular forms of behaviour. However, in my mind, most of the strange actions committed by schizophrenia patients are due entirely to a state of psychosis.

Schizophrenia, as a disease, has been strongly associated with six adverse outcomes. Outcomes in the areas of violence, victimization, self-harm, substance abuse, homelessness, and unemployment may be common. These outcomes also relate to each other, in that one outcome can act as a risk factor for another (Kooyman *et al*, 2007). However, long-term outcomes are of most importance to psychiatrists. Factors such as the choice of medicines, the duration of untreated psychosis, the impact of a relapse on long-term outcome, the limited efficacy of psychopathological treatments, and mortality due to suicide or other causes are of utmost importance. Thus, a proven health advocate may be needed to aid the patient with other forms of adverse outcomes.

In Germany, a study comparing mental illnesses to physical illnesses reveals that patients with mental disorders are more significantly excluded within their society. Areas of exclusion include the job market, work income, and intimate relationships. Researchers assert that this is especially true for persons with schizophrenia or alcohol addiction (Richter *et al*, 2006). Therefore, in some societies, schizophrenia is a greater target of societal stigmas when compared to other forms of illness.

In the United States, the average life span of a schizophrenia patient is 20% lower than that of the average citizen. One possible explanation may be based on the possibility that schizophrenia is a syndrome of accelerated aging. In fact, scientists have associated schizophrenia with a number of anatomical and physiological abnormalities outside of the brain. These abnormalities may contribute towards a decreased life expectancy. This hypothesis was derived through the established syndromes of accelerated aging and by the sharing of risk factors between schizophrenia and other age-related conditions (Kirkpatrick *et al*, 2008). In effect, this theory may be quite plausible if it is true that all schizophrenia patients will be further affected by a decrease in lifespan.

The dopamine system could be vulnerable to aging as well. This may be due to the observed loss of dopamine receptors and transporters over the average person's life span. Researchers have linked midbrain dopamine synthesis to rewarded-related prefrontal activity. They have also demonstrated that healthy aging induces functional alterations within the reward system, and have identified a change from a positive to a negative correlation between midbrain dopamine synthesis and prefrontal activity. This seems to indicate the existence of an age-dependent dopaminergic tuning mechanism for cortical reward processing. It also indicates a possible alteration of key neural circuits during healthy ageing (Dreher *et al*, 2008).

From my perspective, patients with schizophrenia may have a shorter life span for other reasons. When I experienced rapid thoughts during a state of psychosis, the speed of my normal thought processes had increased in an exponential fashion. As a result, I believe that the brain may be dangerously overworked in schizophrenia. If the brain is overworked during a state of extreme psychosis, this could explain a possible accelerated aging process. Thus, from my lay perspective, hyperfunction within the brain may somehow contribute towards a shorter life span in the schizophrenia patient.

A study conducted in Austria associates a reduced life expectancy, in patients with mental illness, to comorbid somatic illnesses. These researchers have uncovered evidence which suggests that patients with severe mental illnesses also have worse physical health, when compared to the average citizen within developed countries. They claim that the physical health of the psychiatric patient is often neglected, and that cardiovascular disease is the main cause of premature deaths (Fleischhacker *et al*, 2008).

Actually, cardiovascular disease is a major cause of death in many developed nations. In the United States of America, it accounts for approximately 50% of all deaths nationwide. The major risk factors associated with cardiovascular disease include obesity, smoking, hypertension, dyslipidemia, and insulin resistance leading to diabetes (Hennekens, 2007). According to some researchers, patients with schizophrenia have alarmingly higher rates of these risk factors when compared to the general population. This may be due to the side effects of an antipsychotic medication, like weight gain or fatigue. However, the use of these medicines, alone, could also increase the individual's risk to develop cardiovascular problems. Second generation antipsychotics have been linked to an increased prevalence of abdominal obesity and dyslipidemia, while both first and second generation antipsychotics have been linked to an increased risk to develop diabetes mellitus type 2 (Scheepers-Hoeks *et al*, 2008).

Conversely, other researchers have found evidence to support the theory that greater body mass index protects against depression, schizophrenia and suicide. In fact, greater body mass index has been associated with a reduced risk of hospitalization for conditions like psychosis, depression and anxiety. Greater body mass index has also been linked to a reduced risk of major psychiatric outcomes (Lawlor *et al*, 2007). From my observations, the side effect of weight gain, due to antipsychotic medications, is quite common. Consequently, it is entirely possible that this side effect may play a positive role in the treatment of schizophrenia and other mental illnesses.

Researchers from Denmark conducted a five-year follow up study on 547 individuals who were diagnosed with first episode schizophrenia. These researchers found a strong association between suicidal thoughts, suicidal plans, previous suicide attempts, depressive symptoms, psychotic symptoms, and young age, to suicidal plans and attempts after both a one and two year follow up period (Bertelsen *et al*, 2007). Additionally, 16 participants eventually died before the end of this study. Therefore, the risk to commit suicide may also be relevant to a reduced life span in the schizophrenia patient.

However, according to other research, cardiovascular disease occurs more frequently, and accounts for more premature deaths than suicide (Hennekens, 2007). Therefore, every schizophrenia patient should be examined for potential problems with his physical health as well.

Dysregulation is another significant problem in schizophrenia. This phenomenon occurs when the patient fluctuates between rigid and unpredictable responses, during decision making processes. According to a study conducted in Switzerland, first episode patients are characterized by a high degree of dysregulation accompanied by low metric entropy and a tendency towards increased mutual information (Cattapan-Ludewig *et al*, 2008).

Furthermore, a crucial mechanism of consciousness is the binding of synchronized and distributed activity within the human brain. Some findings suggest that disturbances in this binding may cause the disintegration of consciousness observed in schizophrenia. This, in turn, can cause disturbances in the reflection of self, and similarly, these dissociated psychic fragments may be experienced as parts of the external world. Scientifically, these disturbances may lead to the disintegration of neural communication. This neurophysiological feature is theorized to be similar to the psychological dissociative processes associated with stress response, and cognitive, affective and neuroendocrine dysregulation (Bob, 2007).

According to researchers from the Czech Republic, random-like processes in the patient have been linked to defects in the organization of semantic memory. These processes were more disorganized and less definable than those of controls, with more semantic links and atypical associations. This suggests that the neural activity in schizophrenia is significantly more chaotic comparatively. Similarities were also drawn between these elements of cognition and chaotic nonlinear dynamical systems. As a consequence, this condition may reflect on a possible neural chaotic process. This increased neural chaos may affect brain processes and cause the random-like disorganization of mental processes (Bob *et al*, 2007a).

Another study suggests that time phenomenology is also disturbed in the schizophrenia patient. In this study, patients required longer delays between stimuli to detect that they were asynchronous. The researchers conclude that this will lead to impairments in the phenomenology of event-structure coding (Giersch *et al*, 2009).

A study of 91 stable outpatients with schizophrenia and 55 healthy controls has drawn a correlation between theory of mind deficits and the residual symptoms of schizophrenia. Theory of mind is an ability to correctly infer the mental states of other persons. Both the social-cognitive and the social-perceptual aspects of theory of mind are impaired in schizophrenia patients. Moreover, these researchers have drawn a correlation between social-cognitive theory of mind abilities with positive and negative symptoms (Bora *et al*, 2008). High negative symptom ratings have been correlated with a poorer recognition of static displays of emotion, while high positive symptom ratings have been associated with a poorer recognition of dynamic displays of emotion (Johnston *et al*, 2008). However, the theory of mind deficit, without persistent negative symptoms, is secondary to the general cognitive dysfunction exhibited by the schizophrenia patient.

The theory of mind along with apophenia, or the tendency to perceive meaning in unrelated events, may serve as a vulnerability marker for schizophrenia. Several researchers from the United Kingdom speculate that over-mentalizing may be underpinned by a hyper-associative cognitive style, linked to an exaggeration of the normal human tendency to attribute mental states. Moreover, they state that perceiving meaning in randomness and, more particularly, attributing mental states where none are indicated may be important elements in the formation of delusional beliefs (Fyfe *et al*, 2008). I would have to agree with their assessment, because the majority of my delusions were generated through an association of random thoughts and the random statements of persons within my physical environment, into one cohesive and united perception.

Another study was conducted on 33 individuals that suffer from a traumatic brain injury, within the United Kingdom. Researchers found that these patients had greater impairments in emotion recognition, 'theory of mind', and cognitive flexibility, when compared to 34 orthopedic control subjects. Increases in behavioural problems were also detected after one year. Nevertheless, the severity of impairments in emotion recognition, the understanding of intentions, and flexibility were unrelated to the severity of any behavioural problems (Milders *et al*, 2008). This may cast doubt on the link that some scientists have placed between theory of mind deficits and social functioning.

Poor premorbid IQ may be a predisposing factor for the development of schizophrenia and other psychoses as well as predictive of poor long-term outcome. A study, conducted in Italy, compares the IQ of 48 patients with schizophrenia and 56 patients with bipolar disorder. The results of this study indicate that low IQ schizophrenia patients have more thought disturbances and positive symptoms, when compared to both high and low IQ patients with bipolar disorder. Low IQ schizophrenia patients also exhibited more cognitive symptoms than high IQ bipolar patients. In addition, no differences were observed between high IQ schizophrenia and low IQ bipolar patients (Stratta *et al*, 2007). Consequently, low IQ may be relevant in thought disorders like schizophrenia, while having a lesser impact in mood disorders like bipolar disorder.

Other cognitive deficits have been observed in the areas of intellectual function, verbal memory and response initiation/inhibition. These deficits, though more subtle, are also present amongst the healthy first-degree relatives of the patient. As a result, specific deficits, such as these, could serve as potential markers in an individual's risk to develop schizophrenia (Groom *et al*, 2008).

The largest study of gender differences, in schizophrenia, was conducted in China. Researchers have discovered that the onset of schizophrenia occurs at a significantly earlier age in male patients, in comparison to female patients. Likewise, late-onset schizophrenia was much more common in females. Male patients received higher daily doses of antipsychotics, and they demonstrated a different pattern of antipsychotic usage. Further, they were more likely to smoke cigarettes, and be single or never married. Male patients were also more likely to demonstrate severe deterioration over time (Tang *et al*, 2007).

Another study indicates that men have more severe negative symptoms, poorer premorbid functioning, and poorer social networks. Likewise, more males abused substances, were unemployed, and lived alone. Researchers have further associated premorbid social adjustment to levels of negative symptoms and number of friends, among this subgroup (Thorup *et al*, 2007).

In contrast, paranoid schizophrenia was more common in females. Female patients had a different pattern of ongoing symptoms and severity and they were more likely to suffer from persistent positive symptoms. Females also had more severe positive and affective symptoms. On a further note, these gender differences were found to be largely consistent with other studies conducted within Western societies (Tang *et al*, 2007).

Women may also suffer from hallucinations that are more severe in nature. Despite demonstrating better scores in functioning, women had poorer self-esteem and they attempted suicide more often. In addition, according to this study, both men and women with first-episode psychosis will demonstrate different psychopathological characteristics and social functioning, which cannot be explained by the older age of onset in women (Thorup *et al*, 2007).

Variation at the age of onset may reflect a variation in cause. Not much else is known about this phenomenon though. Scientists theorize that the effects of pathogen stress, natural selection, sexual selection, migration, life-history profiles, or a combination of these elements may be relevant (Shaner *et al*, 2007). In any case, most doctors currently believe that the cause of schizophrenia is due to a complex combination of multiple factors.

Scientifically speaking, the neurochemical origins of schizophrenia may not necessarily lie in dopamine dysregulation. Most medical professionals define schizophrenia as a disease that is characterized by a number of component causes. These causes can include genetic factors, and early environmental hazards that subtly alter subsequent neurodevelopment. This would then predispose the individual to later stages of dopamine dysregulation. Technically, dopamine dysregulation would then be the final common pathway underlying positive psychotic symptoms. This dysregulation may further play a role in both negative and cognitive symptoms (Di Forti *et al*, 2007).

Structural changes in the brain are also prominent in schizophrenia. Imaging studies have revealed decreases of brain tissue, along with increases in ventricle volumes and cerebrospinal fluid in the schizophrenia patient. Decreases in brain tissue and increases in ventricle volume are known to be continuous for at least 20 years after a chronically ill patient experiences his first symptoms. Moreover, the rate of this progressive decrease in brain tissue is estimated to be at around 0.5% per year. This is twice the rate of healthy control patients, whose decrease in brain tissue is estimated to be approximately 0.2% per year. In the schizophrenia patient, losses of brain volume are most pronounced in the frontal and temporal (gray matter) areas (Hulshoff and Kahn 2008).

Increases in volume have also been observed within the lateral ventricles. These progressive brain changes have been correlated to poor outcome, negative symptoms, and a decline in neuropsychological performance. Theoretically, a continuous pathophysiological process may be occurring

(Hulshoff and Kahn 2008). This is another reason why all schizophrenia patients need to be continually monitored by a medical professional. Psychiatrists need to ensure that the efficacy of their prescription remains constant, especially during times when there are physical changes transpiring within the patient's brain.

Conversely, other scientists believe in the theory that schizophrenia is not a progressively deteriorating illness. In a study conducted in Denmark, patients had an 18% recovery rate, while 13% were institutionalized at a hospital or supported housing unit, after a period of five years. The scientists state that rates of recovery and institutionalization contradict the assumption that the illness deteriorates progressively, since there were no changes in rates observed within a two to five year period (Bertelsen *et al,* 2009).

In the worst case scenario, a schizophrenia patient may not improve while taking his prescribed medicines. These patients are classified as treatment resistant, treatment-refractory, or non-respondent patients. Between 20 to 40 percent of schizophrenia patients fit into this category (Cervera and Seva, 2006). A study conducted on a population in Japan seems to suggest that the serotonin subtype HTR3A may be a possible candidate gene, with respect to the development of treatment resistant schizophrenia (Ji *et al,* 2008).

Forms of treatment resistant schizophrenia are not due either to the severity of one's symptoms or a chronic status. Several factors must be taken into account when diagnosing a patient with this condition. These elements include the nature of the illness, the recognition of possible problems with substance abuse, the determination of whether the patient's symptoms are primary or secondary, and other aspects related to treatment compliance, tolerance, and the presence of minor neurological signs (Cervera and Seva, 2006).

In order to ascertain a proper mode of therapeutic evolution for treatment resistant patients, some guidelines need to be considered. First, psychiatrists must clearly identify the patient's symptoms, and prescribe medications with a suitable dose and duration. Doctors must also use all single therapeutic agents before applying multiple agents. The prevention of extrapyramidal effects by means of an adequate choice during the primary stages of treatment is also crucial. Finally, doctors must determine that their patient's resistance is not due to treatment intolerance, non-compliance to treatment, inappropriate social support or inappropriate psychosocial treatment (Cervera and Seva, 2006).

In contrast, a state of complete remission requires the patient to achieve symptomatic remission according to the Remission in Schizophrenia Working Group severity criteria, functional remission, and a level of adequate subjective well-being for a period of over six months. A study of 2960 schizophrenia patients in Germany was conducted in 2001. The findings of this study indicate that 47% achieved symptomatic remission, 26% achieved functional remission, and 42% achieved a subjective well-being. However, at the end of the year, only 12% reached complete remission, and 35% did not achieve any forms of remission. Further, only 8% of early nonremitted cases achieved a complete remission status. Ninety percent of these patients did not fulfill the combined remission criteria because of a low functional rate and an even lower employment rate (Lambert *et al*, 2006). The researchers observed that each remission component, including complete remission, was mainly predicted by early remission within the first 3 months.

Additionally, first-line treatments through atypical antipsychotics increased the likelihood of complete remission. Similarly, the course of a disorder may depend highly on early outcome (Lambert *et al*, 2006). Hence, early intervention through atypical medicines may be crucial to a state of full remission.

Cognitive behavioural therapy is a further mode of treatment that has positive effects on many forms of psychological problems. Scientists have discovered that CBT is extremely effective in the treatment of unipolar depression, posttraumatic stress disorder, generalized anxiety disorder, panic disorder, some social phobias, and many childhood depressive or anxiety disorders. CBT has also had moderate success in treating marital distress, anger, childhood somatic disorders, and chronic pains. Other researchers have noted that CBT is somewhat superior to antidepressants in the treatment of adult depression, and that it has yielded a large uncontrolled effect size in the treatment of schizophrenia (Butler *et al*, 2006). In view of that, psychological modes of therapy, like CBT, are also significant to the treatment of mental illnesses like schizophrenia.

Hogarty has developed four psychosocial treatments that will aid patients with their recovery from schizophrenia. Major role therapy is designed to be an early precursor to clinical case management. Family psychoeducation is an approach to educate and ally the patient with his family members, to reduce intrafamilial distress. Personal therapy aims to teach patients elements like stress management and affective regulation techniques. Lastly, cognitive enhancement therapy is designed to aid patients with the remediation of social- and nonsocial-cognitive deficits (Eack *et al,* 2007).

Recognizing the prodromal symptoms of schizophrenia in children and adolescents is also extremely important. Educating general practitioners in the field of psychiatry may improve detection and referral rates. Equally, the implementation of early medical detection teams could also reduce delays in the initial assessment and treatment processes. Likewise, public mental health education will also reduce delays in psychiatric diagnoses and treatment.

According to some preliminary studies, atypical antipsychotics can improve symptoms, and delay or prevent the progression of schizophrenia in adolescents (Thomas and Woods, 2006). Some forms of psychotherapies have also been effective. However, the long-term risks and benefits of antipsychotic treatments for adolescents still need to be explored.

From an ethical standpoint, there may be other problems associated with the prescribing of antipsychotic medications for adolescents. Although newer second-generation antipsychotics offer the possibility of an early psychopharmacological intervention, few cases are the real prodromes of schizophrenia. Statistics indicate that no more than 40% of all early interventions turn out to be a true schizophrenia prodrome (Filaković *et al,* 2007). Thus, in some cases, adolescents are prescribed medicines that they really do not need. When this occurs, forms of social stigma can arise as a direct result.

In addition, the true effects of antipsychotic medications on a developing brain are still unknown. Therefore, each individual case of suspected early onset schizophrenia must be addressed with caution. Psychiatrists must properly identify the correct symptoms, and they must also prescribe the best therapy available to treat these symptoms on a discrete and individual basis.

The use of antipsychotic medications during pregnancy also requires further research. One theory links hyperthermia to the development of schizophrenia, within a fetal brain. Hyperthermia is known to cause congenital defects in the central nervous system and other organs. It also causes damage to the developing brainstem, and this has been associated with functional defects. This damage has been further associated with the hypoplasia of parts that undergo active development, during the time of exposure (Edwards, 2007).

Although some studies indicate that there is no direct invasion due to the influenza virus, maternal influenza and other causes of fever during the second trimester of pregnancy are theorized to damage the amygdalohippocampal complex within a fetus (Edwards, 2007). Researchers theorize that familial genetics, season of birth, maternal nutrition, severe stress, and fever medications may act in combination with hyperthermia to cause problems in brain development, within the fetus.

In 2008, a case study was conducted on two women with schizophrenia, who were treated through clozapine. The first test subject had two deliveries while receiving clozapine treatments. The second woman developed schizophrenia after her first child was born. She then became pregnant after clozapine initiation. In both cases, there were no complications with the vaginal deliveries, and the researchers concluded that no specific risks for either the mothers or their children can be attributed to the use of clozapine. However, these researchers also noted that physicians must be aware of the changes in fertility induced by prolactin-sparing drugs (Duran *et al*, 2008). Accordingly, mothers should not breastfeed their children if they are taking clozapine.

Another case report was conducted on a mother who was treated with olanzapine, during the breast-feeding stage. No adverse side effects were noticed, and the mother experienced a rapid improvement in her mental health (Lutz *et al*, 2008). Consequently, olanzapine may be an effective medicine under these circumstances.

Nonetheless, it is possible that antipsychotics may affect neurodevelopment and decrease brain size, at least in rats. Researchers have studied the effects of antipsychotic medicines on caenorhabditis elegans, which is a kind of roundworm. In particular, clozapine, fluphenazine, and haloperidol produced deficits in the development and migration of ALM neurons and axonal outgrowth in PLM neurons. Other antipsychotic drugs, including risperidone, aripiprazole, quetiapine, trifluoperazine and olanzapine, produced modest effects on neuronal development. This study demonstrates the possibility that antipsychotic drugs could affect neuronal migration and axonal outgrowth within a developing nervous system (Donohoe *et al*, 2008).

In Brazil, a study was conducted on 294 patients with schizophrenia and their offspring. The adult offspring had a significantly poorer employment status when compared to the general population. Similarly, fewer male offspring were married in comparison to the average male. Researchers also deduced that the offspring subgroup had social adjustment problems that were markedly reflected in employment and marital status (Terzian *et al*, 2007). Therefore, schizophrenia patients who plan to have a family at some point in the future should take social problems like these into consideration. The individual can potentially adjust his parenting behaviours to directly address these specific social problems.

Group psychotherapies have been created to help the parents of schizophrenia patients as well. These services re-establish a psychic balance and the balance of the whole family system by reducing high expressed emotion. In many cases, their primary emotions are marked by traits of sociability and high self-protection. Other high emotions include fear, sorrow and anger. It is often the case that these emotions will cause parents to become cautious, possess feelings of responsibility, and suffer from guilt (Gruber *et al*, 2006). Accordingly, parents have reported that group psychotherapies were interesting and helpful. These sessions enabled them to overcome the stigma of the disease. Group psychotherapies have further provided parents with knowledge, help, social ties, and a way out with respect to their social isolation.

The caregiver of a sick individual may also feel overwhelmed at times. Caregivers can also experience emotions related to blame, shame or guilt. Grief is another common emotion. In addition, forms of anger may be directed towards the impact of a mental illness. Similar to the patient, a caregiver may also face troubles when accepting the diagnosis of a mental illness. As a result, the affected patient is not always the sole victim of a mental disorder.

In the United States, an interview was conducted on 85 persons of Latin descent, who were caring for an adult with schizophrenia. The aim of the questionnaire was to examine the relationship between caregivers and their sick family members. This study indicates that approximately 75%

of Latinos with schizophrenia live with their families. Elements such as young age and lower levels of education were associated with higher levels of depressive symptoms, in the caregiver (Magaña *et al*, 2007). Higher levels of the patient's symptoms had a similar effect.

According to further studies, the physical and mental health of a caregiver determines levels of burden (Hou *et al*, 2008). In effect, the caregiver's perceived burden mediated the relationship between his depression and the patient's psychiatric symptoms. The caregiver's perceived stigma was also highly associated with depressive symptoms. Low social status is another factor that affects caregivers. Therefore, social interventions may also be necessary for the caregivers of patients with mental illness.

A study of five male and five female caregivers reveals some possible coping techniques. Cognitive, behavioural and emotional therapies were commonly utilized. Other coping mechanisms such as religious, social, and professional support further aided caregivers (Huang *et al*, 2008).

Other researchers have suggested that a new name for schizophrenia may be useful in the education of patients and the general public. The new name would reflect upon a more biopsychosocial conceptualization of the disease. One suggested name is Neuro-Emotional Integration Disorder (NEID). The renaming of schizophrenia subtypes may also be beneficial. Defensive type could replace the paranoid subtype, motoric type could replace the catatonic subtype, and brief neuro-emotional-integration breakdown could replace the brief psychotic episode subtype. Antipsychotic medications could also be referred to as NEI-Enhancing medications (Levin, 2006).

Through this re-labelling, researchers simply wish to stress the fact that schizophrenia is a highly treatable brain disorder. Societal stigmas may also be reduced as a direct result. Other clinical benefits can include improved medication management, improved multifamily group psycho-education, and further improvements in the area of cognitive therapy (Levin, 2006).

In 2002, the Japanese Society of Psychiatry and Neurology changed the Japanese term for schizophrenia from Seishin Bunretsu Byo meaning mind split disease, to the term Togo Shitcho Sho, which translates as integration disorder. This renaming was carried out upon the request from a patient's family group (Sato, 2006). The ambiguity of the old term, recent advances in schizophrenia research, and the deep-rooted negative image of schizophrenia were the main reasons behind this change. Moreover, the main source behind this negative image was due in part to the long-term inhumane treatment of schizophrenia patients.

According to one survey, 78% of those polled used the new term. In addition, 86% of psychiatrists within the Miyagi prefecture found the new term to be more suitable. In their mind, it represents a more modern concept of the disorder (Sato, 2006). In 2004, a Japanese treatment guideline for Togo Shitcho Sho was subsequently developed. Technically, this new label was based on a shift from the Kraepelinian disease concept to a vulnerability-stress model.

Roy additionally believes that the concept of schizophrenia is too vague, and that it therefore should be categorized into newer and more specific subtypes. He observes the fact that the current definitions of schizophrenia include several disorders with distinct causes, which complicates the identification of possible causes. He proposes that the first subtype should include subjects who exhibit the most severe symptoms of psychosis, those who have poorer social functioning prior to the onset of psychosis, and those who have relatives that are also affected with schizophrenia. The second subtype would include subjects with a less severe form of the disorder, including those who have better neuropsychological performance, and those who have relatives that suffer from affective disorders, like depression. According to Roy, researchers will have an increased chance to uncover the true causes of schizophrenia, through these newer subtypes. Better treatment methods, along with an improved diagnostic accuracy may also result (Roy *et al*, 2001).

Several researchers in Israel also criticize the current diagnostic system. One shortcoming they identify is based on a lack of scientific brain-related etiological knowledge of mental disorders. They believe that this latter shortcoming is further hampered by a lack of theoretical framework or language, which translates clinical findings into brain disturbances or insufficiencies. The solution to this problem may be to base a theoretical construct upon insights discovered through neuroscience and neural-computational models. These researchers label this newer and more practical diagnostic system as Brain Profiling (Peled, 2006).

The concept of brain profiling is based on three major dimensions. These dimensions are identified as either a neural complexity disorder, a neuronal resilience insufficiency, or a context-sensitive processing decline. In a neural complexity disorder, there are disturbances occurring to fast neuronal activations in the millisecond range. This dimension also incorporates connectivity and hierarchical imbalances, such as those observed in psychosis. A neuronal resilience insufficiency relates to disturbances that alter slower changes, or long-term synaptic modulations. It further incorporates disturbances to optimization and constraint satisfactions, within the relevant areas of neuronal circuitry. A context-sensitive processing decline is based on the level of internal representations associated with personality disorders (Peled, 2006).

Within the brain profiling system, clinical manifestations are coded 1 for detection, 0 for non-detection, and 0.5 for questionable. These entries will be further grouped according to their presumed neuronal dynamic relationships, and the coefficients determine their relevance to the brain disturbance (Peled, 2006).

Additionally, within this system, scientific predictions regarding etiological factors may be testable through brain imaging investigations. It also provides a more transparent clinical history of the patient, when psychiatrists utilize and study multiple follow-up diagnoses. In comparison to DSM codes, the brain profiling system is also more clinically informative. It may reduce discrimination and stigma because it associates a disorder to the brain and not the individual. It may also improve psychiatry into a more advanced clinical-neuroscience (Peled, 2006).

Along with improvements in psychiatric practices, scientists will also eventually develop improvements in the area of therapeutic medicines. A new approach to the treatment of many illnesses, called network medicine, could advance treatment techniques for schizophrenia as well. In network medicine, the medications produced will selectively target specific molecules within the brain. These new targets are protein-signalling networks. In time, newer therapeutic strategies should give rise to moreefficient and tolerable modes of treatment (Erler and Linding, 2010).

Perhaps having knowledge of famous persons who eventually developed a mental disorder may alleviate some societal stigmas. Probably the most well known person affected by schizophrenia is John Nash. In 1950, when Mr. Nash was 21 years old, he wrote a 27 page dissertation in the field of economics. Nine years later, he developed paranoid schizophrenia and lost his job as a professor at the Massachusetts Institute of Technology. Later in his life, Mr. Nash won the Nobel Prize in Economics for his dissertation (Nobelprize.org, 2008).

The sister of Tennessee Williams, Rose Williams was diagnosed with schizophrenia at a very young age (Disabled World, 2008). Tennessee was an American playwright who lived during the twentieth century. Some of his works include 'The Rose Tattoo', 'Cat on a Hot Tin Roof', and 'The Glass Menagerie'. Perhaps his most famous play is titled 'A Streetcar Named Desire' for which Tennessee eventually won a Pulitzer Prize.

William Chester Minor was also diagnosed with schizophrenia. Born in 1834, Minor was a surgeon who served the Union Army during the American Civil War. After becoming severely ill, he still made valuable contributions towards the creation of the Oxford English Dictionary (Buzzle.com, 2008).

In closing, early detection and treatment is vital with respect to all illnesses, either mental or physical. Longer durations of untreated psychosis will usually result in a worse prognosis, an increased suicide risk, and possible violence.

On the other hand, the philosophical right for freedom gives individuals, who are suspected to be affected by a mental disorder, the right to refuse treatment. In many societies, the patient must pose as a danger to either himself, or to other persons, before involuntary modes of treatment are legally justified.

As a member of a democratic nation, I also recognize and value the principles of freedom and self-determination. However, I also strongly believe that every individual who enters into the preliminary stages of psychosis should be treated for his condition, even in cases where he refuses treatment. From my standpoint, I believe that my duration of psychosis would have been much shorter if I had accepted Dr. Lupton's initial diagnosis. I would also trade some of my personal liberties away, if this prevented the possibility that I would suffer from any permanent forms of brain damage, due to my disease.

In Canada, denying any individual's human right for freedom and autonomy is unconstitutional. Our way of life would be drastically different if persons were not granted the right to live autonomously. Subsequently, I believe in an individual's right for personal autonomy, in the case of euthanasia. In other words, I believe in the right for choice and self-rule, under this specific circumstance. Preserving the ethical integrity of the medical profession may supersede the individual's personal freedoms though. Proponents against the legalization of euthanasia believe that it is morally right to restrict the individual's right for personal autonomy. In a similar fashion, I believe that it is morally right to restrict the individual's personal liberties, if he suffers from extreme, yet treatable thought disturbances. Hence, I believe in the restriction of personal autonomy concerning any individuals who suffer from a correctible mental illness.

In both matters, a conflict of opinion exists with respect to the individual's right to personally and independently choose what happens to his body. However, on a grand scale, human liberties are not an absolute right. Social interests such as the preservation of life and the protection of third parties may take precedence. For example, in one legal ruling, an individual's choice to refuse a blood transfusion on religious grounds was firmly denied. The court involved took into consideration the fact that the individual was a single parent, and that he would be leaving a minor as a ward of the state if he were permitted the right to refuse medical treatment (Medscape Today, 2008).

According to the Canadian Catholic Bioethics Institute, mental health care is compromised when capacity is mistakenly denied or presumed (Kirby and Keon, 2004). Therefore, some patients with a mental illness are capable of making sound decisions, while others are not. However, determining the rational capacity in most patients can be difficult. Patients with a capacity for sound decision-making must have the ability to understand the relevant information concerning treatment, to appreciate the significance of that information, and to reason so as to weigh the available options logically (Kirby and Keon, 2004).

Both non-cognitive functioning, and the individual's emotional state will affect his ability to make sound and rational judgments. For example, feelings of hopelessness can affect a clinically depressed patient, even when he is fully able to comprehend relevant forms of information. Likewise, a delusional state can also affect the schizophrenia patient's decision making in ways that are not clearly related to an absence or loss of cognition. The decision making process in individuals that suffer from substance abuse problems may also be compromised, due to difficulties with their addiction. Similarly, the capacity to make rational decisions may be narrowly focused in patients with eating disorders, and therefore impossible to ascertain (Kirby and Keon, 2004).

In accordance with contemporary medical ethics, patient autonomy is vital. As an element of the Hippocratic Oath, the medical principle do no harm suggests that involuntary modes of treatment will essentially infringe on the personal liberties of the mentally sick. Thus, from an ethical standpoint, no mentally sick individual should ever be forcefully treated for an illness, even when it is in his or her best interests. This is an extremely complicated moral problem though. In my opinion, our health care system has failed when a doctor fails to treat an illness that is treatable. When the patient refuses treatment in this case, he is essentially abusing a fundamental privilege.

In fact, human freedoms are never total and unequivocal, even within democratic societies. For example, in Canada, no persons are permitted the right to purchase firearms. If this privilege were granted, it is highly likely that some individuals may misuse or abuse their right to own a firearm. I believe that a comparable misuse of freedom occurs when the schizophrenia patient chooses to refuse medical treatment.

Hence, I believe that it is morally right to develop mental health laws, with respect to the involuntary treatment of patients that exhibit problems with cognition. From my view of ethics, mental and physical health services should always be delivered in a timely manner. In the case of a psychotic disorder, I propose that at least two psychiatrists should complete a certification process. Once the individual becomes certifiable, it may then become his general practitioner's responsibility to ensure that suitable methods of treatment are examined, and eventually utilized.

Actually, most schizophrenia patients refuse treatment because they are in a state of denial. There are two main factors behind this denial. First, the schizophrenia patient's sense of judgment may be significantly impaired. By definition, schizophrenia is a thought disorder. Thus, psychological elements like cognition, reasoning, and common sense may be impoverished in the patient. When severely ill, the schizophrenia patient will suffer from a diminished intellect, and he will usually be highly irrational. Under these circumstances, the patient should never be granted the authority to make critical life decisions, which may impede his mental health and overall well-being.

On the surface, a potential problem with this mental health care policy may be that some individuals will fear to seek medical help, when first experiencing a state of psychosis. These persons will enter into a state of denial, because they fear that they may be subject to societal stigmas and discrimination. If we deal with the root cause behind this form of denial, we should thereupon solve the problem of personal freedoms and the right to refuse medical treatment. Thus, if we are somehow able to eliminate the existence of social stigmas, we will consequently eliminate the most significant reason behind the patient's refusal for treatment.

Let us view this problem through a thought experiment. If you were diagnosed with an illness like cancer, and the treatment process has a 70% success rate, would you seek treatment? What if you were diagnosed with an illness like AIDS, which may have a 30% treatment success rate? Would you seek treatment under this circumstance? I would assume that the answer to both of these questions would be a yes. If this is true, what differentiates schizophrenia from any other illness? Schizophrenia is a mental disorder, while these other illnesses may be categorized as a physical illness. However, does this factor, alone, have any significance in your choice to seek treatment? I would further assume that most persons would answer no.

In my mind, the only things that differentiate an illness like schizophrenia from an illness like cancer are the elements of negative stereotyping and societal stigma. In the case of cancer, there is no form of shame or intolerance associated with either its diagnosis or treatment. Yet, there is an abundance of societal stigmas tied to almost every aspect in schizophrenia. From one psychiatrist's point of view, the schizophrenia patient's recovery from societal stigmas may be as difficult as a recovery from the illness itself (Diamond, 2006). Therefore, in most cases, when a patient enters into a state of denial, he may be actively neutralizing the progression of internalized stigma.

Now, let us examine the possible outcomes when a schizophrenia patient refuses treatment. According to Hwang, 15% of persons that are treated for a mental health disorder are homeless (Hwang, 2005). In my mind, any patient that refuses treatment will also potentially face homelessness, because he will lack the ability to live an independent way of life. In a small minority of cases, it may be possible for a schizophrenia patient to both refuse treatment and avoid homelessness. However, the majority of patients, who remain in a state of psychosis, will never acquire any forms of formal employment. These individuals will most certainly have to depend on a third party for their basic necessities and everyday living.

Homelessness, then, is a very relevant problem for any individuals who do not acquire any forms of employment. Let us compare this outcome with the outcomes that may result when a patient is involuntarily treated for his illness. Under the latter circumstance, the patient would not face homelessness, though he may be committed into some form of inpatient facility. In this case, the individual's basic necessities will be taken care of. Problems with elements of survival, like food, shelter, and clothing will not surface, nor will they become a source of stress in the patient's life. More importantly though, the individual's mental health will be cared for, and he will not be socially isolated. If you had a choice between living a healthy lifestyle within an inpatient unit or being extremely ill while living on the streets, which would you choose?

From this perspective, involuntary modes of treatment may apparently become a more rational mode of action. In fact, at present times, the schizophrenia patient has no real sensible reason to refuse treatment. If there were a risk of death associated with the administration of antipsychotic medications, then this issue may require some additional consideration. However, the risk of intolerable side effects has been largely addressed through the creation of atypical and third generation antipsychotics. Moreover, from a rational perspective, the effects of fatigue and weight gain should be more preferable than remaining in a state of psychosis.

Then, if irrationality and social stigma are the only reasons behind the patient's refusal for treatment, how can we solve this specific dilemma? In my mind, the creation of a comprehensive health education program, directed towards children during their elementary school years, could combat the prevalence of social stigmas and intolerance. This program can cover topics like exercise, nutrition, sex education, and the dangers linked to smoking, drug or alcohol use. Equally important though, a mature child should also be educated in the area of major health disorders and their warning signs. Under these circumstances, the recognition of prodromal symptoms and the execution of early intervention techniques could best resolve the problem of treatment noncompliance. Therefore, educating our children on the scientific facts of mental illness could effectively negate any fears related to societal stigmas and negative stereotyping.

The element of irrationality, though, may still remain in the schizophrenia patient. When a patient refuses treatment due to a state of psychosis, should we really grant him the right to be fully autonomous? If the patient poses a physical danger to either himself or another person, then involuntary forms of treatment will be justified. However, patients who are innocent in this respect will still technically pose as a danger to themselves, when they refuse treatment. Quintessentially, the individual's mental health will continue to decline, and he may suffer from permanent cognitive defects as a direct result. Likewise, when a patient becomes increasingly more psychotic, he may lose any and all ability to be self-sufficient. When this occurs, a third party will inevitably be needed to help the patient with his basic needs and survival. At this point, though, responsible forms of social intervention will be overdue. From a logical point of view, third party support for persons with a disability should be delivered during the onset of their illness, and not at a time when it is a final option.

Still, there may be another solution to this social problem. When the schizophrenia patient faces involuntary treatment at an inpatient facility or homelessness, we can provide a third option. The creation of a supported housing plan with trained mental health nurses, as caretakers, may also be viable. This can protect the fundamental principles of freedom and personal autonomy, while concurrently addressing the problem of homelessness. In the creation of this prototype, the mental health care system would not infringe on any of the individual's rights, while simultaneously, it would be addressing the problem of homelessness and promoting the concept of voluntary treatment. This project can include a mental health team and outreach workers who will provide as little or as much medical intervention and outpatient support, according to each patient's volition.

In essence, this model would be an inpatient facility without any aspects of forced treatment or rehabilitation. I believe that this type of service is necessary for patients that suffer from treatment resistant forms of mental illness. Therefore, we should only grant patients the right to refuse treatment if they do not respond to any psychiatric or psychological modes of therapy. By providing these persons with a voluntary inpatient unit, we will be addressing the problem of homelessness among a subgroup of patients, who gain no positive benefits when treated through a professional psychiatric team. Hence, a voluntary inpatient unit should be utilized as a last option to provide social support for persons who cannot be helped in any other manner.

From my perspective, the principles of freedom and personal autonomy serve no greater purpose, when applied to persons with schizophrenia or any other treatable forms of cognitive disturbances. Universally, it may be true that no persons would want to be treated for an illness, without their explicit consent. However, it may also be universally true that every individual would want to be treated for an illness, even when there is only a minute chance for success. If this is true, then restricting the individual's basic right for liberty, under this specific circumstance, may be justified. Human rights were created for the betterment of our civilization. When these rights obstruct our growth and well being, they must be re-examined and dynamically reformed.

Several researchers in Australia agree with my point. Their study compares the average duration of untreated psychosis in patients who lived within two types of jurisdictions. The first jurisdiction permits lawful involuntary modes of treatment, only in patients with a dangerousness criterion. The second jurisdiction has other criteria for involuntary modes of treatment. Their research reveals that the average duration of untreated psychosis in the first jurisdiction was 79 weeks, while the average length of untreated psychosis in the second jurisdiction was only 55 weeks (Large *et al*, 2008). I believe that six months of untreated psychosis can only have a negative, and possibly a permanent detrimental impact on a patient's future prognosis.

Indeed, lower lengths of untreated psychosis have been strongly correlated with a reduction in the course of symptoms, enhanced functioning, and improvements in the patient's prognosis. Contrarily, longer lengths of untreated psychosis have been linked to more severe positive and negative symptoms, and poorer social functioning. In Slovenia, a study comparing patients who were treated during the prodromal phase, and patients who were treated following a year of untreated psychosis was conducted. These researchers found that the latter group experienced more symptoms of greater intensity when compared to the early treatment group. The early treatment group also needed lower dosages of antipsychotics, and they required hospitalized care less frequently. A better outcome was also associated with early antipsychotic treatments, and these patients further differed from the other group in several outcome measures (Novak *et al*, 2008). Consequently, I believe that the schizophrenia patient can never truly benefit when he refuses treatment, and that it will always be in his best interests to be treated, even when no formal consent is given.

The risk of permanent brain damage is a further factor that may be correlated to longer lengths of untreated psychosis. In fact, scientists have observed that the schizophrenia patient's brain is in a state of progressive deterioration. According to recent studies, newer atypical antipsychotics, like olanzapine, can prevent losses of grey matter that typically occurs in schizophrenia (schizophrenia.com, 2008). Other studies conducted on olanzapine reveals that it may attenuate brain damage, and that it has further neuroprotective effects on the human brain (Yulug *et al*, 2006).

Other evidence indicates that a lack of insight may occur following brain damage, within the frontal lobe (Pia and Tamietto, 2006). As a result, the judgment of a schizophrenia patient may gradually diminish as he becomes more ill. This further complicates the problem of ethical health care policies and patient autonomy.

For my final point, I would like to stress the fact that a recovery from an illness like schizophrenia is not the same as a cure for schizophrenia. In fact, my recovery and rehabilitation will be a lifelong process. I will still face many challenges both inherent to and as a consequent of schizophrenia. Equally, a relapse may still be possible at some point in my future. The main challenge, in this respect, is to identify any problematic symptoms, before I lose my grasp and perspective of the real world.

Societal stigmas only complicate our mental health care system. Social intolerance is generally spawned through ignorance, and the inclination to discriminate against a social minority. It can be cured through wisdom and benevolence. Healing comes with understanding. A better life comes with determination.

Bibliography

Abbasian C and Power P (2009). A case of aripiprazole and tardive dyskinesia. *J Psychopharmacol.* 2: 214-215.

Adewuya AO and Makanjuola RO (2008). Lay beliefs regarding causes of mental illness in Nigeria: pattern and correlates. Soc Psychiatry Psychiatr Epidemiol. 43: 336-341.

Afshar H, Roohafza H, Mousavi G, Golchin S, Toghianifar N, Sadeghi M and Talaei M (2009) Topiramate add-on treatment in schizophrenia: a randomised, double-blind, placebo-controlled clinical trial. *J Psychopharmacol.* 23: 157-162.

Agid O, Kapur S and Remington G (2008). Emerging drugs for schizophrenia. *Expert Opin Emerg Drugs.* 13: 479-495.

Agius M, Shah S, Ramkisson R, Murphy S and Zaman R (2007). Three year outcomes of an early intervention for psychosis service as compared with treatment as usual for first psychotic episodes in a standard community mental health team. (Preliminary results). *Psychiatr Danub.*19: 10-19.

Allen JA, Yadav PN and Roth BL (2008). Insights into the regulation of 5-HT2A serotonin receptors by scaffolding proteins and kinases. *Neuropharmacology.* 55: 961-968.

AllPscyhONLINE (2008). www.allpsych.com/disorders/dsm.html.

Altamura AC, Bobo WV and Meltzer HY (2007). Factors affecting outcome in schizophrenia and their relevance for psychopharmacological treatment. *Int Clin Psychopharmacol.* 22: 249-267.

Altamura AC and Goikolea JM (2008). Differential diagnoses and management strategies in patients with schizophrenia and bipolar disorder. *Neuropsychiatr Dis Treat.* 4: 311-317.

Altamura AC, Mundo E, Bassetti R, Green A, Lindenmayer JP, Alphs L and Meltzer HY (2007). Transcultural differences in suicide attempters: analysis on a high-risk population of patients with schizophrenia or schizoaffective disorder. *Schizophr Res.* 89: 140-146.

Alves Fda S, Figee M, Vamelsvoort T, Veltman D and de Haan L (2008). The revised dopamine hypothesis of schizophrenia: evidence from pharmacological MRI studies with atypical antipsychotic medication. *Psychopharmacol Bull.* 41: 121-132.

Angermeyer MC and Matschinger H (2005). Labeling--stereotype--discrimination. An investigation of the stigma process. *Soc Psychiatry Psychiatr Epidemiol.* 40: 391-395.

Anisman H, Du L, Palkovits M, Faludi G, Kovacs GG, Szontagh-Kishazi P, Merali Z and Poulter MO (2008). Serotonin receptor subtype and p11 mRNA expression in stress-relevant brain regions of suicide and control subjects. *J Psychiatry Neurosci.* 33: 131-141.

Arango C, Moreno C, Martínez S, Parellada M, Desco M, Moreno D, Fraguas D, Gogtay N, James A and Rapoport J (2008). Longitudinal brain changes in early-onset psychosis. *Schizophr Bull.* 34: 341-353.

Arnsten AF (2007). Catecholamine and second messenger influences on prefrontal cortical networks of "representational knowledge": a rational bridge between genetics and the symptoms of mental illness. *Cereb Cortex.* 17 Suppl 1: 6-15.

Avram AM, Patel V, Taylor HC, Kirwan JP and Kalhan S (2001). Euglycemic clamp study in clozapine-induced diabetic ketoacidosis. *Ann Pharmacother.* 35: 1381-1387.

Babu GN, Subbakrishna DK and Chandra PS (2008). Prevalence and correlates of suicidality among Indian women with post-partum psychosis in an inpatient setting. *Aust N Z J Psychiatry.* 42: 976-980.

Bak M, Krabbendam L, Delespaul P, Huistra K, Walraven W and van Os J (2008). Executive function does not predict coping with symptoms in stable patients with a diagnosis of schizophrenia. *BMC Psychiatry.* 29: 8-39.

Bär KJ, Boettger MK, Schulz S, Harzendorf C, Agelink MW, Yeragani VK, Chokka P and Voss A (2008). The interaction between pupil function and cardiovascular regulation in patients with acute schizophrenia. *Clin Neurophysiol.* 119:2209-2213.

Barak D and Solomon Z (2005). In the shadow of schizophrenia: a study of siblings' perceptions. *Isr J Psychiatry Relat Sci.* 42: 234-241.

Basar-Eroglu C, Schmiedt-Fehr C, Mathes B, Zimmermann J and Brand A (2009). Are oscillatory brain responses generally reduced in schizophrenia during long sustained attentional processing? *Int J Psychophysiol.* 71: 75-83.

BehaveNet. (2008). www.behavenet.com/capsules/disorders/dsm4classification. htm#Sexual.

Beijer U, Andréasson A, Agren G and Fugelstad A (2007). Mortality, mental disorders and addiction: a 5-year follow-up of 82 homeless men in Stockholm. *Nord J Psychiatry.* 61: 363-368.

Bell JS, Aaltonen SE, Bronstein E, Desplenter FA, Foulon V, Vitola A, Muceniece R, Gharat MS, Volmer D, Airaksinen MS and Chen TF (2008a). Attitudes of pharmacy students toward people with mental disorders, a six country study. *Pharm World Sci.* 30: 595-599.

Bell M, Bryson G and Wexler BE (2003). Cognitive remediation of working memory deficits: durability of training effects in severely impaired and less severely impaired schizophrenia. *Acta Psychiatr Scand.* 108: 101-109.

Bell MD, Bryson GJ, Greig TC, Fiszdon JM and Wexler BE (2005). Neurocognitive enhancement therapy with work therapy: Productivity outcomes at 6- and 12-month follow-ups. *J Rehabil Res Dev.* 42: 829-838.

Bell MD, Zito W, Greig T and Wexler BE (2008b). Neurocognitive enhancement therapy with vocational services: work outcomes at two-year follow-up. *Schizophr Res.* 105: 18-29.

Bernstein HG, Braunewell KH, Spilker C, Danos P, Baumann B, Funke S, Diekmann S, Gundelfinger ED and Bogerts B (2002). Hippocampal expression of the calcium sensor protein visinin-like protein-1 in schizophrenia. *Neuroreport.* 13: 393-396.

Bertelsen M, Jeppesen P, Petersen L, Thorup A, Øhlenschlaeger J, le Quach P, Christensen TØ, Krarup G, Jørgensen P and Nordentoft M (2007). Suicidal behaviour and mortality in first-episode psychosis: the OPUS trial. *Br J Psychiatry Suppl.* 51: 140-146.

Bertelsen M, Jeppesen P, Petersen L, Thorup A, Øhlenschlaeger J, Le Quach P, Østergaard Christensen T, Krarup G, Jørgensen P and Nordentoft M (2009). Course of illness in a sample of 265 patients with first-episode psychosis--five-year follow-up of the Danish OPUS trial. *Schizophr Res.* 107: 173-178.

Bertran-Gonzalez J, Bosch C, Maroteaux M, Matamales M, Hervé D, Valjent E and Girault JA (2008). Opposing patterns of signaling activation in dopamine D1 and D2 receptor-expressing striatal neurons in response to cocaine and haloperidol. *J Neurosci.* 28: 5671-5685.

Betensky JD, Robinson DG, Gunduz-Bruce H, Sevy S, Lencz T, Kane JM, Malhotra AK, Miller R, McCormack J, Bilder RM and Szeszko PR (2008). Patterns of stress in schizophrenia. *Psychiatry Res.* 160: 38-46.

Bhattacharjee J and El-Sayeh HG (2008). Aripiprazole versus typical antipsychotic drugs for schizophrenia. *Cochrane Database Syst Rev.* 3:CD006617.

Bipolar Disorder. (2008). www.bipolar.com/what_is_bipolar/signs_and_symptoms.html.

Birchwood M, Trower P, Brunet K, Gilbert P, Iqbal Z, and Jackson C. (2007). Social anxiety and the shame of psychosis: a study in first episode psychosis. *Behav Res Ther.* 45: 1025-1037.

Biswas P, Malhotra S, Malhotra A and Gupta N (2006). Comparative study of neuropsychological correlates in schizophrenia with onset in childhood, adolescence and adulthood. *Eur Child Adolesc Psychiatry.* 15: 360-366.

Blagrove M, Morgan CJ, Curran HV, Bromley L and Brandner B (2009). The incidence of unpleasant dreams after sub-anaesthetic ketamine. *Psychopharmacology (Berl).* 203: 109-120.

Bob P (2007). Consciousness and co-consciousness, binding problem and schizophrenia. *Neuro Endocrinol Lett.* 28: 723-726.

Bob P, Chladek J, Susta M, Glaslova K, Jagla F and Kukleta M (2007a). Neural chaos and schizophrenia. *Gen Physiol Biophys.* 26: 298-305.

Bob P, Susta M, Chladek J, Glaslova K and Fedor-Freybergh P (2007b). Neural complexity, dissociation and schizophrenia. *Med Sci Monit.* 13: HY1-5.

Bob P, Susta M, Glaslova K, Fedor-Freybergh PG, Pavlat J, Miklosko J and Raboch J (2007c). Dissociation, epileptic-like activity and lateralized electrodermal dysfunction in patients with schizophrenia and depression. *Neuro Endocrinol Lett.* 28: 868-874.

Boks MP, Hoogendoorn M, Jungerius BJ, Bakker SC, Sommer IE, Sinke RJ, Ophoff RA and Kahn RS (2008). Do mood symptoms subdivide the schizophrenia phenotype? Association of the GMP6A gene with a depression subgroup.

Am J Med Genet B Neuropsychiatr Genet. 6: 707-711.

Bonnot O, Tanguy ML, Consoli A, Cornic F, Graindorge C, Laurent C, Tordjman S and Cohen D (2008). Does catatonia influence the phenomenology of childhood onset schizophrenia beyond motor symptoms? *Psychiatry Res.* 158: 356-362.

Bonsack C, Montagrin Y, Favrod J, Gibellini S and Conus P (2007). Motivational interviewing for cannabis users with psychotic disorders. *Encephale.* 33: 819-826.

Bora E, Gökçen S, Kayahan B and Veznedaroglu B (2008). Deficits of social-cognitive and social-perceptual aspects of theory of mind in remitted patients with schizophrenia: effect of residual symptoms. *J Nerv Ment Dis.* 196: 95-99.

Bora E, Gökçen S and Veznedaroglu B (2008). Empathic abilities in people with schizophrenia. *Psychiatry Res.* 160: 23-29.

Bostwick JR, Guthrie SK and Ellingrod VL (2009). Antipsychotic-induced hyperprolactinemia. *Pharmacotherapy.* 29: 64-73.

Botha UA, Koen L and Niehaus DJ (2006). Perceptions of a South African schizophrenia population with regards to community attitudes towards their illness. *Soc Psychiatry Psychiatr Epidemiol.* 41: 619-623.

Bozkurt A, Karlidere T, Isintas M, Ozmenler NK, Ozsahin A and Yanarates O (2007). Acute and maintenance electroconvulsive therapy for treatment of psychotic depression in a pregnant patient. *J ECT.* 23: 185-187.

Briegel W (2007). Deletion and schizophrenia in childhood and adolescence. *Z Kinder Jugendpsychiatr Psychother.* 35: 353-358.

Brown AH, Cohen AN, Chinman MJ, Kessler C and Young AS (2008). EQUIP: Implementing chronic care principles and applying formative evaluation methods to improve care for schizophrenia: QUERI Series. *Implement Sci.* 3: 9.

Brunelin J, d'Amato T, van Os J, Cochet A, Suaud-Chagny MF and Saoud M (2008). Effects of acute metabolic stress on the dopaminergic and pituitary-adrenal axis activity in patients with schizophrenia, their unaffected siblings and controls. *Schizophr Res.* 100: 206-211.

Buckley PF, Correll CU and Miller AL (2007). First-episode psychosis: a window of opportunity for best practices. *CNS Spectr.* 12: 1-16

Buckley PF, Mahadik S, Pillai A and Terry A Jr (2007). Neurotrophins and schizophrenia. *Schizophr Res.* 94: 1-11.

Burkhardt A, Rudorf S, Brand C, Rockstroh B, Studer K, Lettke F and Lüscher K (2007). Ambivalences in the relationship of parents towards their schizophrenic or substance dependent adult child: a comparison to their relationships with healthy siblings and to ordinary parent-child-relationships. *Psychiatr Prax.* 34: 230-238.

Butler AC, Chapman JE, Forman EM and Beck AT (2006). The empirical status of cognitive-behavioral therapy: a review of meta-analyses. *Clin Psychol Rev.* 26: 17-31.

Butler RA and Sheridan JL (2007). Highs and lows: patterns of use, positive and negative effects of benzylpiperazine-containing party pills (BZP-party pills) amongst young people in New Zealand. *Harm Reduct J*. 19: 18.

Buzzle.com (2008). www.buzzle.com/articles/famous-people-with-schizophrenia. html.

Caldwell CB and Gottesman II (1992). Schizophrenia--a high-risk factor for suicide: clues to risk reduction. *Suicide Life Threat Behav*. 22: 479-493.

Callaly T, Dodd S, Goodman D, Asgari Y and Berk M (2008). A descriptive interview with 64 patients discharged from an acute-psychiatric-inpatient service. *J Eval Clin Pract*. 6: 990-995.

Canadian Heritage (2008). www.pch.gc.ca/pgm/pdp-hrp/canada/able_e.cfm.

Canadian Mental Health Association (2008). www.cmha.ca/bins/content_page. asp?cid=3-100.

Caqueo Urízar A and Lemos Giráldez S (2008). Quality of life and family functioning in schizophrenia patients. *Psicothema*. 20: 577-582.

Carnahan RM, Reantaso AA, Teegarden BA and Pogue T (2007). Severe Hyperlipidemia Associated With Olanzapine and Quetiapine Use. *The American Journal of Psychiatry*. 164: 1614-1615.

Carroll LS and Owen MJ (2009). Genetic overlap between autism, schizophrenia and bipolar disorder. *Genome Med*. 1: 102.

Carpenter WT Jr (1996). Maintenance therapy of persons with schizophrenia. *J Clin Psychiatry*. 57: 10-18.

Castro-Fornieles J, Parellada M, Gonzalez-Pinto A, Moreno D, Graell M, Baeza I, Otero S, Soutullo CA, Crespo-Facorro B, Ruiz-Sancho A, Desco M, Rojas-Corrales O, Patiño A, Carrasco-Marin E, Arango C and CAFEPS group (2007). The child and adolescent first-episode psychosis study (CAFEPS): design and baseline results. *Schizophr Res*. 91:226-237.

Castro-Fornieles J, Parellada M, Soutullo CA, Baeza I, Gonzalez-Pinto A, Graell M, Paya B, Moreno D, de la Serna E, and Arango C. (2008). Antipsychotic treatment in child and adolescent first-episode psychosis: a longitudinal naturalistic approach. *J Child Adolesc Psychopharmacol*. 18: 327-336.

Cattapan-Ludewig K, Ludewig S, Messerli N, Vollenweider FX, Seitz A, Feldon J and Paulus MP (2008). Decision-making dysregulation in first-episode schizophrenia. *J Nerv Ment Dis*. 196: 157-160.

Centre for Addiction and Mental Health (2008). www.camh.net/About_Addiction_ Mental_Health/Mental_Health_Information/depression_mhfs.html.

Cervellione KL, Burdick KE, Cottone JG, Rhinewine JP and Kumra S (2007). Neurocognitive deficits in adolescents with schizophrenia: longitudinal stability and predictive utility for short-term functional outcome. *J Am Acad Child Adolesc Psychiatry*. 46: 867-878.

Cervera ES and Seva FA (2006). Pharmacological treatment resistant schizophrenia. *Actas Esp Psiquiatr*. 34: 48-54.

Chabungbam G, Avasthi A and Sharan P (2007). Sociodemographic and clinical factors associated with relapse in schizophrenia. *Psychiatry Clin Neurosci*. 61: 587-593.

Charles H, Manoranjitham SD and Jacob KS (2007). Stigma and explanatory models among people with schizophrenia and their relatives in Vellore, south India. *Int J Soc Psychiatry*. 53: 325-332.

Chee CY, Ng TP and Kua EH (2005). Comparing the stigma of mental illness in a general hospital with a state mental hospital: a Singapore study. *Soc Psychiatry Psychiatr Epidemiol*. 40: 648-653.

Chee KY (2009). Outcome study of first-episode schizophrenia in a developing country: quality of life and antipsychotics. *Soc Psychiatry Psychiatr Epidemiol*. 44: 143-150.

Chiou PN, Chen YS and Lee YC (2006). Characteristics of adolescent suicide attempters admitted to an acute psychiatric ward in Taiwan. *J Chin Med Assoc*. 69: 428-435.

Clouth J (2004). Costs of early retirement--the case of schizophrenia. *Psychiatr Prax*. 31: S238-245.

Collip D, Myin-Germeys I and Van Os J (2008). Does the concept of "sensitization" provide a plausible mechanism for the putative link between the environment and schizophrenia? *Schizophr Bull*. 34: 220-225.

Compton MT, Esterberg ML and Broussard B (2008). Causes of schizophrenia reported by urban African American lay community members. *Compr Psychiatry*. 49: 87-93.

Compton MT, Esterberg ML, McGee R, Kotwicki RJ and Oliva JR (2006). Brief reports: crisis intervention team training: changes in knowledge, attitudes, and stigma related to schizophrenia. *Psychiatr Serv*. 57: 1199-1202.

Conrad R, Schilling G, Najjar D, Geiser F, Sharif M and Liedtke R (2007). Cross-cultural comparison of explanatory models of illness in schizophrenic patients in Jordan and Germany. *Psychol Rep*. 101: 531-546.

Cook S, Chambers E and Coleman JH (2009). Occupational therapy for people with psychotic conditions in community settings: a pilot randomized controlled trial. *Clin Rehabil*. 23: 40-52.

Cooke M, Peters E, Fannon D, Anilkumar AP, Aasen I, Kuipers E and Kumari V (2007). Insight, distress and coping styles in schizophrenia. *Schizophr Res*. 94: 12-22.

Corcoran C, Malaspina D and Hercher L (2005). Prodromal interventions for schizophrenia vulnerability: the risks of being "at risk". *Schizophr Res*. 73: 173-184.

Corcoran C, Perrin M, Harlap S, Deutsch L, Fennig S, Manor O, Nahon D, Kimhy D, Malaspina D and Susser E (2009). Incidence of schizophrenia among second-generation immigrants in the jerusalem perinatal cohort. *Schizophr Bull*. 35: 596-602.

Corrigan PW (2006). Recovery from schizophrenia and the role of evidence-based psychosocial interventions. *Expert Rev Neurother*. 6: 993-1004.

Corrigan PW and Watson AC (2007). The stigma of psychiatric disorders and the gender, ethnicity, and education of the perceiver. *Community Ment Health J*. 43: 439-458.

Corrigan PW, Watson AC and Miller FE (2006). Blame, shame, and contamination: the impact of mental illness and drug dependence stigma on family members.

J Fam Psychol. 20: 239-246.

Coton X, Poly S, Hoyois P, Sophal C and Dubois V (2008). The healthcare-seeking behaviour of schizophrenic patients in Cambodia. *Int J Soc Psychiatry.* 54: 328-337.

Cougnard A, Goumilloux R, Monello F and Verdoux H (2007). Time between schizophrenia onset and first request for disability status in France and associated patient characteristics. *Psychiatr Serv.* 58: 1427-1432.

Cougnard A, Grolleau S, Lamarque F, Beitz C, Brugère S and Verdoux H (2006). Psychotic disorders among homeless subjects attending a psychiatric emergency service. Soc *Psychiatry Psychiatr Epidemiol.* 41: 904-910.

Daughters SB, Sargeant MN, Bornovalova MA, Gratz KL and Lejuez CW (2008). The relationship between distress tolerance and antisocial personality disorder among male inner-city treatment seeking substance users. *J Pers Disord.* 22: 509-524.

Dekker N, de Haan L, Berg S, Gier M, Becker H and Linzen DH (2008). Cessation of cannabis use by patients with recent-onset schizophrenia and related disorders. *Psychopharmacol Bull.* 41: 142-153.

DelBello MP, Versavel M, Ice K, Keller D and Miceli J (2008). Tolerability of oral ziprasidone in children and adolescents with bipolar mania, schizophrenia, or schizoaffective disorder. J *Child Adolesc Psychopharmacol.* 18: 491-499.

De Leo D and Klieve H (2007). Communication of suicide intent by schizophrenic subjects: data from the Queensland Suicide Register. *Int J Ment Health Syst.* 1: 6.

De Leo D and Spathonis K (2003). Do Psychosocial and Pharmacological Interventions Reduce Suicide in Schizophrenia and Schizophrenia Spectrum Disorders? *Archives of Suicide Research.* 7: 353 – 374.

De Luca V, Likhodi O, Kennedy JL and Wong AH (2007). Differential expression and parent-of-origin effect of the 5-HT2A receptor gene C102T polymorphism: analysis of suicidality in schizophrenia and bipolar disorder. *Am J Med Genet B Neuropsychiatr Genet.* 144B: 370-374.

De Luca V, Tharmaligam S, Strauss J and Kennedy JL. (2008). 5-HT2C receptor and MAO-A interaction analysis: no association with suicidal behaviour in bipolar patients. *Eur Arch Psychiatry Clin Neurosci.* 258: 428-433.

Deng X, Sagata N, Takeuchi N, Tanaka M, Ninomiya H, Iwata N, Ozaki N, Shibata H and Fukumaki Y (2008). Association study of polymorphisms in the neutral amino acid transporter genes. SLC1A4, SLC1A5 and the glycine transporter genes SLC6A5, SLC6A9 with schizophrenia. *BMC Psychiatry.* 8: 58.

Department of Justice Canada (2008). http://laws.justice.gc.ca/en/notice/index.ht ml?redirect=%2Fen%2FShowFullDoc%2Fcs%2Fe-5.401%2F%2F%2Fen.

Depression Canada (2008). www.depressioncanada.com.

Diamond RJ (2006). Recovery from a psychiatrist's viewpoint. *Postgrad Med.* Spec No:54-62.

Dickerson F, Brown CH, Fang L, Goldberg RW, Kreyenbuhl J, Wohlheiter K and Dixon L (2008). Quality of life in individuals with serious mental illness and type 2 diabetes. *Psychosomatics.* 49: 109-114.

Dickinson D, Gold JM, Dickerson FB, Medoff D and Dixon LB (2008). Evidence of exacerbated cognitive deficits in schizophrenia patients with comorbid diabetes. *Psychosomatics.* 49: 123-131.

Di Forti M, Lappin JM and Murray RM (2007). Risk factors for schizophrenia--all roads lead to dopamine. *Eur Neuropsychopharmacol.* 17: S101-107.

Disabled World (2008). www.disabled-world.com/artman/publish/famous-schizophrenia.shtml.

Docherty NM, St-Hilaire A, Aakre JM and Seghers JP (2009). Life events and high-trait reactivity together predict psychotic symptom increases in schizophrenia. *Schizophr Bull.* 35: 638-645.

Doey T, Handelman K, Seabrook JA and Steele M (2007). Survey of atypical antipsychotic prescribing by Canadian child psychiatrists and developmental pediatricians for patients aged under 18 years. *Can J Psychiatry.* 52: 363-368.

Donohoe DR, Weeks K, Aamodt EJ and Dwyer DS (2008). Antipsychotic drugs alter neuronal development including ALM neuroblast migration and PLM axonal outgrowth in Caenorhabditis elegans. *Int J Dev Neurosci.* 26: 371-380.

Douaud G, Smith S, Jenkinson M, Behrens T, Johansen-Berg H, Vickers J, James S, Voets N, Watkins K, Matthews PM and James A (2007). Anatomically related grey and white matter abnormalities in adolescent-onset schizophrenia. *Brain.* 130: 2375-2386.

Douglas IJ and Smeeth L (2008). Exposure to antipsychotics and risk of stroke: self controlled case series study. *BMJ.* 337: 1227.

Dracheva S, Patel N, Woo DA, Marcus SM, Siever LJ and Haroutunian V (2008). Increased serotonin 2C receptor mRNA editing: a possible risk factor for suicide. *Mol Psychiatry.* 13: 1001-1010.

Drake RE (2007). Management of substance use disorder in schizophrenia patients: current guidelines. *CNS Spectr.* 12: 27-32.

Drake RE, McHugo GJ, Xie H, Fox M, Packard J and Helmstetter B (2006). Ten-Year Recovery Outcomes for Clients With Co-Occurring Schizophrenia and Substance Use Disorders. *Schizophrenia Bulletin.* 32: 464–473.

Dreher JC, Meyer-Lindenberg A, Kohn P and Berman KF (2008). Age-related changes in midbrain dopaminergic regulation of the human reward system. *Proc Natl Acad Sci USA.* 105: 15106-15111.

Dudova I and Hrdlicka M (2008). Successful use of olanzapine in adolescent monozygotic twins with catatonic schizophrenia resistant to electroconvulsive therapy: case report. *Neuro Endocrinol Lett.* 29: 47-50.

Duran A, Ugur MM, Turan S and Emul M (2008). Clozapine use in two women with schizophrenia during pregnancy. *J Psychopharmacol.* 22: 111-113.

Dwivedi Y, Rizavi HS, Teppen T, Sasaki N, Chen H, Zhang H, Roberts RC, Conley RR and Pandey GN (2007). Aberrant extracellular signal-regulated kinase (ERK) 5 signaling in hippocampus of suicide subjects. *Neuropsychopharmacology.* 32: 2338-2350.

Dwivedi Y, Rizavi HS, Zhang H, Mondal AC, Roberts RC, Conley RR and Pandey GN (2009). Neurotrophin receptor activation and expression in human postmortem brain: effect of suicide. *Biol Psychiatry*. 65: 319-328.

Eack SM, Schooler NR, Ganguli R and Gerard E. Hogarty (2007). (1935--2006): combining science and humanism to improve the care of persons with schizophrenia. *Schizophr Bull*. 33: 1056-1062.

Eating Disorders. (2008). www.mirror-mirror.org/.

Edwards MJ (2007). Hyperthermia in utero due to maternal influenza is an environmental risk factor for schizophrenia. *Congenit Anom (Kyoto)*. 47: 84-89.

emedicinehealth (2008). www.emedicinehealth.com/bipolar_disorder/article_em.htm.

England M (2006). Cognitive intervention for voice hearers. *Issues Ment Health Nurs*. 27: 735-751.

Erler JT and Linding R (2010). Network-based drugs and biomarkers. *J Pathol*. 220: 290-296.

Escamilla M, Lee BD, Ontiveros A, Raventos H, Nicolini H, Mendoza R, Jerez A, Munoz R, Medina R, Figueroa A, Walss-Bass C, Armas R, Contreras S, Ramirez ME and Dassori A (2008). The epsin 4 gene is associated with psychotic disorders in families of Latin American origin. *Schizophr Res*. 106: 253-257.

Euthanasia.com (2008). www.euthanasia.com/page4.html.

Evins AE, Mays VK, Rigotti NA, Tisdale T, Cather C and Goff DC (2001). A pilot trial of bupropion added to cognitive behavioral therapy for smoking cessation in schizophrenia. *Nicotine Tob Res*. 3: 397-403.

Favrod J (2004). For a logic of the psychotic experience. *Rev Med Suisse Romande*. 124:15-18.

Favrod J, Pomini V and Grasset F (2004). Cognitive-behavioral therapy for auditory hallucinations resistant to neuroleptic treatment. *Rev Med Suisse Romande*. 124: 213-216.

Fennig S, Horesh N, Aloni D, Apter A, Weizman A and Fennig S (2005). Life events and suicidality in adolescents with schizophrenia. *Eur Child Adolesc Psychiatry*. 14: 454-460.

Ferrari MC, Kimura L, Nita LM and Elkis H (2006). Structural brain abnormalities in early-onset schizophrenia. *Arq Neuropsiquiatr*. 64: 741-746.

Filakovi P, Degmeci D, Koi E and Beni D. (2007). Ethics of the early intervention in the treatment of schizophrenia. *Psychiatr Danub*. 19: 209-215.

Findling RL, Robb A, Nyilas M, Forbes RA, Jin N, Ivanova S, Marcus R, McQuade RD, Iwamoto T and Carson WH (2008). A multiple-center, randomized, double-blind, placebo-controlled study of oral aripiprazole for treatment of adolescents with schizophrenia. *Am J Psychiatry*. 165: 1432-1441.

Fischer SN, Shinn M, Shrout P and Tsemberis S (2008). Homelessness, mental illness, and criminal activity: examining patterns over time. *Am J Community Psychol*. 42 251-265.

Fisher DJ, Labelle A and Knott VJ (2008). Auditory hallucinations and the mismatch negativity: processing speech and non-speech sounds in schizophrenia. *Int J Psychophysiol.* 70: 3-15.

Fitzgerald PB, Montgomery W, de Castella AR, Filia KM, Filia SL, Christova L, Jackson D and Kulkarni J (2007). Australian Schizophrenia Care and Assessment Programme: real-world schizophrenia: economics. *Aust N Z J Psychiatry.* 41: 819-829.

Fleischhacker WW, Cetkovich-Bakmas M, De Hert M, Hennekens CH, Lambert M, Leucht S, Maj M, McIntyre RS, Naber D, Newcomer JW, Olfson M, Osby U, Sartorius N and Lieberman JA (2008). Comorbid somatic illnesses in patients with severe mental disorders: clinical, policy, and research challenges. *J Clin Psychiatry.* 69: 514-519.

Folsom DP, Hawthorne W, Lindamer L, Gilmer T, Bailey A, Golshan S, Garcia P, Unützer J, Hough R and Jeste DV (2005). Prevalence and risk factors for homelessness and utilization of mental health services among 10,340 patients with serious mental illness in a large public mental health system. *Am J Psychiatry.* 162: 370-376.

Fonseca-Pedrero E, Lemos-Giráldez S, Muñiz J, García-Cueto E and Campillo-Alvarez A (2008). Schizotypy in adolescence: the role of gender and age. *J Nerv Ment Dis.* 196: 161-165.

Forbes NF, Carrick LA, McIntosh AM and Lawrie SM (2009). Working memory in schizophrenia: a meta-analysis. *Psychol Med.* 39: 889-905.

Fornells-Ambrojo M and Garety PA (2005). Bad me paranoia in early psychosis: a relatively rare phenomenon. *Br J Clin Psychol.* 44: 521-528.

Fraguas D, de Castro MJ, Medina O, Parellada M, Moreno D, Graell M, Merchán-Naranjo J and Arango C (2008). Does diagnostic classification of early-onset psychosis change over follow-up? *Child Psychiatry Hum Dev.* 39: 137-145.

Frazier JA, McClellan J, Findling RL, Vitiello B, Anderson R, Zablotsky B, Williams E, McNamara NK, Jackson JA, Ritz L, Hlastala SA, Pierson L, Varley JA, Puglia M, Maloney AE, Ambler D, Hunt-Harrison T, Hamer RM, Noyes N, Lieberman JA and Sikich L (2007). Treatment of early-onset schizophrenia spectrum disorders (TEOSS): demographic and clinical characteristics. *J Am Acad Child Adolesc Psychiatry.* 46: 979-988.

Frémaux T, Reymann JM, Chevreuil C and Bentué-Ferrer D (2007). Prescription of olanzapine in children and adolescent psychiatric patients. *Encephale.* 33: 188-196.

Frueh BC, Grubaugh AL, Cusack KJ and Elhai JD (2009). Disseminating evidence-based practices for adults with PTSD and severe mental illness in public-sector mental health agencies. *Behav Modif.* 33: 66-81.

Fruntes V and Limosin F (2008). Schizophrenia and viral infection during neurodevelopment: a pathogenesis model? *Med Sci Monit.* 14: 71-77.

Fullam RS and Dolan MC (2008). Executive function and in-patient violence in forensic patients with schizophrenia. *Br J Psychiatry.* 193: 247-253.

Funayama M and Mimura M (2008). Memory deficits and confabulation. *Brain Nerve.* 60: 845-853.

Fyfe S, Williams C, Mason OJ and Pickup GJ (2008). Apophenia, theory of mind and schizotypy: perceiving meaning and intentionality in randomness. *Cortex.* 44: 1316-1325.

Gallitano-Mendel A, Wozniak DF, Pehek EA and Milbrandt J (2008). Mice lacking the immediate early gene Egr3 respond to the anti-aggressive effects of clozapine yet are relatively resistant to its sedating effects. *Neurop sychopharmacology.* 33: 1266-1275.

García-Bueno B and Leza JC (2008). Inflammatory/anti-inflammatory mechanisms in the brain following exposure to stress. *Rev Neurol.* 46: 675-683.

Gareri P, De Fazio P, Russo E, Marigliano N, De Fazio S and De Sarro G (2008). The safety of clozapine in the elderly. *Expert Opin Drug Saf.* 7: 525-538.

Gauthier JM and Widart F (2008). Mechanisms of indeterminacy between the imaginary and the rational worlds in schizophrenic subjects. *Encephale.* 34: 376-384.

Gebhardt S, Härtling F, Hanke M, Theisen FM, von Georgi R, Grant P, Mittendorf M, Martin M, Fleischhaker C, Schulz E and Remschmidt H (2008). Relations between movement disorders and psychopathology under predominantly atypical antipsychotic treatment in adolescent patients with schizophrenia. *Eur Child Adolesc Psychiatry.* 17: 44-53.

Geitona M, Kousoulakou H, Ollandezos M, Athanasakis K, Papanicolaou S and Kyriopoulos I (2008). Costs and effects of paliperidone extended release compared with alternative oral antipsychotic agents in patients with schizophrenia in Greece: A cost effectiveness study. *Ann Gen Psychiatry.* 7: 16.

Giersch A, Lalanne L, Corves C, Seubert J, Shi Z, Foucher J and Elliott MA (2009). Extended visual simultaneity thresholds in patients with schizophrenia. *Schizophr Bull.* 35: 816-825.

Gioia D (2005). Career development in schizophrenia: a heuristic framework. *Community Ment Health J.* 41: 307-325.

Girard C and Simard M (2008). Clinical characterization of late- and very late-onset first psychotic episode in psychiatric inpatients. *Am J Geriatr Psychiatry.* 16: 478-487.

Goldman M, Marlow-O'Connor M, Torres I and Carter CS (2008). Diminished plasma oxytocin in schizophrenic patients with neuroendocrine dysfunction and emotional deficits. *Schizophr Res.* 98: 247-455.

Granholm E, McQuaid JR, McClure FS, Link PC, Perivoliotis D, Gottlieb JD, Patterson TL and Jeste DV (2007). Randomized controlled trial of cognitive behavioral social skills training for older people with schizophrenia: 12-month follow-up. *J Clin Psychiatry.* 68: 730-737.

Graves RE, Cassisi JE and Penn DL (2005). Psychophysiological evaluation of stigma towards schizophrenia. *Schizophr Res.* 76: 317-327.

Greenstein DK, Wolfe S, Gochman P, Rapoport JL and Gogtay N (2008). Remission Status and Cortical Thickness in Childhood-Onset Schizophrenia. *J Am Acad Child Adolesc Psychiatry.*47: 1133-1140.

Griffiths KM, Nakane Y, Christensen H, Yoshioka K, Jorm AF and Nakane H

(2006). Stigma in response to mental disorders: a comparison of Australia and Japan. *BMC Psychiatry.* 6: 21.

Grinshpoon A and Ponizovsky AM (2008). The relationships between need profiles, clinical symptoms, functioning and the well-being of inpatients with severe mental disorders. *J Eval Clin Pract.* 14: 218-225.

Groom MJ, Jackson GM, Calton TG, Andrews HK, Bates AT, Liddle PF and Hollis C (2008). Cognitive deficits in early-onset schizophrenia spectrum patients and their non-psychotic siblings: a comparison with ADHD. *Schizophr Res.* 99: 85-95.

Gruber EN, Kajevi M, Agius M and Marti -Biocina S (2006). Group psychotherapy for parents of patients with schizophrenia. *Int J Soc Psychiatry.* 52: 487-500.

Haenschel C, Bittner RA, Haertling F, Rotarska-Jagiela A, Maurer K, Singer W and Linden DE (2007). Contribution of impaired early-stage visual processing to working memory dysfunction in adolescents with schizophrenia: a study with event-related potentials and functional magnetic resonance imaging. *Arch Gen Psychiatry.* 64: 1229-1240.

Hafeez ZH and Kalinowski CM (2007). Somnambulism induced by quetiapine: two case reports and a review of the literature. *CNS Spectr.* 12: 910-912.

Hageman I, Pinborg A and Andersen HS (2008). Complaints of stress in young soldiers strongly predispose to psychiatric morbidity and mortality: Danish national cohort study with 10-year follow-up. *Acta Psychiatr Scand.* 117: 148-155.

Haggard P, Martin F, Taylor-Clarke M, Jeannerod M and Franck N (2003). Awareness of action in schizophrenia. *Neuroreport.* 14: 1081-1085.

Hall MH, Taylor G, Salisbury DF and Levy DL (2010). Sensory gating event-related potentials and oscillations in schizophrenia patients and their unaffected relatives. *Schizophr Bull.* 36: doi: 10.1093/schbul/sbq027

Harms MP, Wang L, Campanella C, Aldridge K, Moffitt AJ, Kuelper J, Ratnanather JT, Miller MI, Barch DM and Csernansky JG (2010). Structural abnormalities in gyri of the prefrontal cortex in individuals with schizophrenia and their unaffected siblings. *Br J Psychiatry.* 196: 150-157.

Hauser M, Lautenschlager M, Gudlowski Y, Ozgürdal S, Witthaus H, Bechdolf A, Bäuml J, Heinz A and Juckel G (2009). Psychoeducation with patients at-risk for schizophrenia--an exploratory pilot study. *Patient Educ Couns.* 76: 138-142.

Hausner H, Wittmann M, Haen E, Hajak G and Spiessl H (2008). Psychopharmacoepidemiology: differences in prescribing strategies in the inpatient and outpatient settings. *Psychiatr Prax.* 35: 337-342.

Health Canada (2008). www.hc-sc.gc.ca/hl-vs/iyh-vsv/diseases-maladies/mental-eng.php.

HealthAtoZ (2008). www.healthatoz.com/healthatoz/Atoz/common/standard/transform.jsp?requestURI=/healthatoz/Atoz/ency/multiple_personality_disorder.jsp.

Hennekens CH (2007). Increasing global burden of cardiovascular disease in general populations and patients with schizophrenia. *J Clin Psychiatry.* 68:

4-7.

Henquet C, Di Forti M, Morrison P, Kuepper R and Murray RM (2008). Gene-environment interplay between cannabis and psychosis. *Schizophr Bull.* 34: 1111-1121.

Henry JD, Bailey PE and Rendell PG (2008). Empathy, social functioning and schizotypy. *Psychiatry Res.* 160:15-22.

Heres S, Hamann J, Mendel R, Wickelmaier F, Pajonk FG, Leucht S and Kissling W (2008). Identifying the profile of optimal candidates for antipsychotic depot therapy A cluster analysis. *Prog Neuropsychopharmacol Biol Psychiatry.* 32: 1987-1993.

Hill MK and Sahhar M (2006). Genetic counselling for psychiatric disorders. *Med J Aust.* 185: 507-510.

Hippisley-Cox J, Vinogradova Y, Coupland C and Parker C (2007). Risk of malignancy in patients with schizophrenia or bipolar disorder: nested case-control study. *Arch Gen Psychiatry.* 64: 1368-1376.

Hofer A, Rettenbacher MA, Widschwendter CG, Kemmler G, Hummer M and Fleischhacker WW (2006). Correlates of subjective and functional outcomes in outpatient clinic attendees with schizophrenia and schizoaffective disorder. *Eur Arch Psychiatry Clin Neurosci.* 256: 246-255.

Holliday EG, Mowry BJ and Nyholt DR (2008). A reanalysis of 409 European-Ancestry and African American schizophrenia pedigrees reveals significant linkage to 8p23.3 with evidence of locus heterogeneity. *Am J Med Genet B Neuropsychiatr Genet.* 147B: 1080-1088.

Holthausen EA, Wiersma D, Cahn W, Kahn RS, Dingemans PM, Schene AH and van den Bosch RJ (2007). Predictive value of cognition for different domains of outcome in recent-onset schizophrenia. *Psychiatry Res.* 149: 71-80.

Hong LE, Summerfelt A, Mitchell BD, McMahon RP, Wonodi I, Buchanan RW and Thaker GK (2008a). Sensory gating endophenotype based on its neural oscillatory pattern and heritability estimate. *Arch Gen Psychiatry.* 65: 1008-1016.

Hong MN, Baek GS, Han YH and Kwon MS (2008b). Effects of weight control program on body weight and the sense of efficacy for control of dietary behavior of psychiatric inpatients. *Taehan Kanho Hakhoe Chi.* 38: 533-540.

Hou SY, Ke CL, Su YC, Lung FW and Huang CJ (2008). Exploring the burden of the primary family caregivers of schizophrenia patients in Taiwan. *Psychiatry Clin Neurosci.* 62: 508-414.

Hrdlicka M and Dudova I (2007). Risperidone in adolescent schizophrenic psychoses: A retrospective study. *International Journal of Psychiatry in Clinical Practice.* 11: 273–278.

Huang XY, Sun FK, Yen WJ and Fu CM (2008). The coping experiences of carers who live with someone who has schizophrenia. *J Clin Nurs.* 17: 817-826.

Hulshoff Pol HE and Kahn RS (2008). What happens after the first episode? A review of progressive brain changes in chronically ill patients with schizophrenia. *Schizophr Bull.* 34: 354-366.

Hwang SW (2005). Fifteen per cent of people treated for mental health disorders are homeless. *Evid Based Ment Health.* 8: 118.

Ikebuchi E (2006). Support of working life of persons with schizophrenia. *Seishin Shinkeigaku Zasshi.* 108: 436-448.

Insel TR and Scolnick EM (2006). Cure therapeutics and strategic prevention: raising the bar for mental health research. *Mol Psychiatry.* 11: 11-17.

IsItBipolar (2008). www.isitbipolar.com/mental-illness/.

Jaeger J, Berns S, Douglas E, Creech B, Glick B and Kane J (2006). Community-based vocational rehabilitation: effectiveness and cost impact of a proposed program model. *Aust N Z J Psychiatry.* 40: 452-461.

Jenkins JH and Carpenter-Song E (2005). The new paradigm of recovery from schizophrenia: cultural conundrums of improvement without cure. *Cult Med Psychiatry.* 29: 379-413.

Jenkins JH, Strauss ME, Carpenter EA, Miller D, Floersch J and Sajatovic M (2005). Subjective experience of recovery from schizophrenia-related disorders and atypical antipsychotics. *Int J Soc Psychiatry.* 51: 211-227.

Jenner JA, Rutten S, Beuckens J, Boonstra N and Sytema S (2008). Positive and useful auditory vocal hallucinations: prevalence, characteristics, attributions, and implications for treatment. *Acta Psychiatr Scand.* 118: 238-245.

Ji X, Takahashi N, Saito S, Ishihara R, Maeno N, Inada T and Ozaki N (2008). Relationship between three serotonin receptor subtypes (HTR3A, HTR2A and HTR4) and treatment-resistant schizophrenia in the Japanese population. *Neurosci Lett.* 435: 95-98.

Johnston PJ, Enticott PG, Mayes AK, Hoy KE, Herring SE and Fitzgerald PB (2008). Symptom Correlates of Static and Dynamic Facial Affect Processing in Schizophrenia: Evidence of a Double Dissociation? *Schizophr Bull.* 36: 680-687 first published online October 26, 2008 doi:10.1093/schbul/sbn136

Jorm AF and Griffiths KM (2008). The public's stigmatizing attitudes towards people with mental disorders: how important are biomedical conceptualizations? *Acta Psychiatr Scand.* 118: 315-321.

Jorm AF, Wright A and Morgan AJ (2007). Where to seek help for a mental disorder? National survey of the beliefs of Australian youth and their parents. *Med J Aust.* 187: 556-560.

Kadri N, Manoudi F, Berrada S and Moussaoui D (2004). Stigma impact on Moroccan families of patients with schizophrenia. *Can J Psychiatry.* 49: 625-629.

Kang DH, Kwon KW, Gu BM, Choi JS, Jang JH and Kwon JS (2008). Structural abnormalities of the right inferior colliculus in schizophrenia. *Psychiatry Res.* 164: 160-165.

Kapur S and Remington G (2001). Atypical antipsychotics: new directions and new challenges in the treatment of schizophrenia. *Annu Rev Med.* 52: 503-517.

Katagai H, Yasui-Furukori N, Kikuchi A and Kaneko S (2007). Effective electroconvulsive therapy in a 92-year-old dementia patient with psychotic feature. *Psychiatry Clin Neurosci.* 61: 568-570.

Kelly BD (2005). Structural violence and schizophrenia. *Soc Sci Med.* 61: 721-

730.

Kelly BD (2008). The power gap: freedom, power and mental illness. *Soc Sci Med.* 63: 2118-2128.

Kendi M, Kendi AT, Lehericy S, Ducros M, Lim KO, Ugurbil K, Schulz SC and White T (2008). Structural and diffusion tensor imaging of the fornix in childhood- and adolescent-onset schizophrenia. *J Am Acad Child Adolesc Psychiatry.* 47: 826-832.

Khisty N, Raval N, Dhadphale M, Kale K and Javadekar A (2008). A prospective study of patients absconding from a general hospital psychiatry unit in a developing country. *J Psychiatr Ment Health Nurs.* 15: 458-464.

Kim DH, Maneen MJ and Stahl SM (2009). Building a better antipsychotic: receptor targets for the treatment of multiple symptom dimensions of schizophrenia. *Neurotherapeutics.* 6: 78-85.

Knittel D, Munn G and Simmer E (2008). Prodromal psychosis as an etiology of suicide: a case report and review of the literature. *Am J Forensic Med Pathol.* 29: 238-241.

Kim YS, Cheon KA, Kim BN, Chang SA, Yoo HJ, Kim JW, Cho SC, Seo DH, Bae MO, So YK, Noh JS, Koh YJ, McBurnett K and Leventhal B (2004). The reliability and validity of kiddie-schedule for affective disorders and schizophrenia-present and lifetime version- Korean version (K-SADS-PL-K). *Yonsei Med J.* 45: 81-89.

Kirby MJL and Keon WJ (2004). Mental Health, Mental Illness and Addiction: Overview of Policies and Programs in Canada. {www.parl.gc.ca/38/1/parlbus/commbus/senate/com-e/soci-e/rep-e/report1/repintnov04vol1table-e.htm.}.

Kircher T, Whitney C, Krings T, Huber W and Weis S (2008). Hippocampal dysfunction during free word association in male patients with schizophrenia. *Schizophr Res.* 101: 242-255.

Kirkpatrick B, Messias E, Harvey PD, Fernandez-Egea E and Bowie CR (2008). Is schizophrenia a syndrome of accelerated aging? *Schizophr Bull.* 34: 1024-1032.

Klingberg S, Schneider S, Wittorf A, Buchkremer G and Wiedemann G (2008). Collaboration in outpatient antipsychotic drug treatment: analysis of potentially influencing factors. *Psychiatry Res.* 161: 225-234.

Knittel D, Munn G and Simmer E (2008). Prodromal psychosis as an etiology of suicide: a case report and review of the literature. *Am J Forensic Med Pathol.* 29: 238-241.

Kooyman I, Dean K, Harvey S and Walsh E (2007). Outcomes of public concern in schizophrenia. *Br J Psychiatry Suppl.* 50: 29-36.

Krebs MO and Mouchet S (2007). Neurological soft signs and schizophrenia: a review of current knowledge. *Rev Neurol (Paris).* 163: 1157-1168.

Kumra S and Schulz CS (2008). Editorial: research progress in early-onset schizophrenia. *Schizophr Bull.* 34: 15-17.

Kumra S, Kranzler H, Gerbino-Rosen G, Kester HM, DeThomas C, Cullen K, Regan J and Kane JM (2008). Clozapine versus "high-dose" olanzapine in refractory early-onset schizophrenia: an open-label extension study. *J Child*

Adolesc Psychopharmacol. 18: 307-316.

Kumra S, Oberstar JV, Sikich L, Findling RL, McClellan JM, Vinogradov S and Charles Schulz S (2008). Efficacy and tolerability of second-generation antipsychotics in children and adolescents with schizophrenia. *Schizophr Bull.* 34: 60-71.

Kunikata H, Mino Y and Nakajima K (2005). Quality of life of schizophrenic patients living in the community: the relationships with personal characteristics, objective indicators and self-esteem. *Psychiatry Clin Neurosci.* 59: 163-169.

Kyriakopoulos M and Frangou S (2007). Pathophysiology of early onset schizophrenia. *Int Rev Psychiatry.* 19: 315-324.

Kyriakopoulos M, Vyas NS, Barker GJ, Chitnis XA and Frangou S (2008). A diffusion tensor imaging study of white matter in early-onset schizophrenia. *Biol Psychiatry.* 63: 519-523.

Lai YM, Hong CPH and Chee CYI (2000). Stigma of mental illness. *Singapore Med J.* 42: 111-114.

Lambe EK, Liu RJ and Aghajanian GK (2007). Schizophrenia, hypocretin (orexin), and the thalamocortical activating system. *Schizophr Bull.* 33: 1284-1290.

Lambert M, Schimmelmann BG, Naber D, Schacht A, Karow A, Wagner T and Czekalla J (2006). Prediction of remission as a combination of symptomatic and functional remission and adequate subjective well-being in 2960 patients with schizophrenia. *J Clin Psychiatry.* 67: 1690-1697.

Large MM, Nielssen O, Ryan CJ and Hayes R (2008). Mental health laws that require dangerousness for involuntary admission may delay the initial treatment of schizophrenia. *Soc Psychiatry Psychiatr Epidemiol.* 43: 251-256.

Lawlor DA, Hart CL, Hole DJ, Gunnell D and Davey Smith G (2007). Body mass index in middle life and future risk of hospital admission for psychoses or depression: findings from the Renfrew/Paisley study. *Psychol Med.* 37: 1151-1161.

Lazaratou H, Anagnostopoulos DC, Alevizos EV, Haviara F and Ploumpidis DN (2007). Parental attitudes and opinions on the use of psychotropic medication in mental disorders of childhood. *Ann Gen Psychiatry.* 6: 32.

Lee BH and Kim YK (2008). Reduced plasma nitric oxide metabolites before and after antipsychotic treatment in patients with schizophrenia compared to controls. *Schizophr Res.* 104: 36-43.

Lee PR, Brady DL, Shapiro RA, Dorsa DM and Koenig JI. (2007). Prenatal stress generates deficits in rat social behavior: Reversal by oxytocin. *Brain Res.* 1156: 152-167.

Lee S, Chiu MY, Tsang A, Chui H and Kleinman A (2006). Stigmatizing experience and structural discrimination associated with the treatment of schizophrenia in Hong Kong. *Soc Sci Med.* 62: 1685-1696.

Lee S, Lee MT, Chiu MY and Kleinman A (2005). Experience of social stigma by people with schizophrenia in Hong Kong. *Br J Psychiatry.* 186: 153-157.

Leucht S, Burkard T, Henderson J, Maj M and Sartorius N (2007). Physical illness and schizophrenia: a review of the literature. *Acta Psychiatr Scand.* 116:

317-333.

Levin T (2006). Schizophrenia should be renamed to help educate patients and the public. *Int J Soc Psychiatry.* 52: 324-331.

Lewis DA, Cho RY, Carter CS, Eklund K, Forster S, Kelly MA and Montrose D (2008). Subunit-selective modulation of GABA type A receptor neurotransmission and cognition in schizophrenia. *Am J Psychiatry.* 165: 1585-1593.

Li J, Ran MS, Hao Y, Zhao Z, Guo Y, Su J and Lu H (2008). Inpatient suicide in a Chinese psychiatric hospital. *Suicide Life Threat Behav.* 38: 449-455.

Lieberman JA (2007). Neuroprotection: a new strategy in the treatment of schizophrenia. Neurobiological basis of neurodegeneration and neuroprotection. *CNS Spectr.* 12: 4-6.

Limosin F, Azorin JM, Krebs MO, Millet B, Glikman J, Camus V, Crocq MA, Costentin J and Daléry J (2008). Present data and treatment schedule of aripiprazole in the treatment of schizophrenia. *Encephale.* 34: 82-92.

Limosin F, Loze JY, Philippe A, Casadebaig F and Rouillon F (2007). Ten-year prospective follow-up study of the mortality by suicide in schizophrenic patients. *Schizophr Res.* 94: 23-28.

Lincoln TM, Arens E, Berger C and Rief W (2008). Can antistigma campaigns be improved? A test of the impact of biogenetic vs psychosocial causal explanations on implicit and explicit attitudes to schizophrenia. *Schizophr Bull.* 34: 984-994.

Lincoln TM, Peter N, Schäfer M and Moritz S (2009). Impact of stress on paranoia: an experimental investigation of moderators and mediators. *Psychol Med.* 39: 1129-1139.

Liu JT (2007). Community integrated services for persons with mental illness. *Hu Li Za Zhi.* 54: 11-17.

Liu KW, Hollis V, Warren S and Williamson DL (2007). Supported-employment program processes and outcomes: experiences of people with schizophrenia. *Am J Occup Ther.* 61: 543-554.

Liu SK, Fitzgerald PB, Daigle M, Chen R and Daskalakis ZJ (2009). The relationship between cortical inhibition, antipsychotic treatment, and the symptoms of schizophrenia. *Biol Psychiatry.* 65: 503-509.

Low LF and Draper B (2009). Hospitalization patterns for psychiatric disorders across the lifespan in Australia from July 1998 to June 2005. *Psychiatr Serv.* 60: 113-116.

Lu W, Mueser KT, Rosenberg SD and Jankowski MK (2008). Correlates of adverse childhood experiences among adults with severe mood disorders. *Psychiatr Serv.* 59: 1018-1026.

Lutz UC, Wiatr G, Orlikowsky T, Gaertner HJ and Bartels M (2008). Olanzapine treatment during breast feeding: a case report. *Ther Drug Monit.* 30: 399-401.

Lysaker PH, Beattie NL, Strasburger AM and Davis LW (2005). Reported history of child sexual abuse in schizophrenia: associations with heightened symptom levels and poorer participation over four months in vocational rehabilitation.

J Nerv Ment Dis. 193: 790-795.

Lysaker PH, Bond G, Davis LW, Bryson GJ and Bell MD (2005). Enhanced cognitive-behavioral therapy for vocational rehabilitation in schizophrenia: Effects on hope and work. *J Rehabil Res Dev.* 42: 673-682.

Lysaker PH, Buck KD, Taylor AC and Roe D (2008). Associations of metacognition and internalized stigma with quantitative assessments of self-experience in narratives of schizophrenia. *Psychiatry Res.* 157: 31-38.

Lysaker PH, Davis LW, Warman DM, Strasburger A and Beattie N (2007). Stigma, social function and symptoms in schizophrenia and schizoaffective disorder: associations across 6 months. *Psychiatry Res.* 149: 89-95.

Lysaker PH and Lysaker JT (2010). Schizophrenia and alterations in self-experience: a comparison of 6 perspectives. *Schizophr Bull.* 36: 331-340.

Lysaker PH, Roe D and Yanos PT (2007). Toward understanding the insight paradox: internalized stigma moderates the association between insight and social functioning, hope, and self-esteem among people with schizophrenia spectrum disorders. *Schizophr Bull.* 33: 192-199.

Lysaker PH, Tsai J, Maulucci AM and Stanghellini G (2008). Narrative accounts of illness in schizophrenia: association of different forms of awareness with neurocognition and social function over time. *Conscious Cogn.* 17: 1143-1151.

Lysaker PH, Tsai J, Yanos P and Roe D (2008). Associations of multiple domains of self-esteem with four dimensions of stigma in schizophrenia. *Schizophr Res.* 98: 194-200.

MacDonald AW 3rd, Thermenos HW, Barch DM and Seidman LJ (2009). Imaging genetic liability to schizophrenia: systematic review of FMRI studies of patients' nonpsychotic relatives. *Schizophr Bull.* 35: 1142-1162.

Magaña SM, Ramírez García JI, Hernández MG and Cortez R (2007). Psychological distress among latino family caregivers of adults with schizophrenia: the roles of burden and stigma. *Psychiatr Serv.* 58: 378-384.

Magnezi R, Zrihen I, Ashkenazi I and Lubin G (2007). The cost of preventing stigma by hospitalizing soldiers in a general hospital instead of a psychiatric hospital. *Mil Med.* 172: 686-689.

Mak WW and Wu CF (2006). Cognitive insight and causal attribution in the development of self-stigma among individuals with schizophrenia. *Psychiatr Serv.* 57: 1800-1802.

Mann JJ, Ellis SP, Waternaux CM, Liu X, Oquendo MA, Malone KM, Brodsky BS, Haas GL and Currier D (2008). Classification trees distinguish suicide attempters in major psychiatric disorders: a model of clinical decision making. *J Clin Psychiatry.* 69: 23-31.

Marcinko D, Pivac N, Martinac M, Jakovljevi M, Mihaljevi -Peles A and Muck-Seler D (2007). Platelet serotonin and serum cholesterol concentrations in suicidal and non-suicidal male patients with a first episode of psychosis. *Psychiatry Res.* 150: 105-108.

Marcinko L and Read M (2004). Cognitive therapy for schizophrenia: treatment and dissemination. *Curr Pharm Des.* 10: 2269-2275.

Martens WH (2001). A review of physical and mental health in homeless persons. *Public Health Rev.* 29: 13-33.

Martin V, Huber M, Rief W and Exner C (2008). Comparative cognitive profiles of obsessive-compulsive disorder and schizophrenia. *Arch Clin Neuropsychol.* 23: 487-500.

Marwaha S and Johnson S (2005). Views and experiences of employment among people with psychosis: a qualitative descriptive study. *Int J Soc Psychiatry.* 51 302-316.

Marwaha S, Johnson S, Bebbington P, Angermeyer MC, Brugha T, Azorin JM, Kilian R, Kornfeld A, Toumi M and EuroSC Study Group (2008). Correlates of subjective quality of life in people with schizophrenia: findings from the EuroSC study. *J Nerv Ment Dis.* 196: 87-94.

Marwaha S, Johnson S, Bebbington P, Stafford M, Angermeyer MC, Brugha T, Azorin JM, Kilian R, Hansen K and Toumi M (2007). Rates and correlates of employment in people with schizophrenia in the UK, France and Germany. *Br J Psychiatry.* 191: 30-37.

Masi G, Mucci M and Pari C (2006).Children with schizophrenia: clinical picture and pharmacological treatment. *CNS Drugs.* 20: 841-866.

Mason P, Rimmer M, Richman A, Garg G, Johnson J and Mottram PG (2008). Middle-ear disease and schizophrenia: case-control study. *Br J Psychiatry.* 193: 192-196.

Mattai AA, Tossell J, Greenstein DK, Addington A, Clasen LS, Gornick MC, Seal J, Inoff-Germain G, Gochman PA, Lenane M, Rapoport JL and Gogtay N (2006). Sleep disturbances in childhood-onset schizophrenia. *Schizophr Res.* 86: 123-129.

MayoClinic.com (2008). www.mayoclinic.com/.

McClellan J, Sikich L, Findling RL, Frazier JA, Vitiello B, Hlastala SA, Williams E, Ambler D, Hunt-Harrison T, Maloney AE, Ritz L, Anderson R, Hamer RM and Lieberman JA (2007). Treatment of early-onset schizophrenia spectrum disorders (TEOSS): rationale, design, and methods. *J Am Acad Child Adolesc Psychiatry.* 46: 969-978.

McEvoy JP (2006). Risks versus benefits of different types of long-acting injectable antipsychotcs. *J Clin Psychiatry.* 67: 15-18.

McEvoy JP, Zigman D and Margolese HC (2010). First and second-generation antipsychotics. *Can J Psychiatry.* 55: 144-149.

McEwen BS (2008). Central effects of stress hormones in health and disease: Understanding the protective and damaging effects of stress and stress mediators. *Eur J Pharmacol.* 583: 174-185.

McEwen BS (2007). Physiology and neurobiology of stress and adaptation: central role of the brain. *Physiol Rev.* 87: 873-904.

McGirr A and Turecki G (2008). What is specific to suicide in schizophrenia disorder? Demographic, clinical and behavioural dimensions. *Schizophr Res.* 98: 217-224.

McHugo GJ, Bebout RR, Harris M, Cleghorn S, Herring G, Xie H, Becker D and Drake RE (2004). A randomized controlled trial of integrated versus parallel housing services for homeless adults with severe mental illness. *Schizophr Bull*. 30: 969-982.

McKibbin CL, Twamley E, Patterson TL, Golshan S, Lebowitz B, Feiner L, Shepherd S and Jeste DV (2008). Perceived participation restriction in middle-aged and older persons with schizophrenia. *Am J Geriatr Psychiatry*. 16: 777-780.

McNeil TF, Schubert EW, Cantor-Graae E, Brossner M, Schubert P and Henriksson KM (2009). Unwanted pregnancy as a risk factor for offspring schizophrenia-spectrum and affective disorders in adulthood: a prospective high-risk study. *Psychol Med*. 39: 957-965.

Meadahl M (2009). Brain development. aq. *Simon Fraser University*. 14-17.

MedicineNet.com (2008). www.medicinenet.com/dissociative_identity_disorder/article.htm.

MedlinePlus (2008). www.nlm.nih.gov/medlineplus/ency/article/001523.htm.

Medscape Today (2008). www.medscape.com/viewarticle/417700_4.

Mehler-Wex C, Duvigneau JC, Hartl RT, Ben-Shachar D, Warnke A and Gerlach M (2006). Increased mRNA levels of the mitochondrial complex I 75-kDa subunit. A potential peripheral marker of early onset schizophrenia? *Eur Child Adolesc Psychiatry*. 15: 504-507.

Melamed S, Shalit-Kenig D, Gelkopf M, Lerner A and Kodesh A. (2004). Mental homelessness:locked within, locked without. *Soc Work Health Care*. 39: 209-223.

Melle I, Friis S, Hauff E and Vaglum P (2000). Social functioning of patients with schizophrenia in high-income welfare societies. *Psychiatr Serv*. 51: 223-228.

Melle I, Larsen TK, Haahr U, Friis S, Johannesen JO, Opjordsmoen S, Rund BR, Simonsen E, Vaglum P and McGlashan T (2008). Prevention of negative symptom psychopathologies in first-episode schizophrenia: two-year effects of reducing the duration of untreated psychosis. *Arch Gen Psychiatry*. 65: 634-640.

Meltzer HY (1992). Treatment of the neuroleptic-nonresponsive schizophrenic patient. *Schizophr Bull*. 18: 515-542.

Mental Health Sanctuary (2008). www.mhsanctuary.com/gender/dsm.htm.

Mental Illness Awareness Week (2008). http://www.miaw-ssmm.ca/en/about/what-is-mental-illness.aspx.

Merck. (2008). www.merck.com/mmhe/sec07/ch106/ch106d.html.

Merriam-Webster. (2008). www.merriam-webster.com/dictionary/euthanasia.

MH.com (2008).

Miettunen J, Törmänen S, Murray GK, Jones PB, Mäki P, Ebeling H, Moilanen I, Taanila A, Heinimaa M, Joukamaa M and Veijola J (2008). Association of cannabis use with prodromal symptoms of psychosis in adolescence. *Br J Psychiatry*. 192: 470-471.

Milders M, Ietswaart M, Crawford JR and Currie D (2008). Social behavior following traumatic brain injury and its association with emotion recognition, understanding of intentions, and cognitive flexibility. *J Int Neuropsychol*

Soc. 14: 318-326.

Mittendorfer-Rutz E, Rasmussen F and Wasserman D (2008). Familial clustering of suicidal behaviour and psychopathology in young suicide attempters. A register-based nested case control study. *Soc Psychiatry Psychiatr Epidemiol.* 43: 28-36.

Mood Disorders Society of Canada (2008). www.mooddisorderscanada.ca/quickfacts/index.htm.

Morrens M, Hulstijn W, Lewi P and Sabbe B (2008). Bleuler revisited: psychomotor slowing in schizophrenia as part of a catatonic symptom cluster. *Psychiatry Res.* 161: 121-125.

Mueser KT, Crocker AG, Frisman LB, Drake RE, Covell NH and Essock SM (2006). Conduct disorder and antisocial personality disorder in persons with severe psychiatric and substance use disorders. *Schizophr Bull.* 32: 626-636.

Munk-Olsen T, Laursen TM, Videbech P, Rosenberg R and Mortensen PB (2006). Electroconvulsive therapy: predictors and trends in utilization from 1976 to 2000. *J ECT.* 22: 127-132.

Murphy KC (2002). Schizophrenia and velo-cardio-facial syndrome. *Lancet.* 359: 426-430.

Mymentalhealth.ca (2008). www.mymentalhealth.ca/Home/Learn/TypesofMentalIllness/Schizophrenia/tabid/864/Default.aspx.

Naber D (2008). Subjective effects of antipsychotic drugs and their relevance for compliance and remission. *Epidemiol Psichiatr Soc.* 17: 174-176.

Naeem F, Ayub M, Javed Z, Irfan M, Haral F and Kingdon D (2006). Stigma and psychiatric illness. A survey of attitude of medical students and doctors in Lahore, Pakistan. *J Ayub Med Coll Abbottabad.* 18: 46-49.

National Institute of Mental Health (2008). www.nimh.nih.gov/health/topics/schizophrenia/index.shtml.

Nelson B and Sass LA (2008). The phenomenology of the psychotic break and Huxley's trip: substance use and the onset of psychosis. *Psychopathology.* 41: 346-355.

Neuhaus AH, Luborzewski A, Opgen-Rhein C, Jockers-Scherübl MC and Neu P (2007). Electroconvulsive monotherapy in confusion psychosis: a potential standard regimen? *Pharmacopsychiatry.* 40: 170-171.

Niehaus DJ, Koen L, Galal U, Dhansay K, Oosthuizen PP, Emsley RA and Jordaan E (2008). Crisis discharges and readmission risk in acute psychiatric male inpatients. *BMC Psychiatry.* 8: 44.

Nobelprize.org (2008).

Nordt C, Müller B, Rössler W and Lauber C (2007). Predictors and course of vocational status, income, and quality of life in people with severe mental illness: a naturalistic study. *Soc Sci Med.* 65: 1420-1429.

Novak Sarotar B, Pesek MB, Agius M and Kocmur M (2008). Duration of untreated psychosis and it's effect on the symptomatic recovery in schizophrenia - preliminary results. *Neuro Endocrinol Lett.* 29: 990-994.

Nyamathi A, Nahid P, Berg J, Burrage J, Christiani A, Aqtash S, Morisky D and Leake B (2008). Efficacy of nurse case-managed intervention for latent tuberculosis among homeless subsamples. *Nurs Res*. 57: 33-39.

Olfson M, Mechanic D, Hansell S, Boyer CA, Walkup J and Weiden PJ (2000). Predicting medication noncompliance after hospital discharge among patients with schizophrenia. *Psychiatr Serv*. 51: 216-222.

Onat A, Ozhan H, Esen AM, Albayrak S, Karabulut A, Can G and Hergenç G (2007). Prospective epidemiologic evidence of a "protective" effect of smoking on metabolic syndrome and diabetes among Turkish women-- without associated overall health benefit. *Atherosclerosis*. 193: 380-388.

Opler LA, White L, Caton CL, Dominguez B, Hirshfield S and Shrout PE (2001). Gender differences in the relationship of homelessness to symptom severity, substance abuse, and neuroleptic noncompliance in schizophrenia. *J Nerv Ment Dis*. 189: 449-456.

Oral ET (2007). Stigmatization in the long-term treatment of psychotic disorders. *Neuro Endocrinol Lett*. 28: 35-45.

Oyebode F (2008). The neurology of psychosis. *Med Princ Pract*. 17: 263-269.

Paccaloni M, Pozzan T and Zimmermann C (2004). Being informed and involved in treatment: what do psychiatric patients think? A review. *Epidemiol Psichiatr Soc*. 13: 270-283.

Peled A. (2006). Brain profiling and clinical-neuroscience. *Med Hypotheses*. 67: 941-916.

Perron H, Mekaoui L, Bernard C, Veas F, Stefas I and Leboyer M (2008). Endogenous retrovirus type W GAG and envelope protein antigenemia in serum of schizophrenic patients. *Biol Psychiatry*. 64: 1019-1023.

Petersen L, Thorup A, Øqhlenschlaeger J, Christensen TØ, Jeppesen P, Krarup G, Jørrgensen P, Mortensen EL and Nordentoft M (2008). Predictors of remission and recovery in a first-episode schizophrenia spectrum disorder sample: 2-year follow-up of the OPUS trial. *Can J Psychiatry*. 53: 660-670.

Phillips LK and Seidman LJ (2008). Emotion processing in persons at risk for schizophrenia. *Schizophr Bull*. 34: 888-903.

Pia L and Tamietto M (2006). Unawareness in schizophrenia: neuropsychological and neuroanatomical findings. *Psychiatry Clin Neurosci*. 60: 531-537.

Pirkola S, Sohlman B, Heilä H and Wahlbeck K (2007). Reductions in postdischarge suicide after deinstitutionalization and decentralization: a nationwide register study in Finland. *Psychiatr Serv*. 58: 221-226.

Pomarol-Clotet E, Salvador R, Sarró S, Gomar J, Vila F, Martínez A, Guerrero A, Ortiz-Gil J, Sans-Sansa B, Capdevila A, Cebamanos JM and McKenna PJ (2008). Failure to deactivate in the prefrontal cortex in schizophrenia: dysfunction of the default mode network? *Psychol Med*. 38: 1185-1193.

Pompili M, Amador XF, Girardi P, Harkavy-Friedman J, Harrow M, Kaplan K, Krausz M, Lester D, Meltzer HY, Modestin J, Montross LP, Mortensen PB, Munk-Jørgensen P, Nielsen J, Nordentoft M, Saarinen PI, Zisook S, Wilson ST and Tatarelli R (2007). Suicide risk in schizophrenia: learning from the past to change the future. *Ann Gen Psychiatry*. 6: 10.

Pompili M, Lester D, Innamorati M, Tatarelli R and Girardi P (2008). Assessment and treatment of suicide risk in schizophrenia. *Expert Rev Neurother*. 8:

51-74.

Postrado LT and Lehman AF (1995). Quality of life and clinical predictors of rehospitalization of persons with severe mental illness. *Psychiatr Serv.* 46: 1161-1165.

Pradhan BK, Chakrabarti S, Nehra R and Mankotia A (2008). Cognitive functions in bipolar affective disorder and schizophrenia: comparison. *Psychiatry Clin Neurosci.* 62: 515-525.

Prasad KM, Sanders R, Sweeney J, Montrose D, Diwadkar V, Dworakowski D, Miewald J and Keshavan M (2009). Neurological abnormalities among offspring of persons with schizophrenia: relation to premorbid psychopathology. *Schizophr Res.* 108: 163-169.

Prasad SE, Howley S and Murphy KC (2008). Candidate genes and the behavioral phenotype in 22q11.2 deletion syndrome. *Dev Disabil Res Rev.* 14: 26-34.

Prince M, Patel V, Saxena S, Maj M, Maselko J, Phillips MR and Rahman A (2007). No health without mental health. *Lancet.* 370: 859-877.

Prouteau A and Doron J (2008). Cognitive predictors of the community functioning dimensions in schizophrenia: state of the art and future directions. *Encephale.* 34: 360-368.

psychiatryonline (2008). www.psychiatryonline.com/resourceTOC. aspx?resourceID=1.

PsychNet-UK (2008). www.psychnet-uk.com/dsm_iv/dissociative_identity_disorder.htm.

Psychology Today (2008). www.psychologytoday.com/conditions/did.html.

PSYweb.com (2008). psyweb.com/Mdisord/DSM_IV/jsp/dsm_iv.jsp.

Public Health Agency of Canada (2008). www.phac-aspc.gc.ca/publicat/miic-mmac/index-eng.php.

R dulescu AR and Mujica-Parodi LR (2008). A systems approach to prefrontal-limbic dysregulation in schizophrenia. *Neuropsychobiology.* 57: 206-216.

Rajarethinam R, Upadhyaya A, Tsou P and Upadhyaya M (2007). Caudate volume in offspring of patients with schizophrenia. *The British Journal of Psychiatry.* 191: 258-259.

Rajarethinam RP, DeQuardo JR, Nalepa R and Tandon R (2000). Superior temporal gyrus in schizophrenia: a volumetric magnetic resonance imaging study. *Schizophr Res.* 41: 303-312.

Ran MS, Chan CL, Chen EY, Xiang MZ, Caine ED and Conwell Y (2006). Homelessness among patients with schizophrenia in rural China: a 10-year cohort study. *Acta Psychiatr Scand.* 114: 118-123.

Rassovsky Y, Horan WP, Lee J, Sergi MJ and Green MF (2010). Pathways between early visual processing and functional outcome in schizophrenia. *Psychol Med.* May 19: 1-11.

Redlich AD (2004). Law & Psychiatry: Mental illness, police interrogations, and the potential for false confession. *Psychiatr Serv* 55: 19-21.

Redlich AD, Steadman HJ, Robbins PC and Swanson JW (2006). Use of the criminal justice system to leverage mental health treatment: effects on treatment adherence and satisfaction. *J Am Acad Psychiatry Law.* 34: 292-

299.

Remington G, Kwon J, Collins A, Laporte D, Mann S and Christensen B. (2007). The use of electronic monitoring (MEMS) to evaluate antipsychotic compliance in outpatients with schizophrenia. *Schizophr Res*. 90: 229-237.

Remschmidt H, Martin M, Fleischhaker C, Theisen FM, Hennighausen K, Gutenbrunner C and Schulz E (2007). Forty-two-years later: the outcome of childhood-onset schizophrenia. *J Neural Transm*. 114: 505-512.

Ricciardi A, McAllister V and Dazzan P (2008). Is early intervention in psychosis effective? *Epidemiol Psichiatr Soc*. 17: 227-235.

Richter D, Eikelmann B and Reker T (2006). Work, income, intimate relationships: social exclusion of the mentally ill. *Gesundheitswesen*. 68: 704-707.

Ringen PA, Melle I, Birkenaes AB, Engh JA, Faerden A, Vaskinn A, Friis S, Opjordsmoen S and Andreassen OA (2008). The level of illicit drug use is related to symptoms and premorbid functioning in severe mental illness. *Acta Psychiatr Scand*. 118: 297-304.

Ritsner MS, Ratner Y, Gibel A and Weizman R (2007). Positive family history is associated with persistent elevated emotional distress in schizophrenia: evidence from a 16-month follow-up study. *Psychiatry Res*. 153: 217-223.

Rosen A (2007). Return from the vanishing point: a clinician's perspective on art and mental illness, and particularly schizophrenia. *Epidemiol Psichiatr Soc*. 16: 126-132.

Rosenberg SD, Lu W, Mueser KT, Jankowski MK and Cournos F (2007). Correlates of adverse childhood events among adults with schizophrenia spectrum disorders. *Psychiatr Serv*.58: 245-253.

Rosenheck R, Leslie D, Keefe R, McEvoy J, Swartz M, Perkins D, Stroup S, Hsiao JK, Lieberman J and CATIE Study Investigators Group (2006). Barriers to employment for people with schizophrenia. *Am J Psychiatry*. 163: 411-147.

Ross RG, Heinlein S, Zerbe GO and Radant A (2005). Saccadic eye movement task identifies cognitive deficits in children with schizophrenia, but not in unaffected child relatives. *J Child Psychol Psychiatry*. 46: 1354-1362.

Roy MA, Mérette C and Maziade M (2001). Subtyping schizophrenia according to outcome or severity: a search for homogeneous subgroups. *Schizophr Bull*. 27: 115-38.

Sajatovic M and Jenkins JH (2007). Is antipsychotic medication stigmatizing for people with mental illness? *Int Rev Psychiatry*. 19: 107-112.

Salkever D, Slade E and Karakus M (2006). Differential effects of atypical versus typical antipsychotic medication on earnings of schizophrenia patients : estimates from a prospective naturalistic study. *Pharmacoeconomics*. 24: 123-139.

Salkever DS, Karakus MC, Slade EP, Harding CM, Hough RL, Rosenheck RA, Swartz MS, Barrio C and Yamada AM (2007). Measures and predictors of community-based employment and earnings of persons with schizophrenia in a multisite study. *Psychiatr Serv*. 58: 315-324.

Saravanan B, Jacob KS, Deepak MG, Prince M, David AS and Bhugra D (2008). Perceptions about psychosis and psychiatric services: a qualitative study from Vellore, India. *Soc Psychiatry Psychiatr Epidemiol.* 43: 231-238.

Sato M (2006). Renaming schizophrenia: a Japanese perspective. *World Psychiatry.* 5: 53-55.

Scheepers-Hoeks AM, Wessels-Basten SJ, Scherders MJ, Bravenboer B, Loonen AJ, Kleppe RT and Grouls RJ (2008). Schizophrenia and antipsychotics associated with the metabolic syndrome. An overview. *Tijdschr Psychiatr.* 50: 645-654.

schizophrenia.com (2008). www.schizophrenia.com/szfacts.htm.

Schomerus G, Heider D, Angermeyer MC, Bebbington PE, Azorin JM, Brugha T and Toumi M (2008). Urban residence, victimhood and the appraisal of personal safety in people with schizophrenia: results from the European Schizophrenia Cohort (EuroSC). *Psychol Med.* 38: 591-597.

Schomerus G, Heider D, Angermeyer MC, Bebbington PE, Azorin JM, Brugha T, Toumi M and European Schizophrenia Cohort (2007a). Residential area and social contacts in schizophrenia. Results from the European Schizophrenia Cohort (EuroSC). *Soc Psychiatry Psychiatr Epidemiol.* 42: 617-622.

Schomerus G, Kenzin D, Borsche J, Matschinger H and Angermeyer MC (2007b). The association of schizophrenia with split personality is not an ubiquitous phenomenon: results from population studies in Russia and Germany. *Soc Psychiatry Psychiatr Epidemiol.* 42: 780-786.

Schooler N, Rabinowitz J, Davidson M, Emsley R, Harvey PD, Kopala L, McGorry PD, Van Hove I, Eerdekens M, Swyzen W, De Smedt G and Early Psychosis Global Working Group. (2005). Risperidone and haloperidol in first-episode psychosis: a long-term randomized trial. *Am J Psychiatry.* 162: 947-953.

Schooler NR (2006). Relapse prevention and recovery in the treatment of schizophrenia. *J Clin Psychiatry.* 67: 19-23.

Schultze-Lutter F, Ruhrmann S and Klosterkötter J (2009). Early detection of psychosis - establishing a service for persons at risk. *Eur Psychiatry.* 24: 1-10.

Schwartz-Stav O, Apter A and Zalsman G (2006). Depression, suicidal behavior and insight in adolescents with schizophrenia. *Eur Child Adolesc Psychiatry.* 15: 352-359.

Seeman MV (2007). Symptoms of schizophrenia: normal adaptations to inability. *Med Hypotheses.* 69: 253-257.

Serper M and Berenbaum H (2008). The relation between emotional awareness and hallucinations and delusions in acute psychiatric inpatients. *Schizophr Res.* 101: 195-200.

Shaner A, Miller G and Mintz J (2007). Evidence of a latitudinal gradient in the age at onset of schizophrenia. *Schizophr Res.* 94: 58-63.

Shimizu E, Imai M, Fujisaki M, Shinoda N, Handa S, Watanabe H, Nakazato M, Hashimoto K and Iyo M (2006). Maintenance electroconvulsive therapy (ECT) for treatment-resistant disorganized schizophrenia. *Prog Neuropsychopharmacol Biol Psychiatry.* 31: 571-573.

Shoval G, Sever J, Sher L, Diller R, Apter A, Weizman A and Zalsman G (2006). Substance use, suicidality, and adolescent-onset schizophrenia: an Israeli

10-year retrospective study. *J Child Adolesc Psychopharmacol.* 16: 767-775.

Smith M, Hopkins D, Peveler RC, Holt RI, Woodward M and Ismail K (2008). First-v. second-generation antipsychotics and risk for diabetes in schizophrenia: systematic review and meta-analysis. *Br J Psychiatry.* 192: 406-411.

Sodhi M, Wood KH and Meador-Woodruff J (2008). Role of glutamate in schizophrenia: integrating excitatory avenues of research. *Expert Rev Neurother.* 8: 1389-1406.

Spence W, Mulholland C, Lynch G, McHugh S, Dempster M and Shannon C (2006). Rates of childhood trauma in a sample of patients with schizophrenia as compared with a sample of patients with non-psychotic psychiatric diagnoses. *J Trauma Dissociation.* 7: 7-22.

Spitzer C, Vogel M, Barnow S, Freyberger HJ and Grabe HJ (2007). Psychopathology and alexithymia in severe mental illness: the impact of trauma and posttraumatic stress symptoms. *Eur Arch Psychiatry Clin Neurosci.* 257: 191-196.

Srinivasan L and Tirupati S (2005). Relationship between cognition and work functioning among patients with schizophrenia in an urban area of India. *Psychiatr Serv.* 56: 1423-1428.

Stanford University (2008). http://plato.stanford.edu/entries/affirmative-action/#2.

Stargardt T, Weinbrenner S, Busse R, Juckel G and Gericke CA (2008). Effectiveness and cost of atypical versus typical antipsychotic treatment for schizophrenia in routine care. *J Ment Health Policy Econ.* 11: 89-97.

Startup M, Startup S and Sedgman A (2008). Immediate source-monitoring, self-focused attention and the positive symptoms of schizophrenia. *Behav Res Ther.* 46: 1176-1180.

Statistics Canada (2008). www.statcan.gc.ca/pub/89-628-x/2008007/c-g/5201147-eng.htm.

Steinberg L (2008). A social neuroscience perspective on adolescent risk-taking. *Dev Rev.* 28: 78-106.

Steinberg ML, Williams JM, Steinberg HR, Krejci JA and Ziedonis DM (2005). Applicability of the Fagerström Test for Nicotine Dependence in smokers with schizophrenia. *Addict Behav.* 30: 49-59.

Steinert T, Bergbauer G, Schmid P and Gebhardt RP (2007). Seclusion and restraint in patients with schizophrenia: clinical and biographical correlates. *J Nerv Ment Dis.* 195: 492-496.

Stratta P, Riccardi I, Daneluzzo E, Tempesta D, Stzuglia F, Tomassini A and Rossi A (2007). Does premorbid IQ have a pathoplastic effect on symptom presentation in schizophrenic and bipolar disorders? *Encephale.* 33: 733-737.

Suzuki K, Awata S, Takano T, Ebina Y, Takamatsu K, Kajiwara T, Ito K, Shindo T, Funakoshi S and Matsuoka H (2006). Improvement of psychiatric symptoms after electroconvulsive therapy in young adults with intractable first-episode schizophrenia and schizophreniform disorder. *Tohoku J Exp Med.* 210: 213-220.

Suzuki K, Shindo T, Katsura M, Takamatsu K, Ebina Y, Takano T, Awata S and Matsuoka H (2007). Resolution of catatonia by successful seizure induction via electroconvulsive therapy with electrodes applied bilaterally to the parietotemporal region. *J ECT*. 23: 103-105.

Suzuki K, Takano T, Ebina Y, Takamatsu K, Awata S and Matsuoka H (2007). Continuation electroconvulsive therapy to prevent relapse of schizophrenia in relapse-prone patients. *J ECT*. 23: 204-205.

Szubert S, Florkowski A and Bobi ska K (2008). Impact of stress on plasticity of brain structures and development of chosen psychiatric disorders. *Pol Merkur Lekarski*. 24: 162-165.

Tang YL, Gillespie CF, Epstein MP, Mao PX, Jiang F, Chen Q, Cai ZJ and Mitchell PB (2007). Gender differences in 542 Chinese inpatients with schizophrenia. *Schizophr Res*. 97: 88-96.

Tao FB, Xu ML, Kim SD, Sun Y, Su PY and Huang K (2007). Physical activity might not be the protective factor for health risk behaviours and psychopathological symptoms in adolescents. *J Paediatr Child Health*. 43: 762-767.

Taylor PJ (2008). Psychosis and violence: stories, fears, and reality. *Can J Psychiatry*. 53: 647-659.

Taylor S (2007). Electroconvulsive therapy: a review of history, patient selection, technique, and medication management. *South Med J*. 100: 494-498.

Terzian AC, Andreoli SB, de Oliveira LM, de Jesus Mari J and McGrath J (2007). A cross-sectional study to investigate current social adjustment of offspring of patients with schizophrenia. *Eur Arch Psychiatry Clin Neurosci*. 257: 230-236.

Thewissen V, Bentall RP, Lecomte T, van Os J and Myin-Germeys I (2008). Fluctuations in self-esteem and paranoia in the context of daily life. *J Abnorm Psychol*. 117: 143-153.

Tirapu-Ustárroz J and Muñoz-Céspedes JM (2005). Memory and the executive functions. *Rev Neurol*. 41: 475-484.

Thomas LE and Woods SW (2006). The schizophrenia prodrome: a developmentally informed review and update for psychopharmacologic treatment. *Child Adolesc Psychiatr Clin N Am*. 15: 109-133.

Thorup A, Petersen L, Jeppesen P, Ohlenschlaeger J, Christensen T, Krarup G, Jorgensen P and Nordentoft M (2007). Gender differences in young adults with first-episode schizophrenia spectrum disorders at baseline in the Danish OPUS study. *J Nerv Ment Dis*. 195: 396-405.

Torchalla I, Albrecht F, Buchkremer G and Längle G (2004). Homeless women with psychiatric disorders -- a field study. *Psychiatr Prax*. 31: 228-235.

Torrey EF. Surviving Schizophrenia: A manual for families consumers and providers. 3rd ed.. HarperCollins Publishers, London. 1995.

Trémeau F, Antonius D, Cacioppo JT, Ziwich R, Jalbrzikowski M, Saccente E, Silipo G, Butler P and Javitt D (2009). In support of Bleuler: objective evidence for increased affective ambivalence in schizophrenia based upon evocative testing. *Schizophr Res*. 107: 223-231.

Tsuang J and Fong TW (2004). Treatment of patients with schizophrenia and substance abuse disorders. *Curr Pharm Des*. 10 2249-2261.

van Haren NE, Cahn W, Hulshoff Pol HE and Kahn RS (2008). Schizophrenia as a progressive brain disease. *Eur Psychiatry*. 23: 245-254.

van Haren NE, Hulshoff Pol HE, Schnack HG, Cahn W, Mandl RC, Collins DL, Evans AC and Kahn RS (2007). Focal gray matter changes in schizophrenia across the course of the illness: a 5-year follow-up study. *Neuropsychopharmacology*. 32: 2057-2066.

Vance A, Hall N, Casey M, Karsz F and Bellgrove MA (2007). Visuospatial memory deficits in adolescent onset schizophrenia. *Schizophr Res*. 93: 345-349.

Vaskinn A, Sundet K, Friis S, Simonsen C, Birkenaes AB, Jónsdóttir H, Ringen PA and Andreassen OA (2008). Emotion perception and learning potential: mediators between neurocognition and social problem-solving in schizophrenia? *J Int Neuropsychol Soc*. 14: 279-288.

Ventegodt S, Kandel I and Merrick J (2008). Clinical holistic medicine: avoiding the Freudian trap of sexual transference and counter transference in psychodynamic therapy. *Scientific World Journal*. 8: 371-383.

Ventegodt S, Kandel I and Merrick J (2007). First do no harm: an analysis of the risk aspects and side effects of clinical holistic medicine compared with standard psychiatric biomedical treatment. *ScientificWorld Journal*. 7: 1810-1820.

Veronese A, Vivenza V, Nosè M, Cipriani A, Tansella M and Barbui C (2008). Understanding antipsychotic non-classical prescriptions: a quantitative and qualitative approach. *Epidemiol Psichiatr Soc*. 17: 236-241.

Vickar GM, North CS, Downs D and Marshall DL (2009). A randomized controlled trial of a private-sector inpatient-initiated psychoeducation program for schizophrenia. *Psychiatr Serv*. 60: 117-120.

Vitiello B (2009). Combined cognitive-behavioural therapy and pharmacotherapy for adolescent depression: Does it improve outcomes compared with monotherapy? *CNS Drugs*. 23: 271-280.

Volkow ND, Wang GJ, Telang F, Fowler JS, Goldstein RZ, Alia-Klein N, Logan J, Wong C, Thanos PK, Ma Y and Pradhan K (2009). Inverse association between BMI and prefrontal metabolic activity in healthy adults. *Obesity (Silver Spring)*. 17: 60-65.

Voracek M (2007). Genetic factors in suicide: reassessment of adoption studies and individuals' beliefs about adoption study findings. *Psychiatr Danub*. 19: 139-53.

Vorstman JA, Chow EW, Ophoff RA, van Engeland H, Beemer FA, Kahn RS, Sinke RJ and Bassett AS (2009). Association of the PIK4CA schizophrenia-susceptibility gene in adults with the 22q11.2 deletion syndrome. *Am J Med Genet B Neuropsychiatr Genet*. 150B: 430-433.

Vrijenhoek T, Buizer-Voskamp JE, van der Stelt I, Strengman E; Genetic Risk and Outcome in Psychosis (GROUP) Consortium, Sabatti C, Geurts van Kessel A, Brunner HG, Ophoff RA and Veltman JA (2008). Recurrent CNVs disrupt three candidate genes in schizophrenia patients. *Am J Hum Genet*. 83: 504-510.

Vyas NS, Hadjulis M, Vourdas A, Byrne P and Frangou S (2007). The Maudsley early onset schizophrenia study. Predictors of psychosocial outcome at 4-year follow-up. *Eur Child Adolesc Psychiatry.* 16: 465-470.

Waghorn G, Lloyd C, Abraham B, Silvester D and Chant D. (2008). Comorbid physical health conditions hinder employment among people with psychiatric disabilities. *Psychiatr Rehabil J.* 31: 243-246.

Walterfang M, Wood AG, Reutens DC, Wood SJ, Chen J, Velakoulis D, McGorry PD and Pantelis C (2008). Morphology of the corpus callosum at different stages of schizophrenia: cross-sectional study in first-episode and chronic illness. *Br J Psychiatry.* 192: 429-434.

Wang SH, Rong JR, Chen CC, Wei SJ and Liu KC (2007). A study of stress, learned resourcefulness and caregiver burden among primary caregivers of schizophrenic adolescents. *Hu Li Za Zhi.* 54: 37-47.

Warman DM, Grant P, Sullivan K, Caroff S and Beck AT (2005). Individual and group cognitive-behavioral therapy for psychotic disorders: a pilot investigation. *J Psychiatr Pract.* 11: 27-34.

WD (2008). www.wrongdiagnosis.com/m/mental_illness/subtypes.htm.

WebMD (2008). www.webmd.com/mental-health/mental-health-types-illness.

Weiser M, van Os J, Reichenberg A, Rabinowitz J, Nahon D, Kravitz E, Lubin G, Shmushkevitz M, Knobler HY, Noy S and Davidson M (2007). Social and cognitive functioning, urbanicity and risk for schizophrenia. *Br J Psychiatry.* 191: 320-324.

Weiten W. Psychology Themes & Variations. Brooks/Cole Publishing Company. United States. 1995.

Wenger T and Fürst S (2004). Role of endogenous cannabinoids in cerebral reward mechanisms. *Neuropsychopharmacol Hung.* 6: 26-29.

Werner P, Aviv A and Barak Y (2008). Self-stigma, self-esteem and age in persons with schizophrenia. *Int Psychogeriatr.* 20: 174-187.

Wheeler A, Humberstone V and Robinson G (2009). Outcomes for schizophrenia patients with clozapine treatment: how good does it get? *J Psychopharmacol.* 23: 957-965.

Wilson TW, Rojas DC, Teale PD, Hernandez OO, Asherin RM and Reite ML (2007). Aberrant functional organization and maturation in early-onset psychosis: evidence from magnetoencephalography. *Psychiatry Res.* 156: 59-67.

Wong EH, Nikam SS and Shahid M (2008). Multi- and single-target agents for major psychiatric diseases: therapeutic opportunities and challenges. *Curr Opin Investig Drugs.* 9: 28-36.

Wundsam K, Pitschel-Walz G, Leucht S and Kissling W (2007). Psychiatric patients and relatives instruct German police officers - an anti-stigma project of "BASTA - the alliance for mentally ill people". *Psychiatr Prax.* 34: 181-187.

Wykes T, Newton E, Landau S, Rice C, Thompson N and Frangou S (2007). Cognitive remediation therapy (CRT) for young early onset patients with schizophrenia: an exploratory randomized controlled trial. *Schizophr Res.*

94: 221-230

Xiang YT, Weng YZ, Li WY, Gao L, Chen GL, Xie L, Chang YL, Tang WK and Ungvari GS. (2007). Efficacy of the Community Re-Entry Module for patients with schizophrenia in Beijing, China: outcome at 2-year follow-up. *Br J Psychiatry*. 190: 49-56.

Xu B, Roos JL, Levy S, van Rensburg EJ, Gogos JA and Karayiorgou M (2008). Strong association of de novo copy number mutations with sporadic schizophrenia. *Nat Genet*. 40: 880-885.

Yamada K, Hattori E, Iwayama Y, Toyota T, Ohnishi T, Iwata Y, Tsuchiya KJ, Sugihara G, Kikuchi M, Okazaki Y and Yoshikawa T (2009). Failure to confirm genetic association of the CHI3L1 gene with schizophrenia in Japanese and Chinese populations. *Am J Med Genet B Neuropsychiatr Genet*. 150B: 508-514.

Yamada K, Watanabe K, Nemoto N, Fujita H, Chikaraishi C, Yamauchi K, Yagi G, Asai M and Kanba S (2006). Prediction of medication noncompliance in outpatients with schizophrenia: 2-year follow-up study. *Psychiatry Res*. 141: 61-69.

Yang LH (2007). Application of mental illness stigma theory to Chinese societies: synthesis and new directions. *Singapore Med J*. 48: 977-985.

Yang LH, Kleinman A, Link BG, Phelan JC, Lee S and Good B (2007). Culture and stigma: adding moral experience to stigma theory. *Soc Sci Med*. 64: 1524-1535.

Yücel M, Solowij N, Respondek C, Whittle S, Fornito A, Pantelis C and Lubman DI (2008). Regional brain abnormalities associated with long-term heavy cannabis use. *Arch Gen Psychiatry*. 65: 694-701.

Yulug B, Yildiz A, Hüdaoglu O, Kilic E, Cam E and Schäbitz WR (2006). Olanzapine attenuates brain damage after focal cerebral ischemia in vivo. *Brain Res Bull*. 71: 296-300.

Zafar SN, Syed R, Tehseen S, Gowani SA, Waqar S, Zubair A, Yousaf W, Zubairi AJ and Naqvi H (2008). Perceptions about the cause of schizophrenia and the subsequent help seeking behavior in a Pakistani population - results of a cross-sectional survey. *BMC Psychiatry*. 8: 56.

Zaw FK (2006). ECT and the youth: catatonia in context. *Int Rev Neurobiol*. 72: 207-231.

Zhang ZJ, Hao GF, Shi JB, Mou XD, Yao ZJ and Chen N (2008). Investigation of the neural substrates of voice recognition in Chinese schizophrenic patients with auditory verbal hallucinations: an event-related functional MRI study. *Acta Psychiatr Scand*. 118: 272-280.

Zhu B, Ascher-Svanum H, Faries DE, Peng X, Salkever D and Slade EP (2008). Costs of treating patients with schizophrenia who have illness-related crisis events. *BMC Psychiatry*. 8: 72.

Lightning Source UK Ltd.
Milton Keynes UK
14 January 2011

165741UK00001B/51/P